Sociogenesis Reexamined

Willibrord de Graaf   Robert Maier
Editors

Sociogenesis
Reexamined

Springer-Verlag
New York Berlin Heidelberg London Paris
Tokyo Hong Kong Barcelona Budapest

Willibrord de Graaf, PhD
Robert Maier, PhD
Department of General Social Sciences
Faculty of Social Sciences
Universiteit Utrecht
P.O. Box 80.140
3508 TC Utrecht, The Netherlands

Library of Congress Cataloging-in-Publication Data
Sociogenesis reexamined : with 7 figures / [edited by] Willibrord de
    Graaf, Robert Maier.
        p.   cm.
    Includes bibliographical references and index.
    ISBN 0-387-94276-9. -- ISBN 3-540-94276-9
    1. Social psychology. 2. Developmental psychology. I. De Graaf,
Willibrord. II. Maier, Robert.
HM251.S68717   1994
302--dc20   94-1169

Printed on acid-free paper.

Production managed by Laura Carlson; manufacturing supervised by Jacqui Ashri.
Camera-ready copy prepared by the editors.
Printed and bound by Braun Brumfield, Ann Arbor, MI.
Printed in the United States of America.

9 8 7 6 5 4 3 2 1

ISBN 0-387-94276-9 Springer-Verlag New York Berlin Heidelberg
ISBN 3-540-94276-9 Springer-Verlag Berlin Heidelberg New York

Contents

List of Figures and Tables

Contributors

Viveka Adelswärd, University of Linköping, Department of Communication Studies, 58183 Linköping, Sweden

Ed Elbers, University of Utrecht, Department of General Social Sciences, P.O. Box 80140, 3508 TC Utrecht, The Netherlands

Claire Farrer, University of Ghent, Blandijnberg 2, 9000 Ghent, Belgium

Christiane Gillièron, Université de Genève, Faculté de Psychologie, 9, route de Drize, 1227 Carouge, Switzerland

Willibrord de Graaf, University of Utrecht, Department of General Social Sciences, P.O. Box 80140, 3508 TC Utrecht, The Netherlands

Michèle Grossen, University of Neuchâtel, Séminaire de Psychologie, Espace Louis-Agassiz 1, 2000 Neuchâtel, Switzerland

Kuno Lorenz, Universität des Saarlandes, Fachbereich 5, 6600 Saarbrücken, Germany

Robert Maier, University of Utrecht, Department of General Social Sciences, P.O. Box 80140, 3508 TC Utrecht, The Netherlands

Ivana Marková, University of Stirling, Department of Psychology, Stirling, FK9 4LA, Scotland

Anne-Nelly Perret-Clermont, University of Neuchâtel, Séminaire de Psychologie, Espace Louis-Agassiz 1, 2000 Neuchâtel, Switzerland

Rik Pinxten, University of Ghent, Blandijnberg 2, 9000 Ghent, Belgium

Roger Säljö, University of Linköping, Department of Communication Studies, 58183 Linköping, Sweden

John Shotter, University of New Hampshire, Department of Communication, Durham, NH 03824-3586, USA

Chris Sinha, University of Aarhus, Institute of Psychology, Asylvej 4, 8240 Risskov, Denmark

Jaan Valsiner, University of North Carolina at Chapel Hill, Department of Psychology, Davie Hall, Chapel Hill, NC 27599-3270, USA

René van der Veer, University of Leiden, Department of Education, P.O. Box 9555, 2300 RB Leiden, The Netherlands

Jan de Wolf, University of Utrecht, Department of Anthropology, P.O. Box 80140, 3508 TC Utrecht, The Netherlands

Sociogenesis Reexamined: An Introduction

Willibrord de Graaf and Robert Maier

When starting a center for sociogenetic studies, it was not our intention to propose a project around a clear-cut theoretical framework. The choice for a focus around the idea of sociogenesis was meant to open up some space for an interdisciplinary social scientific approach towards the development of persons in their historical and societal contexts. We strongly believed that much theorizing on human development had eventually ended in the pitfall of the traditional bifurcations between individual and society, between environment and reaction, between dynamic and static approaches. There were, of course, promising perspectives emerging in developmental psychology around the reception of the Russian socio-historical psychologists and the introduction of social psychological theories. And the same could be said about the interest of sociologists and anthropologists in developmental theories. But we felt that the elaboration of a conception of human development as an inherently social process could gain a lot from opening up the borders between disciplines and scientific cultures. The creation of a new world order should not be left to politicians!

One of the first activities we undertook was to organize an opportunity for exchange and theoretical confrontation on the theme of mechanisms in sociogenesis.[1]

Thus we hoped to make a start on the refinement and reworking of the concept of sociogenesis. In this introduction we shall circumscribe two possible branches in defining sociogenesis as a useful guide in mapping existing approaches. Incidentally we already hint at questions which remain to be solved, but we also try to offer some more systematic perspectives for research in this field. Finally we present the results of our meeting on the mechanisms in sociogenesis: we have placed the different contributions to this book in their respective places in the two branches of sociogenesis, and in the ways that they propose elaborations and innovations in the study of sociogenesis.

---

[1] This was done in the form of a workshop, organized at the Rijksuniversiteit Utrecht in December 1990. We would like here to thank the KNAW (Koninklijke Nederlandse Academie voor Wetenschappen), the Royal Dutch Academy of Sciences, and the Faculty of Social Sciences of the Rijksuniversiteit Utrecht for their financial support.

We knew that in Europe, at least, the concept of sociogenesis was explicitly linked to the scholarly works of Norbert Elias, and particularly in the field of sociology. Less known was the use of this notion by the Russian psychologist Lev Vygotsky when he referred to the development of the higher mental functions. In a more loose way, the notion could be found to point at the crossroads of ontogenesis and phylogenesis (see Cairns & Cairns, 1988), or at any socio-historical condition influencing human development (Bain, 1983).

Although the concept of sociogenesis is used in numerous ways, it is possible to delineate two main interpretations. One regards the developmental process as social, and tries to conceptualize psychological functions as originating in social practices and structures. The other refers to the socio-historical formation of the modern mind and modern man, and tries to analyze the structural changes in society in their effect on psychological functioning.

The former definition of sociogenesis already has a long history in social science, although not under that name. In recent years there has not only been a growing interest in the works of Vygotsky (1896-1934), but also in those of G.H. Mead (1863-1931). And undoubtedly, these scientists were both active in the field of psychology and sociology, and were familiar with the writings of, for instance, Baldwin, Bühler and James. This is not the place to map the context of their times and the specific influences they underwent, but it goes without saying that the proposition (and its specific elaboration) of the primary social character of individual development has been part of the social sciences, although mostly in the margin. We shall present these two theorists as typical for this branch of sociogenesis, together with the ethogenic approach of R. Harré, who, since the end of 1970 has formulated a theory which was, partly directly, partly with hindsight, inspired by these two authors.

Mead based his conception of the social basis of the self in a Darwinian framework of the necessary adaptation of human beings to their surroundings. In the social group the individual human being learns to organize his impulses, and in that process consciousness and the self develop. In a sense Mead can be said to be concerned with the problem of order and cohesion (and his notion of "the generalized other" has been strongly coined this way by others). At the same time, he rejected the idea of the organism as a passive recipient: individuals act differently upon their environment and therefore perceive identical stimuli in different ways. Thus, the possibility of human intelligence in affecting the social order is a necessary part of the adaptation of the human species.

This evolutionary grounded conception of human activity as a primary social one finds its corollary in the development of the self. Mutual adjustment in the social group presupposes social communication. This communication starts with gestures, and in the process of signalling and responding, the individual learns to reflect upon his own reactions: in what ways were they appropriate? This self-reflection creates self-consciousness, and later, in the acquiring of language, makes the formation of the subjective attitude when internalizing the attitudes and meanings of the social group possible. Language plays a crucial role in the development of the self, and continues to do so even when we are "privately" thinking: thinking is a kind of internal conversation within the self. The self consists of two sides, the "me," which is the object of reflection, and the reflecting "I." The "me" is the way the self sees itself in the eyes of the others, and the "I" is the way the self looks at itself and its activities. It is not possible to describe these two sides as autonomous entities. The self, as the process of consciousness, cannot be an object of itself: at the very moment the "I" reflects on itself it becomes "me."

This brief summary of some of Mead's central concepts is sufficient to suggest a few strong and weak points. Mead is convincing in his effort to underline the social nature of development as the growth of a meaningful acting individual and to point at the central constituting role of language in this process. He fails, however, to be more specific about the transition from gesture to language, and thus about the mechanisms of internalization, and he cannot theorize the relation of this "micro-social" process to "macro-social" and/or historical developments.

It is precisely the cornerstone of Marxist theorizing to stress the significance of historically specific processes for the formation of human relations. And in post-revolutionary Russia, attempts were made to grasp the implications of the proposition "the concrete individual is to be seen as the ensemble of the social relations" for psychological theory. In the socio-historical school the social character of development was conceptualized as the transition from socially and culturally shared practices and capacities to individually appropriated psychological actions and cognitions by means of the process of internalization. Or, in Vygotsky's terms, every human function comes to stage twice: firstly as a social, interpersonal activity, and secondly as an internalized social relation, as a higher psychological function. The Marxist emphasis on history and dialectics was translated in the idea that human development could only be understood as the process in which active human beings interact with their cultural environment and thus, with the assistance of others, construct their solutions for (developmental) tasks. Vygotsky presents two important mediating factors in this process: tools and language (signs). Tools are used to produce changes in the physical world; signs are used to influence the behavior of others or of oneself. The first one of these is rather contested (see van der Veer in this book) and the second is more well known and accepted: speech is the crucial vehicle for the transmission of the cultural heritage. In the exchange of verbal symbols, the child learns the meanings of objects, including itself. It starts by stating names as a guidance for its own activities and ends with inner conversations and meanings of words. The rise of consciousness is the product of this transition to "silent and abstract speech," whereby reflection on own responses is part of the internalization of cultural values and operations. Like the Meadian self, Vygotsky is proposing a person who is always the co-constructed result of interaction.

The problems with his formulations are the distinction between lower and higher mental functions, and his characterization of these lower functions as biological and not also social. Furthermore, he does not articulate the relations of ontogenetic micro-social processes to changing societal formations, and he seems to presuppose scientistic norms in his picture of the growth of knowledge. But Vygotsky's approach is rather strong in that it opens (by way of the zone of proximal development) the possibility for analyzing the cultural context of instruction as part of the problem of learning.

Harré is the strange liaison between the Vygotsky theory based in Marxism and the societally, rather abstract, approach of Mead (see Harré, 1986 and 1987). While recognizing the practical-political orders in society, Harré confines himself to an elaboration of the person as a social construct. He places his approach in the dramaturgical tradition of Goffman and, although not explicitly, in the ethnomethodological school. The central assumption is that personal being must be understood by the accounts individuals give of their actions and the rules or conventions which they follow. In this process individuals learn to develop a theory about what it is to be a person, to have a self, within which they can order their experiences. This learning process takes place in conversations, as the principal mode of life. In conversations, psychological and social reality is constructed. So development starts within this public-collective domain of conversations, moral order(s) and material practices. Becoming a person means, then, to appropriate in the private, individual domain some of these public forms of speaking. This learning process is accomplished in joint action between the developing child and its carers. In this process people develop their sense of subjectivity, and learn to express themselves in the ongoing conversation, its rules and in the practical order within which it takes place. Children are treated as persons, and, accordingly, start (by imitating the ways of being a person) to treat the people around them as persons. This "axiom of development" does not suppose any core of inner self, but instead shows how selves are socially created.

Although aiming at a thoroughly social explanation of psychological functioning, Harré seems to end with some of the same shortcomings mentioned for Mead and Vygotsky, especially where he does not analyze the relations of material practices and moral orders and the developmental processes in specific local situations. Moreover, his conception of personal being risks falling apart in two conflicting presuppositions: on the one hand, persons intentionally and meaningfully create their social order, and on the other hand, it is this social order that bestows individuals with the competencies for intentional acting.

The sociogenetic branch we have depicted here with the help of three theories provides us with the inspiring perspective of analyses of development as a truly social dynamic. It hints at the complex ways in which development is the product of joint activity, that means, is the ongoing process of mutual construction of psychological reality. However, the problem remains that this "micro-sociogenesis" is barely connected with social processes of economic and political power, and in some ways seems to produce a world of communication and action which is cut off from the world of material and bodily practices. These questions will be taken up after the following considerations on the second branch of sociogenesis.

There is a different line of questioning which gave meaning to the sociogenetic problematic. Central here is the understanding of how modern man achieved his apparently evident growth in the twists of evolution and history. Sociogenetic thinking has been informed by this, at times rather murky, source. Let us consider this influence, adopting, to begin with, a rather polemic perspective.

The white man of the north seems to be at a stage of development unreached until then, and from this perspective—the highest evidently—he tries to order the preceding ones. Hierarchical classifications of groups and individuals belonging to them is the appropriated method, and once these classifications are established a diversity of explanations offer themselves for explaining the hierarchical differences.

Formulated more crudely, it is the story of the self-glorification of modern man, conceived for quite some time as white, and of European or Caucasian extraction. It is the story of the emergence of modern man. We should not be ashamed to consider these sources of sociogenetic thinking, even if they were quite frequently tinted with a racist flavor. How can we be sure of avoiding similar pitfalls if we do not explicitly take into account and confront the motives which have been so self-evident and powerful in the past centuries?

Two different versions of the story of the development of the supremacy of the most developed human group have circulated. The first parted from a common origin; it was monogenic: there were just one Adam and one Eve, or one common biological origin after Darwin. But conditions, such as the climate, and the particular efforts in order to adapt and to reproduce themselves, explain the emergence of the known differences. The other version postulated different points of departure. There were several couples named Adam and Eve, and the races, with their various qualities and limitations, have different origins. This is the polygenic conception, which was, for example, still defended in the last century by Louis Agassiz in the United States. Darwinian wisdom led to new polygenic insights. At the beginning of this century, German and English anthropologists and biologists (Klaatsch, 1920, or Hartl and Gates) thought that the different races went back to different apes: the "whites" to the chimpanzee, the "yellows" to the orangoutang, and the "blacks" to the gorilla. Evidently, the chimpanzee was seen as the brightest big ape, whereas the gorilla....

These two versions can also be combined. In 1962, Coon, an American anthropologist, who was also president of the American Anthropological Association, published a new chapter of these stories. "Whites," "blacks" and others originated from different races of the *homo erectus*, and living in different climates, they developed in different directions. The "whites," and to a lesser extent the "yellows" lived in a cold climate, and natural selection pushed them to develop more highly a form of intelligence that was based on technical inventions. This theory has been reformulated in recent years by a South African biologist (J. Hofmeyr) and by some right-wing French biologists, who, under a pseudonym, published a book in 1977 with the title *Race and Intelligence*.

This is not the place to argue against such conceptions. It goes without saying that many scientists (such as Gould or Cavalli-Sforza) have confronted these conceptions very strongly. We only want to point out these patterns of thought which, for a long time, fitted so well with the Zeitgeist, and which continue to supply the reservoirs of many folk theories.

We have limited ourselves to trace some quite filthy and nasty roots of sociogenetic thinking. By doing this, we can clearly identify some of the early characteristics of the sociogenetic language.

First of all, there is a powerful rhetoric, speaking on a super-macro level. Origins, conditions of development, general factors which influence this development, clear hierarchies, and definite valuation are the ingredients of this rhetoric.

Secondly, these conceptions use a crude, realistic style. They tell the story as it was and is. The perspective of the creator, and certainly the perspectives of the "spoken about" is excluded completely. In other words, methods and concepts are used as neutral instruments.

Thirdly, these conceptions merge individual and society. The individual stands for the group, the group is the agglomeration of the individuals. One can stand for the other without any metaphoric intention.

Theories of development of this century break more or less completely with these very problematic conceptions. If we can only applaud the good intentions motivating these breaks, we must also register the following consequences: Several of the old roots can grow quite astonishing offsprings in these theories. In Freud's conception of development one can identify doubtful bits of recapitulation (for example, see Gould), in other theories, like the one of Piaget, normative forms of hierarchy have been pointed out, for example by Kessen. A different problem arises in the theoretical framework of Vygotsky, who is one of the few who formulated explicitly sociogenetic questions. He appeals to a conception of history which advances in a linear way with great, decisive steps. The direction is one of scientific progress and of social emancipation. Such a conception also reproduces, therefore, some of the problematic aspects of a hierarchical order of human societies.

These theories may avoid the evident pitfalls of the old rhetoric, but at the same time they are becoming blind; a sociogenetic outlook seems almost absent. Maybe Freud's theory, which grows quite a number of the offsprings from the old roots, is, because of this fact, the most problematic, but also the most inspiring one.

In short, these theories appear cleaner, scientifically more elaborated and legitimated. But at the same time they no longer dare to reformulate the great questions, which have not been wiped out by this disciplined silence.

The various evolutionary theories formulated in social theory are, in general, much more civilized than the racist stories already mentioned. These theories have, however, the same characteristics of the powerful rhetoric of racist thinking. They dare to reformulate the big questions, which at times are barely more civilized than the racist brothers and sisters. But in this disciplinary arena, there is much less of a break than in psychology, and therefore we find here more of an explicit discussion about the values and the problems of the naive sociogenetic questions.

A central point of these approaches is the problem of how modern societies and modern man developed. Modern should be understood as industrial, capitalist, democratic, rational or something like that. Different theories address specific aspects of this problem: some ask if there are natural, general laws of social development, and if some final stage can be anticipated. Marxist thinking, but also Spencer with his social Darwinism, belong to this category.

Other theories confront the issue of violence. Does social development necessarily proceed by rather violent steps, or is there a possibility to conceive this development as a peaceful, orderly occurrence? In other words, can modern societies not be pictured as relatively harmonious systems, which proceed with some rationality and which are able to handle dysfunction by orderly, peaceful means. The work of Durkheim, Schumpeter, Weber and definitely that of Parsons can be read as answers to these questions.

These theories try to answer these kind of global questions, but to a large extent the focus on ontogenetic processes is lost. Modern individuals are pictured as being socialized and this process of socialization is conceived as functional to the global, social dynamic. This disciplinary blindness has its price: these theories presuppose individuals which are, to begin with, endowed with biological or psychological dispositions which favor their unproblematic, functional socialization. S. Moscovici has pointed out these presuppositions in a very detailed study of the theories of Durkheim, Simmel, and Weber.

We should mention here the approach of Elias, who explicitly used the term sociogenesis. According to his theory, the recent development of modern man can be written in the form of a few, bulky chapters, meaning, that this development can be conceptualized in terms of a few, big stages. The transformation of the social system on the one hand, and metamorphosis of social and private individuals go hand in hand. There are global changes which influence and are influenced by the specific variations of the makeup of individuals. These interactions are explained by a constant interplay of operations of domination and assimilation, of imitation and emancipation. Modern individuals live in nation states; they have internalized the former external forms of control. This conception still stimulates many researchers, but at the same time the globality and the linearity of this conception is heavily contested, for example by Duerr.

Be it the horrors of world wars and the associated cruelties, the never diminishing occurrence of poverty and misery in the world or the despair to ever reach the summit of civilization based on science or all of these factors, in any case the old questions surrounding the evidence of "modern man" cannot be asked anymore in a straightforward way. We can diagnose a rather radical transformation of outlook: before, an ascending line seemed evident, the summit had either been reached already or it could at least be visualized. The direction pursued and eventually the further steps to be undertaken were, in principle, not problematic. Now, we find another landscape of problems: there is not *one* summit, and anyway it was never reached. On the contrary, there are many valleys and mountains. Different individuals and social and cultural groups not only pursue different goals, they also use a great variety of approaches in order to reach the chosen goals.

In other words, the presuppositions of well-known evolutionary theories are no longer accepted as such. The simple hierarchy and linearity assumed by these theories is rejected, and therefore also the associated value systems. Foucault and also Giddens are known spokesmen of such a critique. Modern man has no longer any reason to glorify himself; on the contrary, if this image is not altogether rejected, modern man becomes a dreary and gloomy figure, with numerous psychiatric troubles.

To analyze the doom of this figure, and to find a suitable therapy, is one of the lines of actual questioning, pursued for example by Sennet or Lasch. We find this line quite unsatisfactory; we would prefer to suggest analyzing the shortcomings of questions associated with the self-glorification of "modern man." Then it might no longer be necessary to understand and to repave the loss of this identity.

Another line takes the multiplicity of goals and means which social groups and individuals pursue seriously. The problem, then, is to accept either a complete relativity, or to search for measures and instruments which would permit comparison of these differences, to find ways to translate, at least partially, the various approaches one into another, or to look at the underlying conditions of variations and at the laws of development which could help to understand these multiplicities. Also the questions involving a critical analysis of the viewpoint of the analyst and of his/her interests belong here.

We might mention the approach of Foucault, who works out an approach that belongs here. Motivated by actual problems he departs from explicit questions concerning the emergence of these problems. In these areas, he attempts to analyze the historically specific conditions of discourse formations and/or of power arrangements which might explain the shape and the identity of individuals and of their "problems."

In this part we have traced one particular background of the sociogenetic question. It is the story of the rise and the fall of "modern man." According to us, this background permits the understanding, the (rhetorical) force, and the straightforwardness of the sociogenetic problematic. But at the same time we become acquainted with all the doubts, the shame, and the suspicions which are associated with the sociogenetic line of questioning.

However, such considerations cannot be avoided. Only by considering this background can we acknowledge the potentialities of the sociogenetic approach. At the same time, these considerations, presented quite superficially here, when elaborated upon in more detail, should enable the appalling and dreadful pitfalls which surrounded the elaboration of sociogenetic theory to be avoided. Thus, we might undertake the task to (re-)situate the sociogenetic line of questioning.

From the preceding remarks we can easily distill some negative indications concerning research perspectives in sociogenesis. It appeared as problematic if one separates systematically micro from macro approaches. For example, learning studied exclusively in a micro-environment might have various meanings when considered in its global settings. In the short overview of the work of Harré, we have also identified another problem: if we separate strictly (as far as methodology and concepts are concerned) the mental from the material, we risk ending up in very relativist space. A similar omission concerns biology: without taking into account the fact that humans are biological organisms, we might also end up in this space. On the other hand, reducing all phenomena to biology is not satisfactory within a sociogenetic perspective.

Another lesson concerns the nature of the models used. Models of development which presuppose a simple, straightforward linearity and hierarchy are not necessarily problematic, but we have to be extremely careful not to reproduce the old murky conceptions such as racism or an innocent idea of progress.

Our aim here is not to offer a complete program of research in sociogenesis. We limit ourselves to indicate some possible and promising lines of investigation: Investigations of the transformations of the spatial and temporal settings of development and learning in different areas of competence in history. For example, adolescents spend much more time at school now than in former times. What are the consequences of this change for the content of what they learn and for the forms of instruction. We might also consider the changing ways students deal with this new learning context. More generally, we might ask the question if various forms of learning arise and if individuals construct in their development different "forms of knowledge" associated with these learning contexts.

Another promising line concerns the actions of developing individuals. These actions might be conceived as pre-structured by the social context which discriminates between acceptable and non-acceptable actions. Such a view can be found in Bourdieu's work as well as in post-Vygotskian research. Therefore, we should focus the research on the creative potentialities of individuals in development. But in this case we might miss the social embedding of these actions completely. Comparative methods seem indicated in order to be able to take into account the various interactions of both sides. We know that this problem has, in principle, been resolved conceptually, by terms such as "duality of structure and agency" (Giddens) or the "structure structurante" expression of Bourdieu, which comes, by the way, from Piaget. These solutions sound wonderful, however, a concrete, and empirical illustration and elaboration is still missing.

Presentation

Part 1: Theoretical and Historical Foundations of Sociogenesis

The old problem as to whether social behavior governs individual behavior or the other way around, is attacked by Kuno Lorenz on a conceptual level. Taking the concepts of competition (as an instance of individual behavior) and cooperation (as an instance of social behavior) he attempts to show, starting with the Greeks, how a theory of progress based on notions of rationality and morality has been developed. In this line of thinking the direction is from competition towards cooperation. An alternative account is a theory of decline, in which social competition spoils "natural" cooperation.

Transgressing this pair of opposites is the thinking of Herder. He situates the cultural process as a process of education in which individual distinction goes together with social coherence. Sociality refers to cooperation by means of individual contributions and rationality is competition by way of individual distinction grounded in a community. From this perspective, competition and cooperation are no longer in opposition to each other but are complementary.

The account by Ivana Marková aims at showing how the dialogism of Bakhtin offers the possibility to study mind and language in their development and change. This dialogism reaches further than cognitivism, because it situates the totality of human activity as a social-historical phenomenon. Dialogism pertains to the relations between agents, cognitivism to individuals. To elucidate dialogism as an epistemological approach to the sociogenetic study of language, Marková points to its historical roots in religious thinking and in Hegel. From there she reconstructs how the conception of language as a mental tool in intersubjectivity has originated, and in what ways Vygotsky and Bakhtin differ in their respective, more semiotic and dialogic, approaches. By referring to Rubinstein and the problem of instruction, Marková indicates how language is not just a tool but is already a meaningful definition of the problem. Following this line, Marková concludes by drawing attention to the possible relations between language (as a system of signs) and speech (as the dialogical process), thought (as cultural knowledge) and thinking (as the individual process). In this way Marková wants to demonstrate that language and thought are relatively stable products of history, while continuously being changed by the participating individuals. There exists a co-genetic logic in the relation between individual and culture: both develop together, mutually influencing each other.

Jaan Valsiner starts his argument with the observation that the social formation of psychological functions has been paid lip service for more than a century, but that genuine theoretical models to explain how this could proceed remain absent. He ascribes this state of affairs to uni-directional approaches which suppose that development means the gradual learning and acceptance of the social world by the individual. But how the social becomes personal remains unexplained. In the bi-directional approach, learning, the transmission of culture, is a dynamic process in which all participants (learners and teachers) change the content of what is learned. Or to phrase it in Valsiner's medical metaphor of "contagion," the cultural message can, as a virus, be altered, resisted or accepted. Cultural transmission as the process in which the person builds his own personal culture out of the collective culture, is always a process of co-construction. This means that it is goal-directed but not predictable, that it depends on the current state of the developing person and on the actual constraints of the learning situation. This implies, according to Valsiner, the existence of the person as a concept in theoretical discourse: there is a separation between person and society but this has to be conceived as an "inclusive separation," in which individual psychological functions are the result of systemic interactions between person and society. But it also implies that novelty is always the possible outcome of this process of co-construction. A "bounded indeterminacy" exists which points to the active role of the person who is appropriating the world, that is, is constructing his/her personal culture. Methodologically, Valsiner's perspective on sociogenesis stresses the necessity to look for the periods of fluidity or chaos in development, because it is probably there and then that novelty is being constructed.

Part 2: New Conceptual Approaches

The argument of John Shotter concerns the ways in which the study of sociogenesis itself needs to be analyzed as a sociogenesis of the relationship between theory and practice. Shotter takes his stand in a Wittgensteinian approach regarding the relationship between language and thought. If there is no unambiguous reference in language to reality, how can we then say something of common interest about reality?

For Shotter it is necessary to distinguish two types of sociogenetic relationship between practice and theory. One form concerns the equilibration of practice to theory, and points at the styling of theory as a straightforward result of systematic efforts while forgetting all the impasses, failures, etc. which took place in the development of theory. The other form implicates the equilibration of theory to practice, and shows how effective practices are constructed as practices and not as instances of theory. So to understand these relationships Shotter proposes a third form of sociogenesis—not as a theory of mechanism—in analyzing what he calls sensory topics. These are the shared understandings people develop when sharing the same feelings in shared conditions. Sensory topics form together the common sense, the imaginary universal which lends meaning to the particular, local topos. Because these sensory topics are constantly in flux they have to be seen as temporary "generative potentials," offering the possibility for novelty.

In his contribution "Iconology and Imagination: Explorations in Sociogenetic Economics," Chris Sinha explores the limitations of the cognitivist paradigm, which neglects the context and which is unable to provide a satisfactory account of human epigenetic development. According to Sinha, the strength of the cognitivist view is based on historical factors such as monetary exchange and the use of general equivalences. However, recognizing these influences opens the possibility of overcoming the limitations of the cognitivist paradigm and of elaborating a sociogenetic theory which no longer underestimates the role of social context and of the imaginary.

The contribution by René van der Veer, "The Concept of Sociogenesis in Cultural-Historical Theory," explores how Vygotsky introduced the concept of sociogenesis in his theory, relying particularly on Janet. Discussing the relevant features of this theory and the "forbidden color" experiment, van der Veer concludes that Vygotsky at times used a concept of culture and a view of internalization which were too narrowly defined. Because of these limitations a rather inadequate view of human sociogenesis emerges with internal inconsistencies. Suggestions are made as to how to overcome these limitations.

In the contribution "Questioning the Mechanisms of Sociogenesis," Robert Maier examines (a) Conceptual problems relating to development and sociogenesis. If sociogenesis has to have any meaning, it affects development in a major way. Therefore, development becomes a category which is affected by the cultural and historical context; (b) If the organism is conceived of as being a developing, active agent, how can it be affected by social and historical contexts? By socio-cultural actions-systems, which are specific for each period and context. In other words, the social systems of actions, acting on actions of individual organisms are a serious candidate for the mechanisms of sociogenesis.

Part 3: Analysis of Existing Theoretical Frameworks

In the chapter "The Constructive Function of Language in the Baby's Development from Sensorimotor Adaptation to Humanity," Christiane Gillièron attempts to complement the Piagetian account of sensorimotor development. Words do not only point to things, but also to cultural constructs. Speaking of language offers two references to sociogenesis. First of all, language development presupposes interactions, most objects are, after all, cultural constructs. Secondly, language is at the basis of the creation and permanency of cultural objects, and as such it has a crucial role in shaping our "Umwelt." However, there really is a difference in the way language comes to babies and the way it came to the species.

The contribution "On Learning and Tradition: A Comparative View" is written by two anthropologists, Rik Pinxten and Claire Farrer, who have investigated the Apache and the Navajo cultures. In particular, they present the practices of learning in these two cultures. Confronting their findings with a sociogenetic approach—in Vygotskyan terms or otherwise—two points are stressed: firstly, that in Western cultures history plays an important role, which is not the case in oral cultures, and secondly, that an analysis of the learning processes of other cultures, such as the Apache and the Navajo, may help to broaden and to correct the models of sociogenesis presented so far.

Several theories have been developed to overcome the split between individual and society and to deal with the problem of the socio-historical construction of subject-forms while leaving space for subjects as actors of change. Willibrord de Graaf discusses in his contribution two of these theories: the theory of social representations of S. Moscovici and the reflexive sociological approach of P. Bourdieu. He analyses these theories in two aspects: their epistemological assumptions and their statements on action and structure. Both Bourdieu and Moscovici offer strong arguments for a (self-) reflexive position to science in order to deal with common sense experience. But their explanation of the acting subject looks rather "over-socialized." The concepts of habitus and social representation seem to refer to structures which "inhabit" human beings. The dynamic potential of these concepts as sociogenetic mechanisms could be enhanced by elaborating the contradictions which they now tend to overlook.

Part 4: Empirical Case Studies

The contribution "Becoming a Conscientious Objector: The Use of Arms and Institutional Accounting Practices," by Viveka Adelswärd and Roger Säljö, explores the argumentation in the case of constrained institutional communications. According to the authors of this contribution, communication is neither an individual act, nor completely determined by features in the situation or social structure. A subtle interplay of adapted arguments and justifications is characteristic of the interviews which are analyzed. The agency of the individual and the constraints of socio-cultural institutions have to be conceptually accounted for if we want to understand human communication in complex societies.

In discussing Vygotsky's theory of sociogenesis, Ed Elbers points to the problem that his emphasis on transmission of culture seems to exclude the possibility of cultural change. But in other writings Vygotsky indicates that the developing child is not simply introduced into existing cultures but is itself active in defining its environment, in constructing meanings. Elbers describes studies which show how the process of internalization is always a "joint regulation" between children and carers, and thus stresses the importance of the contribution of the child in its own development. In addition, Elbers takes up Vygotsky's theory of play which singles out the role-playing as a way of learning what roles are and as preparation for future life. So play manifests both the spontaneous contribution of the child as its importance for reproduction of culture.

In offering a study of pretend play, Elbers elaborates his discussion on the meaning of play as a way in which children reflect on rules and thus anticipate real-life conditions. Elbers concludes that this anticipation creates new adjustments by children to the official culture, and so can lead to adjustments of this culture. It is here, according to Elbers, that the principle for cultural change can be found.

In the chapter "Psycho-social Perspective on Cognitive Development," by Michèle Grossen and Anne-Nelly Perret-Clermont, the relevance of the notions of "socio-cognitive conflict" and of "intersubjectivity" for sociogenesis is discussed. Recognizing limitations in the theories of Vygotsky and Piaget, the authors discuss in detail one experiment which combines adult-child and child-child interactions in the case of a cognitive task. The interrelations between the intersubjective space, the social and the cognitive competencies which are exhibited in this experiment necessitate a reformulation of the concept of sociogenesis.

From the anthropological point of view, Jan de Wolf discusses in what ways sociogenesis implies psychogenesis and vice versa. He does so by examining the possible explanations of circumcision rituals in biologistic, sociologistic and psychologistic terms. Referring to Harris, who made the distinction between the concepts of individual, person and self, de Wolf analyses how circumcision practices can be understood in this threefold distinction, but then again the problem remains as to how these concepts can be brought together. De Wolf proposes that Goffman's concept of character can be used to elucidate the circumcision rituals as the crossroads of self and society. To undergo circumcision is to show oneself as a true member of society, and at the same time the circumcision ritual offers the other members of society the restatement of the shared rules and values. Participation in circumcision rituals is the affirmation of character, the proof of taking an action which is decisive and consequential, and the empathic involvement of others gives the opportunity to identify oneself with the symbolic necessity as expressed in the circumcision. Although this may be a solution to the problem of linking sociogenesis and psychogenesis, the question remains, as de Wolf himself notices, in what ways concepts like person or self can be used as universal tools in understanding other cultures or are necessarily bound to western scientific schemes of analysis and evaluation.

References

Agassiz, L. (1859), *An essay on classification*. London.

Bain, B. (ed.) (1983), *The sociogenesis of language and human conduct*. New York: Plenum Press.

Cairns, R.B. & B.D. Cairns (1988), The sociogenesis of concepts. In N. Borger et al. (eds.), *Persons in context. Developmental processes*. New York: Cambridge University Press.

Cavalli-Sforza, L.L. (1981), *Cultural transmission and evolution: A quantitative approach*. Princeton, NJ: Princeton University Press.

Coon, C.S. (1963), *The origin of races*. London.

Duerr, H.P. (1988), *Nackheit und Scham. Der Mythos vom Zivilisationsprozess*. Frankfurt/M: Suhrkamp Verlag.

Elias, N. (1969), *Über den Prozess der Zivilisation. Sociogenetische und psychogenetische Untersuchungen* (second edition). Bern, München: Francke Verlag.

Gould, S.J. (1977), *Ontogeny and phylogeny*. New York: Cambridge University Press.

Harré, R. (1986), The step to social constructionism. In M. Richards & P. Light (eds.), *Children of social worlds*. Cambridge: Polity Press.

Harré, R. (1987), Persons and selves. In A. Peacocke & B. Gillet (eds.), *Persons and personality*. Oxford: Basil Blackwell.

Klaatsch, H. (1920), *Der Werdegang der Menschheit und die Entstehung der Kultur*.
  Berlin: Bong.

Moscovici, S. (1988), *La machine à faire des dieux*. Paris: Fayard.

Part 1

Theoretical and Historical Foundation of Sociogenesis

1. Competition and Cooperation: Are They Antagonistic or Complementary?

Kuno Lorenz

At the root of questions concerning the development of social behavior in human beings, we are confronted with a presupposition which, in my opinion, exerts a considerable influence upon the conceptual framework of sociogenetic studies.

I am referring to the questionable assumption that by some crucial experiment(s) we may eventually decide whether, in the last resort, individual behavior governs social behavior or vice versa; and this decision does not depend on how theories answer to the problem of distinguishing between genetic and environmental determination. Rather, it is connected with the rivalry between sociology and psychology as to which type of theories should count as being fundamental to the explanation of human behavior.

In this situation I would like to make an attempt to circumvent rival claims by opting for a kind of interdependence between individual and social behavior, which involves starting with a conceptual analysis of the relevant terms. But instead of treating individuation and socialisation directly I want to restrict myself to a more special case, which may throw some light on how to proceed in general.

I have chosen competition as a *prima facie* case of individual behavior, and cooperation as a similar *prima facie* case of social behavior, and the title of my contribution could easily be understood as if I were to consider that these two kinds of behavior are, by themselves, the driving forces for developing individual and social behavior in general.

Of course, this line of reasoning would make it impossible to retain the correct boundaries between empirical research and conceptual investigation. A philosopher's contribution cannot start by selecting certain phenomena as candidates for an answer to the inquiry into the mechanisms of sociogenesis, and then proceed by attempting to find out whether they have been well chosen or not.

Only the positive sciences, psychology and sociology in particular, might pursue such a line of empirical research, though they would certainly start in a far more sophisticated manner.

My task is of a different nature. I am not looking for phenomena which may count as competitive or cooperative activities—*finding* phenomena—but I am rather using "competitive" and "cooperative" as conceptual tools as applied to activities, which means, that I have to construct two appropriate kinds of activities—*inventing* phenomena—such that they may serve, in the terminology of Wittgenstein's *Philosophical Investigations*, as measuring rods, as a means of comparison, with which to identify ongoing activities in terms of competitiveness or cooperativeness.

Philosophical inquiry is a reflexive activity, but nonetheless inseparably linked to positive activity. Finding and inventing phenomena belong together, even though division of labour tends to make us think otherwise.

In order to understand the two notions "competition" and "cooperation," which are usually understood as "pursuing individual interests" and "pursuing common interests," respectively, it is useful to go back in history to where ideas about becoming human have been spelled out in terms of a cultural process starting from a state of nature. One of the oldest documents still available is the myth attributed by Plato to the sophist Protagoras and included in Plato's dialogue *Protagoras* (320c8—323c2). Here we find a tale in which human beings come into existence in two distinct steps.

In the first step, technical abilities are acquired to compensate for natural deficiencies—they appear individually as a character of the species and make its members able to survive collectively as natural beings. The whole realm of τέχναι, which includes the arts, and religious rites as well, is available on this level. But there is a second step, which is understood as the advent of rationality in its full sense of practical abilities to provide for political units of self-government: honesty or justness (δίκη) and modesty or respect (αἰδώσ) lead to solidarity (φιλία).

These language dependent abilities, arising from mutual recognition, cannot be exercised except through individual distinction and social coherence. Any such social individual leads a life governed by reason—a rational being.

Here we have found the backbone necessary for guaranteeing the original equivalence of the two ancient "definitions" of man: a rational animal (ζῷον λογον ἔχον) and a social animal (ζῷον πολιτικόν). Two remarks should be added: First, the Platonic separation of non-rational, or not-yet-rational, poietical activities from rational practical activities—I have expressed this by using the Aristotelian distinction of poiesis (producing something with an external aim in mind) and praxis (doing something for its own sake) (Bien, 1973)—relegates every action not governed by a general law (in Aristotelian terminology: an action which is not its own aim) to a sphere of merely natural as well as cultural exigencies, which means that it is not truly human, not truly civilized. Late offshoots of this Platonic move may be identified easily, for example, as being Kant's insistence on the undetectability of actions based on morality (Kambartel, 1989) and, still later, as being Habermas' dichotomy of actions into those which are rational (!) with respect to means and ends, and those which serve mutual communication (Habermas, 1981). Competitive ("amoral") behavior seems to precede the more developed stage of cooperative ("moral") behavior, even though the notion of rationality is no longer understood as being restricted to the area of moral legislation (Hegselmann, 1988).

Secondly, the additional Aristotelian separation of rationality as an ability to theorize from sociality as an ability to lead a good life, gradually gives way to a similar developmental bifurcation into a primary level of mere acting, or better still: behavior, and a secondary level of deliberate activity, that is, actions guided, or at least accompanied by, speaking or thinking. Taking both remarks together, we arrive at speaking, on the level of competitive behavior, to be a case of strategic activity without any communicative value.

Whether using language for establishing consensus or showing activity according to a consensus, either characterization of a human group as civilized is part of a progress theory of the cultural process, the progress being measured in terms of complexity of (group) organization, such that Hobbes' *bellum omnium contra omnes* is the initial stage.

In addition to this widespread and influential picture, there is also an alternative account of the cultural process in terms of a decline theory: on the basis of an *aetas aurae*, a natural state of paradisiac existence for each individual—well known from Rousseau's forceful descriptions—an ever increasing consciousness develops and spoils the ability to act spontaneously. Natural individual creativity is hampered by social pressures which are derived from conscious activity both for and against others, and the decline can be measured by the losses in (self-)production (Lorenz, 1990).

Here it seems that both competitive and cooperative behavior impose constraints on a primordial uninhibited way of autarkic living. The Stoic slogan *"secundum naturam vivere,"* though never forgotten, has been audibly resuscitated in these days of growing ecological consciousness, but, of course, without its original pledge for individual self-sufficiency: rather than moving from "barbaric" competition to "civilized" cooperation, as the cultural process is viewed in progress theories, we have here the call to reverse the cultural process leading, according to decline theorists, from natural cooperation, possibly including cooperation with non-human nature as well, to cultural competition.

In both cases competitive behavior is judged to be inferior to cooperative behavior—we may see this as the consequences of the two contradictory traditional assumptions: that man is, by nature, bad (pre-supposition of progress theories) or man is, by nature, good (presupposition of decline theories), but obviously such a moral preoccupation acts as an antidote for the need to argue for either case, or even for other alternatives.

Luckily, there is one author who indeed takes up this issue and uses arguments against both versions or, even better, emends both versions in such a way that neither "good" and "bad" nor "true" and "false" are used descriptively with respect to available phenomena, but as reflexive terms for passing philosophical judgments by reconstructing the objects in question in the way I explained in the beginning. The author I am referring to, and who will act as a guide to solve my title question, is Herder. He seems to have been the first in history to become aware of the *conceptual* relation which holds between the two characterizations of human beings occurring in Protagoras' myth: they are deficient beings, insofar as they lack sufficient protection against inanimate nature and do not possess effective weapons against animals, and they are proficient beings insofar as they have both poietical and practical abilities. For these two abilities, Herder uses the terms "freedom" and "reason," respectively (Abhandlung, 1960).

It is by exercising these abilities that humans define their deficiencies, and therefore it is wrong to treat the relation between proficiency and deficiency as an empirical one of compensation.

The point becomes even clearer if we turn to the details of the interdependence between being proficient and being deficient.

Herder defines the cultural process neither by progress nor by decline, but by a process of education. In fact, in the ninth book of his *Ideen zur Geschichte der Menschheit* (Part II, 1785), he uses a dialogue model of teaching and learning to identify items of a cultural process, inasmuch as both "doing" and "suffering," terms used to characterize the two roles in a teaching and learning process, always occur together. And since every individual being educated by his elders and educating his offspring plays both parts, it is individual distinction together with social coherence, that is competitiveness against a common background and cooperativeness split up into individual approaches, which defines the process of education.

Reason as the ability to organize, and freedom as the ability to produce appear, when exercised, on the side of "doing" as proficiency, and on the side of "suffering" as deficiency. According to Herder, that is why tradition may include errors (deficiency of reason) and why something evil may occur among the items somebody chooses (deficiency of freedom) (Lorenz, 1990).

We can already see here the differences to both an understanding of competition merely as fixing and pursuing individual interests, and cooperation merely as establishing and pursuing common interests. Such an understanding of sociality and rationality in terms of individual and common interests, respectively, has turned the reflexive use of sociality and rationality, which up to Aristotle was the outcome of a self-characterization of humans, into the positive use of describing pre-existing properties of humans. It was Hannah Arendt who first clearly demonstrated how, by translating the Greek term "πολιτικόν" into the Latin term *sociale*, such a change of meaning has led to conceptual confusion throughout our tradition today (Arendt, 1958). Yet, it was not this fact alone which had this effect, but one has to take into account another important feature due to the Stoic replacement of πολιτικόν by κοινόν: sociality was no longer restricted to the second Protagorean level of reason-guided ways of living but is understood as also pervading the first level of "natural" abilities.

It is this insight, together with the recognition that also rationality—not limited to means-ends rationality—is required for exercising first-level poietical activities which made Herder confident of being right in re-establishing the reflexive use of sociality and rationality, but not throughout the whole range of human activities.

Here, "sociality" (Herder's "freedom") does not refer to the fight among individual interests whether understood in the intentional setting of a (cultural) "fight for power" or reduced to explanations by a causal theory to account for the Darwinian "fight for survival," but to social coherence both in acting and speaking, which is cooperation *by means of* individual contributions: Realizing that everyone must invent his own way of life and his own world view, provides the opportunity for the gradual development of sociality, which may also be called solidarity to use a term more akin to the Greek term φιλία (friendship) which had served the same purpose as mentioned above.

Likewise "rationality" (Herder's "reason") no longer refers to the ability of acting according to common interests, even if "common" is not restricted to some group interests but refers to full-fledged moral generality. Instead, it signifies individual distinction on all levels which is competition *grounded in* a community of acting and speaking (as a paradigm of rational behavior everyone acknowledges: competition by argumentation). Realizing how one's own way of living and one's own world view is found amidst shared activities, is an actualization of another step on the way towards individuality.

Traditionally, from antiquity via Kant to the present day, we are accustomed to speak here of self-determination as the task of reason; but, as reason is said to be concerned with the universal and not with the particular, self-determination is understood as the deliberate submission to universal laws, that is, as the creation of the universal human and not as an universal task to be carried out individually.

It is not difficult to understand why such vexations have occurred. They are unavoidable, I think, when one forgets that individuality and sociality are but stages in a process which is simultaneously a process of individuation and of socialization, the one which had been conceptualized by Herder as the education process. An account which starts with a set of ready-made individuals who have their own preferences and beliefs, because otherwise there is no opportunity to either determine or explain any of the different competitive or cooperative relations among them (these qualifications are understood in the positive sense of fight among individual interests and activity in the common interest, respectively), and also not any one of those relations which count as preceding or following them, such as deliberation, negotiation, arbitration, etc., can no longer apply the concept of self-determination or autonomy to human individuals, but only to the whole species of humans. Among individuals, then, there are only external—natural or cultural—relations of exerting influence on one another—a clear case of heteronomy.

Of course, the process of education I referred to as an alternative must again not be understood in the positive sense of educating, neither in the intentional framework of given educational aims, nor in the causal framework of social engineering.

It has to be a process of *self*-education, where both sides in the process of teaching and learning change their ways of life and their world views by a further step of both individual distinction and social coherence.

The dialogue model for reconstructing the context of non-verbal and verbal activity, that is, the ways of life and the world views (for better visualization you may think of Wittgenstein's famous language-game in the first paragraphs of his *Philosophical Investigations*) clearly shows that, at first, non-verbal activity counts as social, yet verbal activity counts as individual, and if you stop here, non-verbal activity is treated merely as (objective) behavior and verbal activity merely as (subjective) expression.

You have to proceed through one further step of reflection, that is, of reconstruction, and you arrive at the semiotic aspect of non-verbal activity—actions have (subjective) sense (e.g., as explicated by Max Weber's theory of intentions (Weber, 1966)—and at the pragmatic aspect of verbal activity—speaking has (objective) meaning (as explicated, e.g., by the pragmatic maxim of C.S. Peirce (Scherer, 1984): now, non-verbal activity shows its individual aspect and verbal activity its social aspect.

Ways of life and world views can be comprehended only if seen in both their individual and their social aspects. Self-education is not striving for a balance between guiding and letting grow, but setting up limits against becoming influenced: being guided is countered by acting, making use of individual knowing-how, and growing is countered by invoking the knowledge of social norms, the common aspect of activity.

Individuality, a difference between individuals on the level of reflection, can be recognized only within some common activity, sociality, an equality of individuals on the level of reflection, can be performed only by being conscious of the different approaches within the same common activity.

Therefore, we may conclude: the antagonism between competition and cooperation, taken descriptively, changes into the complementarity of competition and cooperation if understood reflexively.

It is just one process, educating self and other, which, from different perspectives, leads to both individuation and socialization.

References

Abhandlung über den Ursprung der Sprache [1772] (1960), In E. Heintel (ed.), *Johann Gottfried Herder. Sprachphilosophische Schriften.* Hamburg: Meiner.

Arendt, H. (1958), *The Human Condition.* Chicago: University of Chicago Press. p. 22ff.

Bien, G. (1973), *Die Grundlegung der politischen Philosophie bei Aristoteles.* Freiburg/ München: Alber.

Habermas, J. (1981), *Theorie des kommunikativen Handelns I-II*. Frankfurt/M: Suhrkamp. espec. I, chap. III.

Hegselmann, R. (1988), Ist es klug, moralisch zu sein? In D. Henrich, R.P. Horstmann (eds.), *Metaphysik nach Kant?* Stuttgarter Hegelkongress 1987. Stuttgart.

Kambartel, F. (1989), Autonomie, mit Kant betrachtet. Zu den Grundlagen von Handlungstheorie und Moralphilosophie. In F.Kambartel (ed.), *Philosophie der humanen Welt*. Frankfurt/M.: Suhrkamp.

Lorenz, K. (1990), *Einführung in die philosophische Anthropologie*. Darmstadt: Wissenschaftliche Buchgesellschaft. (espec. chap. 2.2).

Lorenz, K. (1990), *Einführung in die philosophische Anthropologie*. Darmstadt: Wissenschaftliche Buchgesellschaft. pp. 65-69.

Scherer, B.M. (1984), *Prolegomena zu einer einheitlichen Zeichentheorie. C.S. Peirce's Einbettung der Semiotik in die Pragmatik*. Stauffenburg: Tübingen.

Weber, M. (1966), *Soziologische Grundbegriffe*. Stauffenburg: Tübingen.

2. Sociogenesis of Language: Perspectives on Dialogism and on Activity Theory

Ivana Marková

Introduction

Due to the increasing interest in Bakhtin's work by students and researchers in the social sciences and humanities, much attention has recently been focused on *dialogism* as an epistemological approach to the study of mind and language (e.g., Holquist, 1990; Marková, 1990; Wertsch, 1990, 1991). Dialogism appears to offer an epistemology that is suited, significantly more than mainstream *cognitivism*, to the study of mind and language as *social phenomena* in their change and development. Like cognitivism, dialogism crosses the boundaries between disciplines, capturing interest of scholars in such diverse subjects as linguistics, sociology, communication, psychology, anthropology and literature. Unlike cognitivism, however, the concerns of dialogism reach far beyond those of the cognitive aspects of mind and language. Dialogism encompasses the totality of human agency and conceives it as situated in socio-historical phenomena and in culture. While the focus of *cognitivism* is on the *individual, dialogism*, by definition, concerns the relationships *between* human agents. Such relationships can be those between the self and other, the individual and society, or those between some aspects of human social activities, with language and communication being considered as the most fundamental among them.

As an epistemological approach to the study of mind and language, dialogism can contribute to the theory of *sociogenesis of language* at different levels, such as socio-historical and cultural, ontogenetic and microgenetic. In this chapter, when discussing the concepts of dialogism and activity in psychological research, I will emphasize the importance of the recognition of these different levels in the study of language and thought. In addition, I shall point to some conceptual and terminological problems arising from ambiguous or unclear formulation of questions about the relationship between language and thought. In discussing these issues I shall focus mainly on the work of M.M. Bakhtin (1895-1975), L.S. Vygotsky (1896-1934), and S.L. Rubinstein (1889-1960).

From the Origins of Dialogism to Bakhtin

Today, dialogism is associated primarily with the name of the Russian scholar Mikhail Bakhtin. Dialogism, however, was a subject of keen interest and study of the religiously oriented neo-Kantian philosophers of the 1920s, and the term *dialogism* was probably coined by Rosenstock (1924) in his treatise on applied psychology.

Toward the end of the last century, while return to Kant dominated much of German philosophy, dissatisfaction was expressed by many neo-Kantians with the metaphysics of the transcendental ego. According to this metaphysics, human subjectivity and rationality were located solely in the transcendental self (ego), the nature of which was conceived as universal, timeless and rational. Its critics felt that the transcendental self was divorced from actual human existence and from the life experience of real people, their emotions and concerns. Instead, the neo-Kantians, alongside philosophers such as Kierkegaard and Buber, were concerned with the *dialogical principle*, as they called it, of the mutuality between the self and other. Much inspiration for dialogism came from Jewish orthodox religion. This was very clearly expressed by Hermann Cohen, the founder of the Marburg School of neo-Kantianism. Cohen (1971) maintained that the dialogical principle of selfhood, by which he understood the mutual relation between I and Thou, is fundamental in Jewish Orthodox religion. It would be unthinkable to talk about the ethical self and to mean the individual self alone. The self is always involved in moral action and that can be defined only in terms of I and Thou, a relationship that is unending. This fundamental relationship between I and Thou is established and maintained through speech and communication, a position so emphatically expressed by Buber in his *Ich und Du* (1923). Buber here pinpoints the "sphere of between" as an essential category (*Urkategorie*) of human reality. The dialogical principle and dialogism were also extensively studied by other neo-Kantians such as Rozenzweig (1921) and Ebner (1921). Indeed, dialogism and the dialogical principle of the neo-Kantians have sometimes been claimed to be the most significant bridges connecting philosophy and religion in this century (Michnak, 1968). In contrast to the individualism of the Kantian transcendental ego, the dialogical approach has thus drawn attention to the social nature of humankind. Language and communication have thus been elevated to become the fundamental epistemological principles for its study.

In addition to the religious resources of dialogism, and in spite of its being a basically anti-Hegelian movement, dialogism in general and neo-Kantianism particularly assimilated much of Hegel's thought. Namely, they absorbed his social dialectic of the dyadic relationship between the self and other and his ideas concerning the social nature of self-consciousness, including his claim that humanity relies on the acknowledgment of human beings by each other. The main thrust of Hegel's social dialectic was to show how the self, in the complex journey of self-education, achieves self-consciousness through mutual interaction with other human beings and through acknowledgement of each other. Self-consciousness, reflexive knowledge, and the mind are not *naturally given* to human beings, but arise in *socio-historical and cultural* processes through life-and-death struggle, work, and self-education. According to Hegel (1805-1806/1976), there are two characteristics comprising the essence of humanity: first, the capacity to recognize others for what they are, and second, the desire to be recognized by others. Self-consciousness results from this process of mutual recognition and it can exist only to the extent that it has been created in interdependence with other consciousnesses. For example, Hegel writes in his *Phenomenology of Spirit* (1807, pp. 110, 112): "Self-consciousness achieves its satisfaction only in another self-consciousness..."I" that is "We" and "We" that is "I"...they *recognize* themselves as *mutually recognizing* one another." This phrase of Hegel's, expressing the dialogical principle of the reflexive and social nature of human consciousness, has been repeated in many variations by numerous scholars of different philosophical and psychological orientations. Here are but a few examples:

The individual does not contain in himself the essence of human being, neither as a moral being nor as a thinking being. The essence of human being is contained only within the community, in the unity of person with person....(Feuerbach, 1843)

My sense of myself grows by imitation of you, and my sense of yourself grows in terms of my sense of myself. (Baldwin, 1897, p. 15)

[An individual] becomes an object to himself only by taking the attitudes of other individuals towards himself within a social environment or context of experience and behavior in which both he and they are involved. (Mead, 1934, p. 138)

Self-consciousness refers to the ability to call out in ourselves a set of definite responses which belong to the others of the group. (Mead, 1934, p. 277)

Whatever the construction, the knowledge of other and the knowledge of self are parallel, and the task of understanding early social cognition must be the task of studying self, other and their interaction. (Lewis & Brooks-Gunn, 1979, p. 240)

The mechanism of knowing oneself (self-awareness) and the mechanism for knowing others are one and the same. (Vygotsky, 1979, p. 29)

I am aware of myself and become myself only through recognition of myself for the other, through the other and with the help of other. The most important acts, constitutive of self-consciousness, are determined by their relation to another consciousness. (Bakhtin, 1986a, p. 329-30)

Clearly, even Bakhtin expressed himself in a very Hegelian way although at various places in his writings he referred to Hegel's "monologism" (cf. for example, Bakhtin, 1986a, p. 384). Bakhtin was well acquainted with Buber's work, even before his university years, and he was also strongly influenced by the neo-Kantians of the Marburg school, in particular by Cohen and Kagan (Clark & Holquist, 1984). It can be assumed that the dialogical principle was also close to Bakhtin's own religious inclinations and his Russian Orthodox faith.

One can conclude this section by pointing out that Bakhtin's dialogism was part of the *Zeitgeist* of the dialogically oriented movement in the early part of this century. Bakhtin's dialogism, however, went far beyond the claims of the mutuality between self and others in speech and communication. Having argued that "language and the word are almost everything in human life," (Bakhtin, 1986a, p. 118) he kept on elaborating this thesis to its very limits throughout his life work. For Bakhtin, all human sciences are by definition dialogical and he put dialogue and dialogism in the center of their subject matter.

Activity and the Notion of a "Tool" in Philosophy

The reflexive and social theory of the self in which language and communication play an essential role has, since the eighteenth century, been part of a more general trend that viewed human beings as agents. Human agency first became an important aspect of epistemology through Kant's claims that objects as we know them must conform to our own concepts (Kant, 1781, B xvi-xviii) and that the mind gives laws to nature (ibid., A 127). This can be interpreted to mean that it is our mind and the activity of thought processes that determine the kind of world we perceive.

In Hegel's epistemology human agency took on an even more fundamental role. As the start Hegel made important claims concerning different kinds of relationships between agents and objects. The relationship between an animal and an object is direct, immediate, and impulsive. The animal *consumes* the object in order to live. In contrast, the approach of human beings towards objects is by nature reflexive and mediated through tools and instruments. Human beings have a capacity for work, that is, for creating, manipulating, and reconstructing objects in their environment (Hegel, 1971, p. 437). In order to transform an object from what it is into something different, one needs to take a distant look at that thing; in other words, one must reflect upon one's action. Sometimes one has to wait for a long time for the results of one's actions. Hegel characterized work as desire in abeyance or in waiting.

Using physical tools and instruments to change their physical environment is but one feature of the reflexive nature of human beings. Equally important, people also intersubjectively interact with other human beings, that is, with objects that are equal to themselves in having intellect and in using mental tools such as logical reasoning and language. Just as physical tools *mediate* between people and nature, so do mental tools *mediate* between people themselves. Analyzing language as a mental tool *mediating* intersubjective activities, Hegel pointed out that human speech is very different from animal "speech." In his view, human speech has developed from gestures, physical signs, and from mimicry, a position that was later on elaborated by Wundt (1916). Language is the most important of mental tools. It is, as Hegel called it, an *ideal instrument* because it is through language that people express their recognition of each other.

When Hegel discussed speech as an ideal instrument of intersubjectivity, he did not say explicitly whether he meant language as a socio-cultural product or speech in face-to-face interaction. However, it can be inferred from the views he expressed in the *System der Sittlichkeit* (1971) that he meant language in the former sense. However, in the *Phenomenology of Spirit* (1807/1977) he made a brief comment about the ontogenetic acquisition of speech, and it is certainly clear from the master and slave passage that it is through speaking in face-to-face interaction that interactants acknowledge each other.

It is important to bear in mind that Hegel used the term *mediation* (*Vermittlung*) with respect to the human use of physical and mental tools. This was in contrast to the "immediacy" of animals. It is my view that in his sense "mediation" could almost be substituted by the term *reflexion*. To reflect means to consider one's possibilities of choice and the implications of one's choices for one's activities and their impact. To reflect means to act with one's goal in mind. Physical and mental tools, therefore, are results of reflexive, that is intelligent, reasoning and of the particular intentions of their creator.

Semiotics and Dialogue

A number of scholars have recently drawn attention to similarities between Vygotsky's and Bakhtin's approaches to the study of activity, language and speech, and in particular, to their emphasis on semiotics (Wertsch, 1990, 1991; Lee, 1985; Kozulin, 1990; Brushlinski & Polikarpov, 1990). Wertsch, moreover, has emphasized Vygotsky's and Bakhtin's socio-historical and cultural approach to the study of mind. While the similarities between Vygotsky's and Bakhtin's views cannot be ignored, I will raise here some issues focusing on the differences between these two scholars. Analysing these differences I hope to clarify certain conceptual and terminological problems in the research concerning the relationship between language and thought. The differences between Vygotsky's and Bakhtin's positions, in my view, are encapsulated in the fact that Vygotsky's starting point for the study of language was *semiotics* while for Bakhtin it was *dialogue*.

Vygotsky argued that the only correct way of exploring consciousness is by the methods of semiotics. He maintained that a word is a microcosm of human consciousness (Vygotsky, 1986, p. 256). Higher mental processes such as cognition, logical memory and selective attention, are "mediated" by semiotic tools. These tools range from simple signs, for example, words, to complex semiotic systems, such as literary creations, and interactive relationships with other human beings.

Let us consider Vygotsky's conception of the word as a sign and a mental tool. Before the child acquires language, a word, for him or her, is a stimulus from the *outside*: it is, first, the parents and other caretakers who, by the word, direct and control the child's activities. Only later on, when the child masters the language, can that word effect the child's activities from *within*. A series of experiments by Vygotsky, Luria, and their students on the role of speech in the regulation of normal and abnormal behavior (Luria, 1961) support these claims. In this sense, a word, in Vygotsky's and Luria's experiments, is conceived to be a ready-made mental tool mediating action. It instigates an action in the child but does not itself change in this process, just as a physical tool does not change its form when used upon an object. Indeed, a hammer would not be a good hammer if it did not resist the nail, because it could not be used for the same purpose again.

Having become a sign regulating action, the same word can "mediate" repeatedly the same kind of action because the user (whether a listener if the word comes from outside or a speaker if the person uses it him- or herself) now associates the word with certain commitments, responsibilities, or relationships. The phrase "a mental tool mediating action," therefore, conveys what is intended to be made known. The term "mediating" in this phrase means "facilitating" or "triggering off" action. Thus it appears that while the term "mental tool" preserves its Hegelian meaning, the term "mediating" does not. In Vygotsky's and Luria's experiments, "mediating" is not meant to convey "reflexion," that is the opposite of "immediacy."

The important feature of Vygotsky's theory was his distinction between the natural and social stage in human ontogenesis. He characterized the pre-verbal child as being in the natural stage. At this stage the child's activities are similar to those of an animal, being immediate rather than mediated. When discussing these stages Vygotsky used the term "mediation" in its original Hegelian sense. It is only when the child acquires speech and other kinds of symbols and signs that these semiotic mediators start directing the child's activities, which then become truly human. That is to say, they stop being immediate and become mediated (Vygotsky, 1986; see also Brushlinski &

Polikarpov, 1990, pp. 48-50). I shall borrow here a quotation, cited by Brushlinski and Polikarpov (1990, p. 50), of Varshava's and Vygotsky's definition of these two stages, which was published in the Psychological Dictionary in Moscow, 1931:

> from the moment the child masters language, the whole inner development of the child changes from the animal phase (biological) into a proper human (social) phase. It is language that lifts the child towards the whole mental experience of humankind and enables the development of his or her higher mental functions (generalization, judgment, computation and so on).

One cannot leave unnoticed, in this and other claims of Vygotsky, the direct influence of Hegel's ideas in the *System der Sittlichkeit*, including the use of terms such as "mediation," "physical tool," "instrument," and "mental tool." However, while Hegel's analysis of tools and mediation was a part of his socio-historical and cultural analysis of the development of humankind, that is of the process of cultural and social genesis, in Vygotsky's work this Hegelian kind of analysis was applied to ontogenesis. Vygotsky, of course, also spoke about language in its socio-cultural context as Wertsch (1985, 1990, 1991) and others have emphasised. However, it was in human ontogenesis concerned with the study of action, language, and thought, and in his distinction between the natural and social stage in child development that Vygotsky used "tools," "instruments" and "mediation" as explanatory concepts. This makes his argument a bit difficult to digest today. While such views were quite common amongst child psychologists in the 1920s (cf. Brushlinski & Polikarpov, 1990), they are certainly out of fashion in the 1990s. Our knowledge of child development today is based on the assumption that a newborn baby is fully equipped for intersubjectivity and that she or he functions from birth as a social human being (cf. Newson, 1977, Trevarthen, 1979, Marková, 1987).

Vygotsky's main concern was to explain the emergence of the social stage in child development, and it was in this context that the well-known Vygotsky-Piaget controversy took place and that Vygotsky expressed his views concerning the function of egocentric and inner speech. According to Vygotsky, all internal higher mental processes, such as selective attention, logical memory, verbal thought, and concept formation, have their origin in forms that are *external* to the child's cognition. They first exist for the child as interactional, that is behavioral, processes that have social purposes before they become the child's own *inner*, that is cognitive processes. Vygotsky's argument for this transition from outer to inner is very similar to that of George Herbert Mead (1934). Mead, too, maintained that the origin of gestures in a social act can be explained without bringing in the individual's inner processes such as intentionality or awareness. Gestures in interaction serve as social stimuli even before they become internalized, that is, even before the individual is able to *reflect upon* them. In the same vein, Vygotsky argued that, "when we speak of a process, 'external' means 'social.' Any higher mental function was external because it was social at one point before becoming an internal, truly mental function" (1981, p. 164). Nevertheless, in spite of the considerable similarity in the way Mead and Vygotsky explained the process of internalization, there is an important terminological dissimilarity between them revealing an underlying conceptual difference. Mead made it quite clear that it is *reflexivity*, that is the ability to become an *object* to itself, that makes for a human dialogue. It is a characteristic of such dialogues of symbolic or significant gestures that the interactants attribute the same meanings to their vocal and verbal gestures. Reflexivity in Mead's sense means constructing one's own point of view on the basis of one's own and the other person's perspectives; or of constructing the meaning of a word or of an utterance from one's own and the other's perspectives. Vygotsky, instead, uses Hegel's term "mediation" to account for internalization. However, neither he nor his followers make it clear what precisely mediation is. As I have argued above, "mediation" can mean different things in different Vygotskian contexts.

Bakhtin's position with respect to semiotics was very different from that of Vygotsky. Bakhtin maintained that, "Semiotics deals primarily with the transmission of ready-made communication using a ready-made code. But in live speech, strictly speaking, communication is first created in the process of transmission, and there is, in essence, no code" (1986a, p. 147).

Today, Bakhtin is often referred to as a semiotician (e.g., Lee, 1985), but the above quote shows no evidence that he would wish to be labelled in this way. Although Bakhtin frequently spoke about a word as a sign, he was critical of Saussure's semiotics at various places in his writing (cf. for example Vološinov, 1973; Bakhtin, 1986). Apart from the criticism of semiotics for being concerned with a ready-made code, he was also critical of Saussure for ignoring *speech genres* (Bakhtin, 1986a, p. 81). Bakhtin's focus on living speech, rather than on relatively stable language codes, was clearly expressed, for example, in Vološinov: "The meaning of a word is determined entirely by its context. In fact, there are as many meanings of a word as there are contexts of its usage" (Vološinov, 1973, p. 79). It was because of this position that Veltruský, one of the most important semioticians of the Prague school, expressed his dissatisfaction with what he called the extreme position of Vološinov, totally ignoring the relatively stable features of word meaning potential (Veltruský, 1976, p. 136). Of course, there is ample evidence in Bakhtin's writing that he fully acknowledged that language also has relatively stable, societal aspects that are embodied in grammar and the meaning potential of words. He also fully recognized the importance of the science of linguistics. However, Bakhtin made clear his position that linguistics cannot deal with all the aspects of language and in particular that it is not equipped to deal with face-to-face speech and communication (Bakhtin, 1984, p.

150ff.). And it is in dialogue that Bakhtin's interest lies.

Bakhtin's analysis of the word is very different from that of Vygotsky. He never considered a word as a sign on its own but only as belonging, jointly, to the speaker and the listener. Moreover, words do not belong to speakers and listeners as a dyad. First, there is the speaker's meaning, and second, there is the listener's meaning, which these two participants each bring into the dialogue; and then there is the final meaning as the participants' joint perspective. Bakhtin spoke about discourse as "a three-role drama (it is not a duet but a trio)" (Bakhtin, 1986, p. 359). In other words, the meaning of a word in each context lies somewhere *between* the speaker and listener as their joint product. Words and utterances are always jointly constructed by speakers and audiences, even if the audience is only imaginery.

For Bakhtin, a word is always double-directed. By this he means that it is directed, at the same time, both at the object of speech and at another person. It is only in its relations to another person's speech that a word manifests its truly dialogical relationships, such as its hidden polemics, irony, or parody. In such concrete cases the word cannot be a ready-made sign. Its meaning changes as a person uses it for his or her own purposes; by asking a question the speaker problematizes another person's word; a word is never neutral, it evaluates another person's word; it is used to master another person's word. (Bakhtin, 1984, p. 162). For example, one can repeat another's word as closely as possible, in order to imitate and gain control over the other's word. Or, one can repeat the other's word not to imitate it but to problematize it or to put on it a different meaning and thus to appropriate it.

There is, however, no basic disagreement between Vygotsky's and Bakhtin's positions with respect to language. Rather, their positions are complementary and the differences discussed in this section are ones of emphasis rather than of principle. Vygotsky's aim was to explain the *social* nature of inner speech and of the processes involved in the internalization of the higher mental functions. However, without making it self-evident, the notion of language he used for this purpose was that of a relatively stable system of signs or, to use Bakhtin's expression, of ready-made codes of semiotics. Vygotsky's approach to language was more *object-related* than *person-related*. Of course, the object-relatedness of Vygotsky's approach was social in the sense that it was in the context of dialogue—whether adult with child or child with him- or herself—that this object-relatedness took place. However, the intellectual tasks that Vygotsky explored, such as learning, cognition, and problem-solving, were lacking in Bakhtin's heteroglossia and hidden polemics, and it was these very characteristics of language that, for Bakhtin, defined the dialogicity of speech. Vygotsky and Bakhtin were simply exploring different things.

For Vygotsky, once the child reaches the social stage, acting upon objects is social acting because it is acting mediated by word and thought. From this point of view it is a dialogical activity. However, for Bakhtin, acting upon objects was a monological activity. Following Dilthey, Bakhtin argued that the study of objects belongs to natural science and, as such, requires causal explanation. In contrast, human interaction, as it is studied by the human sciences, is always dialogical and a subject of understanding and interpretation (rather than causal explanation). In contrast, as a Hegelian scholar, Vygotsky did not make any fundamental distinction between the subjects of the natural and human sciences: "The mastery of nature and the mastery of behaviour are mutually related (because) in the course of man's transformation of nature, his own nature changes as well" (Vygotsky, 1983, p. 90). Although the differences between Vygotsky's and Bakhtin's positions are ones of emphasis and not of substance, it is important that they be borne in mind when asking questions about the relationship between language and thought. Neither Vygotsky nor Bakhtin were interested in getting involved in a Sausserean problem.

Language and Activity Theory

One of Vygosky's contemporaries was S.L. Rubinstein. Before the Soviet Revolution he studied philosophy, sociology, anthropology, and natural sciences in Marburg under the neo-Kantians. He was a very sophisticated philosopher and psychologist who was well read in all the modern philosophical and psychological trends of his time. While for Vygotsky the starting point for the study of consciousness was semiotics, for Rubinstein it was activity. Curiously, Rubinstein's work has not been discussed, in the context of the Soviet activity theory, as much as that of the "troika" Vygotsky-Luria-Leontjev (for an excellent comparison on the subject of activity theory and language between Vygotsky, Rubinstein, and Bakhtin, see Brushlinski & Polikarpov, 1990) which, in my opinion, is undeserving.

There are many similarities between the activity theories of Vygotsky and Rubinstein. They were both concerned with the study of human consciousness, with the study of processes rather than products, and with the relationship between language and thought. But for Vygotsky the point of departure was *semantics*, whereas for Rubinstein it was an *activity theory*. These differences in their points of departure are not only ones of emphasis but also of different theoretical assumptions. I shall bring them out by comparing the manner in which Vygotsky and Luria on the one hand, and Rubinstein on the other, conceptualized *instruction* in learning and problem-solving situations.

In the Vygotsky-Luria research on learning, concept formation and problem-solving, the role of instruction was linked to the child's developmental stages. For example, the role of instruction was shown to be crucial in the studies on the zone of *proximal development*. By instructing the child properly, the tutor can induce him or her to use skills and abilities that otherwise would not be activated. Socially provided assistance in the form of instruction is essential in child development, enabling the child to take full advantage of his or her intellectual potentialities. Vygotsky (1978) explained that the basic characteristic of appropriate instruction is that it leads to *internalization* of processes which until now have only been available externally, that is through relationships with other people. This is a reference, again, to the internalization of higher mental processes. As Valsiner (1988, p. 147) clarifies it, only if instruction is timed properly can it be effective in the sense of facilitating the "integration of the instructed function into the child's own action schemes, and the internalizing of it into his cognitive schemata (making use of Piaget's (1979) terminology here)." One can see that this theorizing leans upon the semiotic nature of language. Instruction, which is a matter of words, functions as a semiotic mediator of the child's mental activity and stimulates its internalization. Indeed, it is at this very point, i.e. when higher mental processes become internalized, Vygotsky (1986) argues, that language and thought, which originally started from two different genetic roots, are finally brought together. From now on thought becomes verbal and speech rational (Vygotsky, 1986, p. 83). This intertwining of language and speech also signifies the end of the natural stage and the beginning of the social stage in child development.

Rubinstein's approach to the question of the relationship between language and thought was theoretically more sophisticated. He pointed out that the question of this relationship itself has often been ambiguously formulated: the relationship between language and thought usually being considered either from the functional or the genetic point of view (Rubinstein, 1957). In the former case, the question concerns thinking or thought that has already been genetically accomplished. In the latter case it concerns an inquiry as to whether language and speech are necessary preconditions for the emergence of thought in historical evolution or in ontogenetic development. It could be added that "genetic" can mean not only ontogenetic and historical but also phylogenetic, socio-cultural, or microgenetic. And of course, one can supply different answers about the relationship between language and thought depending on what kind of genesis is meant.

Having made the distinction between language as a historical and cultural category and speech as an activity of the individual, Rubinstein (1958, p. 45) argued that the intellectual activity of the individual is not the outcome of internalization of external influences. Such a position would ignore the socio-historical nature of human thought (this argument must have been directed at Vygotsky). According to Rubinstein each cognitive activity, before it becomes internalized, must already have a well established internal basis. It is thus implied that a newborn baby must already be biologically and socially predisposed for verbal thought. Rubinstein made it clear that he did not deny the existence of internalization processes. However, internalization must be conceptualized as a *consequence* and not as a *mechanism* of intellectual development (Rubinstein, 1958, p. 45).

Rubinstein takes the same theoretical point of view with respect to the role of *instruction* in learning and problem-solving. Instruction is not just a verbal stimulus for the child; it is already a verbal thought in terms of which the given problem is defined. Therefore, it is already the beginning of the analysis of that problem. In other words, one and the same problem can be defined in different ways thus leading to different kinds of analysis, depending on how it is verbally formulated. From this point of view, instruction not only directs the individual to a particular mental activity, it also re-formulates the problem itself. It is a figure-ground relationship, constantly re-defined by the thinking and speaking human agent. The instruction affects the thought and the thought has an effect on the way the problem is verbally re-formulated. Rubinstein characterized his own theoretical approach as that of *analysis through synthesis*.

Rubinstein's arguments, that one often cannot find the solution of a given problem because it was formulated in a certain way and a particular mental set established, are similar to those of Kuhn (1962). In his *Structure of Scientific Revolutions*, Kuhn gave numerous examples of problems in the history of science that could have been solved several centuries earlier if they had been formulated differently or if certain philosophical assumptions had not been made. In Rubinstein's case, too, the formulation of a problem could misguide the solver by drawing attention to irrelevant features of the problem situation. In his empirical research Rubinstein used certain kinds of problems to prove his point: these were problem-solving puzzles and mathematical problems. He showed that these were differences in problem-solving processes arising from whether the instruction directed the solver's attention to relevant or irrelevant aspects of the problem-situation. Rubinstein (1958) believed that there is no essential difference between problem-solving puzzles in the laboratory on the one hand, and creative tasks in the arts and science on the other. In creative and scientific problems irrelevant information exists naturally, being a necessary part of the situation. In psychological experiments and in education it is the researcher or the tutor who misleads his or her subjects or pupils by presenting them with inappropriate instruction.

Vygotsky, too, as we have seen above, argued that the quality of instruction and its proper timing are decisive as to whether the child will solve the task in question. However, there is an important difference between Vygotsky's and Rubinstein's theorizing on this point. In Vygotsky's experiments the instruction is a *verbal sign* (and it must be an effective sign) *mediating* the motor or mental task and facilitating *internalization* of the relevant higher mental processes. In other words, the task of the instruction is to bring language and thinking together. In contrast, in Rubinstein's experiments the solver is given not only a verbal sign, but a *verbal thought* defining the problem in one way rather than in another. One might perhaps think that the difference between Vygotsky's and Rubinstein's approach is not sufficient to justify a detailed discussion of their cases. However, it is an important difference. In Vygotsky's case, language and thought are brought together by means of instruction. In Rubinstein's case, speech already involves thinking (although, as Rubinstein (1957) himself points out, speaking does not mean thinking!) because thinking is a specific characteristic of human speech. It is wrong, he argued, to talk about thinking as one of the functions of speech as is sometimes done (e.g., Bűhler, 1928).

These considerations also show that the question about the relationship between language and thought, or speech and thinking, must clearly specify whether one means language as a relatively stable system of signs possessed by society, or speech in face-to-face dialogue: whether one means thought as a stock of knowledge circulated in the given culture or thinking as an activity of a single individual. We shall now turn to these questions in some detail.

Thought/Thinking and Language/Speech

Humboldt (1836) drew attention to the internal relations between language as social possession and as individual expression. As a social possession, language may be conceived as a stock of words and a system of rules that, over the course of millennia, have stabilized themselves so as to exert an invisible power over individuals. At the same time, however, each person expresses him- or herself in language as if it peculiarly belonged to him or her. In this sense, language lives only through actual speech and individual use. Every speech action, therefore, is the result of interaction between language as a collective and cultural property and the individual's idiosyncratic expression. Humboldt's distinction between language and speech was later taken up by various scholars (e.g., Potebnja, 1913; Mathesius, 1911). However, it was Saussure's explicit elaboration of the social/individual dichotomy of *langue* and *parole* that stimulated so much interest, criticism and inspiration for language oriented social science.

Just as, for heuristic purposes, one can distinguish between language and speech, so one can distinguish between thought, i.e. knowledge as a socio-historical category, and thinking as an individual process. By knowledge I mean a very broad range of social phenomena, from scientific knowing, to shared and collective representations of things and events, and to traditions and myths passed on over generations. All of these social forms of knowledge have, inevitably, their expressions in the thinking processes of individual human beings.

Knowledge and thought circulate in society mostly through their verbal forms. Indeed, it is through language that knowledge obtains its seemingly fixed and objectified character (Rommetveit, 1990). It would be ludicrous, therefore, even to attempt, artificially, to consider them as independent entities and to ask questions about language separately from thought and vice versa. Yet questions about the relationship between language and thought are frequently asked and they are legitimate questions. However, to answer them properly one must clarify whether it is the social or the individual realization of language and thought that is the focus of enquiry. In the remainder of this chapter we shall draw attention to four possible relationships between language, thought, speech, and thinking and to the implications of such relationships for psychological theory and research.

(a) *Language as a System of Signs and Knowledge as a Cultural Category*
Individuals are born into the language of their community and into various systems of socially shared knowledge, beliefs, traditions, and myths. These socially formed systems of knowledge, whether one calls them "collective representations" (Durkheim, 1898) or "social representations" (Moscovici, 1984), are adopted by individuals just like the systems of "facts" of the physical and social reality in which they live. Moreover, just as natural facts have their names, say, "wind" or "stars," so do social "facts" have their names, say, "democracy," "idiot" or "crime." Often, things are thought to be what they are because of how they are called. Saying that something is "X" is not just placing that thing into a particular category. Saying that something is X also provides an explanation of that thing and an evaluation of it. Vygotsky (1986, p. 222) referred to children's explanations of the names of objects by their attributes. For example, the child explains that a cow is called "cow" because it has horns, or a calf is called "calf" because it has small horns, and so on. However, even adults make very close associations between names and the properties of objects to which they refer. Numerous efforts to re-name particular social phenomena convey the belief that the change of a name will remove the stigma or the negative evaluation attached to the thing in question (Moscovici, 1984; Marková & Jahoda, 1992).

Words, therefore, are signs evoking particular associations. Since much of what we say is said unreflexively, i.e. without awareness of the implications of particular meanings and labels for other people (Goffman, 1968), language as a system of signs perpetuates conservative images about social phenomena, knowledge, and beliefs. Often, a social phenomenon may have already changed, yet its name may have remained the same. For example, political changes are not accompanied immediately by changes of particular political terms. Thus, "democracy" in a previously totalitarian regime and "democracy" in a market economy are the same labels for different social phenomena. In a period of social change the label may still evoke associations with the previous regime. One cannot take it for granted that in the countries of Eastern and Central Europe the term "democracy" that was associated with "people's democracy" in the past regime now has similar associations to those in the West. Similarly the term "equality" may still be associated with equality in possessions and not with equalities in choices and opportunities people are given. Thus, language is a conservative semiotic tool; it perpetuates prejudice, evokes images, and in order to change one's images, it has to be brought to awareness. The less aware we are of its power, the greater its effect (Moscovici, 1984).

Research into the relationship between language as a system of signs and knowledge as a historical category is one of the focuses of research examining social representations in present European social psychology, sociology, and media studies. It raises important questions, for example about the nature of prejudice, about labeling of disadvantaged social groups, about semantic networks of political terms, and about the ways mass media write about AIDS, crime, or quality of life.

(b) *Language as a System of Signs and Individual Thinking*
It is this relationship that was explored in the typical Vygotsky and Luria experiment. Here it is the word, the ready-made sign that, in a tool-like manner, controls and directs the individual's thinking in a given situation. Since this case has already been discussed in detail, we shall not dwell on it again. As Vygotsky and Luria themselves emphasized, this research raises important questions not only in the field of child psychology but also in the areas of learning difficulties and neural and motor disorders.

(c) *Speech and Thought (or Knowledge as a Cultural Category)*
This relationship is a complex one because it involves at least two different cases. First, one can be asking about the effect of culturally shared knowledge upon the individual's speech/thinking (verbal thought). For example, one can ask in what ways existing social representations of a particular social phenomenon, say, of drug use, gender, or national identity, are reflected in the individual's (or individuals') verbal thought. This is different from (a) because in that case the relationship under investigation was, in a sense, disembodied. In (a) one is concerned with the study of the relationships within two relatively stable semiotic systems: language labels and knowledge as a cultural phenomenon. In (c), however, one is focusing on the relationship between knowledge as a cultural phenomenon and the individual's mental activities as molded by their mental environment. In this case, shared knowledge imposes itself on the individual as a power affecting his or her verbal thought.

However, one can pose the question about the relationship between the individual's verbal thought and knowledge as a cultural category in a different manner. Now we focus on the individual as an agent of social change.

Whether a creative individual and scientist like Darwin or Einstein, or a leader of a pressure group, he or she influences changes in shared knowledge and beliefs and raises public awareness, thus facilitating social change. A pressure group may persistently seek to awake public awareness concerning the stigmatizing use of certain words in order to stop public prejudice and change collective representations of a particular phenomenon. There are many examples of such cases in the language related to the handicapped. Recently, terms like "mongol," "low-grade," or "mentally handicapped," have been discarded and substituted by other terms such as "person with learning difficulties" or "exceptional child." These are direct attempts, through speech, to change social representations.

(d) Speech and Thinking

This relationship is the one in which Bakhtin was particularly interested. It involves individuals in a face-to-face dialogue or in a dialogical situation in a broader sense, such as reading a text, in which case the dialogue proceeds between the speaker and an absent audience. This paradigm also includes Rubinstein's experiments in which speech and thinking co-determine each other. The emphasis of these experiments is on the hermeneutic relationship between what is said and how it can be interpreted.

Finally, it is important to emphasize once again that these four kinds of relationships between language and thought have heuristic value only. Speech and thinking are always embedded in their historical and cultural contexts and cannot be separated from them. Moreover, one cannot simply categorize the situations involving the study of language and thought in one of the four groups according to some external criteria. The nature of their relationship is given solely by the definition of the problem under study.

Conclusion

Dialogism has recently been re-defined as a socio-cognitive approach to human cognition and communication (Marková and Foppa, 1990; 1991; Rommetveit, in press). The important feature of dialogism is its concern with the social, cultural and historical embeddedness of all human phenomena. Dialogism, therefore, is closely linked to both kinds of problems delineated by Willibrord de Graaf (this volume) as the main concerns of sociogenesis: the socio-historical construction of subject-forms and the corresponding variations in psychic development. Indeed, the four types of relationships between language and thought discussed in this chapter also refer to these two kinds of concerns of sociogenesis. Both language and thought are relatively stable products of history and culture, yet constantly changed and developed by individuals in the course of use.

The fundamental feature of dialogism, relevant to sociogenesis, is its underlying logic of internal relations, that is, dialectic (Bakhtin, 1986) or co-genetic logic (Rommetveit, 1990; in press). According to this logic of triadic development, every phenomenon, be it an organism, a speech action or a single word, has its "outside." The phenomenon and its "outside" complement each other, both being parts of the same whole. They are defined in terms of each other, just as are figure and ground, and each determines what the other is and how it functions in time. The phenomenon, for example, the individual's cognition, and its "outside," for example, the relevant cultural environment, co-develop together. The individual affects its environment and the environment has its effect on the individual. They are internally related, mutually influencing each other. The intelligibility of the term "individual cognition" in the dyad "individual-culture" is dependent on the intelligibility of its counterpart, "culture." If one component of the dyad undergoes change or development, the logic of their internal relationship is such that the other component also undergoes change or development. If sociogenesis takes as its goal examination of the relationships between individual and culture, then co-genetic logic is essential to this project. Although there are still some strong voices emphasizing the study of biological genesis of language without sociogenesis (Pinker and Bloom, 1991), they are now being strongly tempered (Premack, 1991, Lewontin, 1991). The last two decades have certainly renewed interest in dialogism and intersubjectivity, and the signs are that this interest will continue. It is within this context that clarity of questions about the cultural and individual nature of language and thought can be a vital factor in encouraging progress in this area of study.

Note

I adopt Holquist's (1990) view that the book on *Marxism and the Philosophy of Language*, signed by Vološinov, was essentially Bakhtin's work.

References

Bakhtin, M.M. (1984), *Problems of Dostoevsky's Poetics*. C. Emerson (ed. and trs.), Minneapolis, MN: University of Minnesota Press.
Bakhtin, M.M. (1986a), *Speech Genres and Other Late Essays*. C. Emerson and M. Holquist (eds.), V. McGee (trs), Austin, TX: University of Texas Press.
Baldwin, J.M. (1897), *Social and Ethical Interpretations in Mental Development*. London: Macmillan.
Buber, M. (1922), *Ich und Du*. Berlin: Schockenverlag. R.G.Smith (trs.), Edinburgh; T.

and T. Clark, 1937; New York: Charles Scribner, 1937.

Brushlinski, A.V. and Polikarpov, V.A. (1990), *Myschlenije i Obschcenije* [Thinking and Communication]. Minsk: Universitetskoje.

Clark, K. and Holquist, M. (1984), *Mikhail Bakhtin.* Cambridge, MA: Harvard University Press.

Cohen, H. (1971), *Reason and Hope: Selections from Hermann Cohen's Jewish Writings,* E. Josspe (trs.), New York: Norton.

Durkheim, E. (1898), Representations individuelles et representations collectives. *Revue de Metaphysique et de Morale,* VI, 273-302.

Ebner, F. (1921), *Das Wort und die geistigen Realitäten: pneumatologische Fragmente.* Innsbruck: Brenner-Verlag.

Feuerbach, L. (1843), *Principles of the Philosophy of the Future.* M.H. Vogel (trs.), New York: Bobbs-Merrill.

Goffman, E. (1968), *Stigma.* Harmondsworth: Penguin.

Hegel, G.W.F. (1805-06), *Jenaer Systementwurfe III.* In G.W.F. Hegel, *Gesammelte Werke,* 8, Hamburg: Felix Meiner, 1976.

Hegel, G.W.F. (1807), *Phenomenology of Spirit.* A.V. Miller (trs.), Oxford: Clarendon Press, 1977.

Hegel, G.W.F. (1971), *System der Sittlichkeit.* In Jenaer Schriften, Berlin: Irrlitz.

Holquist, M. (1990), *Dialogism: Bakhtin and His World.* London: Routledge.

Humboldt, von W. (1836), *Linguistic Variability and Intellectual Development.* G.C. Buck and F.A. Raven (trs.), Coral Gables, FL: University of Miami Press, 1971.

Kant, E. (1781), *Critique of Pure Reason.* N.K. Smith (trs.), London: Macmillan; New York: St Martin's Press, 1929.

Kozulin, A. (1990), *Vygotsky's Psychology.* Hemel Hempstead: Harvester Wheatsheaf.

Kuhn, T.S. (1962), *The Structure of Scientific Revolutions.* Chicago: University of Chicago Press.

Lewis, M. and Brooks-Gunn, J. (1979), *Social Cognition and the Acquisition of Self.* New York and London: Plenum Press.

Lee, B. (1985), Intellectual origins of Vygotsky's semiotic analysis. In J.V. Wertsch (ed.) *Culture, Communication and Cognition.* Cambridge and London: Cambridge University Press.

Lewontin, R.C. (1990), How much did the brain have to change for speech? Commentary on Pinker and Bloom, *Behavioral and Brain Sciences,* 13, 740-41.

Linell, P. (1991), Dialogism and the orderliness of conversation disorders. In J. Brodin and E.Bjorck-Akesson (eds.), *Methodological Issues in Research in Augmentative and Alternative Communication.* Stockholm: The Swedish Handicap Institute.

Luria, A.R. (1961), *The Role of Speech in the Regulation of Normal and Abnormal Behaviour.* Oxford and New York: Pergamon Press.

Marková, I. (1987), *Human Awareness.* London: Hutchinson Education.

Marková, I. (1990), Introduction. In I. Marková and K. Foppa (eds.), *The Dynamics of Dialogue.* Hemel Hempstead: Harvester Wheatsheaf.

Marková, I. and Foppa, K. (eds.) (1990), *The Dynamics of Dialogue.* Hemel Hempstead: Harvester Wheatsheaf.

Marková, I. and Foppa, K. (eds.), (1991), *Asymmetries in Dialogue.* Hemel Hempstead: Harvester Wheatsheaf.

Marková, I. and Jahoda, A. (In press). Why is the earth called 'earth'? In Baron, S. (ed). *Community Normality and Difference: Meeting Special Needs*. Aberdeen University Press.

Mathesius, V. (1911), O potencialnosti jevu jazykovych, *Vestnik Kralovske Ceske Spolecnosti Nauk*.

Mead, G.H. (1934), *Mind, Self and Society*. Chicago: University of Chicago Press.

Michňák, K. (1968), *Metafyzika Subjektivity* [The Metaphysics of Subjectivity]. Acta Universitatis Carolinae Philosophica et Historica, Monographia XXIII, Prague: The Charles University Press.

Moscovici, S. (1984), The phenomenon of social representations. In R.M. Farr and S. Moscovici (eds.), *Social Representations*. Cambridge and London: Cambridge University Press.

Newson, J. (1977), An intersubjective approach to the systematic description of mother-infant interaction. In R.H. Schaffer (ed.), *Studies in Mother-Infant Interaction*. London and New York: Academic Press.

Pinker, S. and Bloom, P. (1990), Natural language and natural selection. *Behavioral and Brain Sciences*, 13, 707-784.

Potebnja, A. (1913), *Mysl i Yazyk* [Thought and Language]. Kharkov: Gosudar stvennoe Izdatelsvto Ukrainy.

Premack, D. (1990), On the coevolution of language and social competence, Commentary on Pinker and Bloom, *Behavioral and Brain Sciences*, 13, 754-56.

Rommetveit, R. (1990), On axiomatic features of a dialogical approach to language and mind. In I. Marková and K. Foppa, *The Dynamics of Dialogue*. Hemel Hempstead: Harvester Wheatsheaf.

Rommetveit, R. (in press), Outlines of a dialogically based social-cognitive approach to human cognition and communication. In A. Heen Wold (ed.), *Dialogical Alternative*. Oslo: Oslo University Press; Oxford: Oxford University Press.

Rosenzweig, F. (1921), *Stern der Erlösung*. Frankfurt: Kauffmann.

Rubinstein, S.L. (1957), *Bitiye i Soznaniye* [Being and Consciousness]. Moscow: Izdatelstvo Akademii Nauk USSR.

Rubinstein, S.L. (1958), *O Myshlenii i Putyach yego Issledovaniya* [On Thinking and its Investigation]. Moscow: Izdavatelstvo Akademii Nauk USSR.

Trevarthen, C. (1979), Communication and cooperation in early infancy: a description of primary intersubjectivity. In Bullowa, M. (ed.), *Before Speech: The Beginning of Interpersonal Communication*. Cambridge and New York: Cambridge University Press.

Valsiner, J. (1988), *Developmental Psychology in the Soviet Union*. Brighton: Harvester.

Varshava, B.E. and Vygotsky, S.L. (1931), *Psichologicheskij Slovar*. Moskva.

Veltruský, J. (1976), Construction of semantic contexts. In L. Matejka and I.R. Titunik (eds.), *Semiotics of Art*. Cambridge, MA: The MIT Press.

Vološinov, V.N. (1973), *Marxism and the Philosophy of Language*. L. Matejka and I.R. Titunik (trs.), New York and London: Seminar Press.

Vygotsky, L.S. (1978), *Mind in Society: The Development of Higher Psychological Processes*. M. Cole (ed.), Cambridge, MA: Harvard University Press.

Vygotsky, L.S. (1979), Consciousness as a problem in the psychology of behavior.

Soviet Psychology, 17, 3-35.

Vygotsky, L.S. (1981), The genesis of higher mental functions. In J.V. Wertsch (ed.), *The Concept of Activity in Soviet Psychology*. Armonk, NY: Sharpe.

Vygotsky, L.S. (1983), Istoriya Rezvitiya Vysshikh Psikhicheskikh Funkcii [The history of the development of higher psychological functions]. In L.S. Vygotsky, *Sobranie Sochinenie* [Collected papers]. Vol. 3. Moscow: Pedagogika.

Vygotsky, L.S. (1986), *Thought and Language*. Cambridge, MA: The MIT Press.

Wertsch, J.V. (1985), *Vygotsky and the Social Formation of Mind*. Cambridge MA: Harvard University Press.

Wertsch, J.V. (1990), Dialogue and dialogism in a socio-cultural approach to mind. In I. Marková and K. Foppa (eds.), *The Dynamics of Dialogue*. Hemel Hempstead: Harvester Wheatsheaf.

Wertsch, J.V. (1991), *Voices of the Mind*. Hemel Hempstead: Harvester Wheatsheaf; Boston MA: Harvard University Press.

Wundt, W. (1916), *Elements of Folk Psychology*. E.L. Schaub (trs.), London: George Allen and Unwin; New York: Macmillan.

3. Bidirectional Cultural Transmission and Constructive Sociogenesis

Jaan Valsiner

Contemporary psychology is remarkable for the discrepancy between the socially promoted beiief in the speedy advancement of the discipline, and the actually very slow progress in the basic ideas and understanding of the pertinent phenomena. The case of sociogenesis is exemplary in this respect: psychologists have been talking about the relevance of the social world for the formation of the psychological functions of persons for over a century, but still there is very little progress in building explicit theoretical models that could explain *how* the individual becomes a person via social relationships.

Indeed, the sociogenetic thinkers have been busy reiterating the main thesis: All (or at least the "higher") psychological functions of human beings are socially constituted. This declaration can be discovered in the work of Pierre Janet (1925, 1926, 1930, see also Van der Veer & Valsiner, 1988, 1992 in press), James Mark Baldwin (1895, 1902, 1930; Cairns, 1992 in press), Josiah Royce (Valsiner & Van der Veer, 1988), George Herbert Mead (1903, 1910, 1934, see also Markova, 1987, 1990a), Lev Vygotsky (Kozulin, 1990; Van der Veer & Valsiner, 1991), as well as others (e.g., Ananiev, 1930; Boodin, 1913; Cairns, 1979, 1985; Gergen, 1991, Markova, 1990b, Shotter, 1990; Wertsch, 1991). These sociogenetic theorists were preceeded in the focus on the social foundations of individual psychological phenomena by the wide social tradition of "animal magnetism" and "hypnotism" in the 19th century (see Janet, 1925, chapter 4).

However, the claims that psychological functions of individual persons are of social origin and/or nature have not solved the problem of sociogenesis. Instead, such claims have created a new "black box" solution (see Bateson, 1972) that, while recurring in scientific and popular science texts, replaces the knowledge of mechanisms of sociogenesis by declarations about the social nature of the human self. The processes of development by way of which the social nature of the construction of the individual person takes place need to be made explicit, but this has not been the case. The usual sociogenetic argument of the 1990s, like its counterpart a century before, carries with it very few specific ideas that could be used to build a model of sociogenesis.

Models of Sociogenesis

Conceptualization of person↔society relationships has always been a complicated matter, organized by the cultural models shared by laypersons and
scientists alike. The existing efforts to explain sociogenesis can be seen to
reflect a restricted range of possible ideas. Three types can be demonstrated to
have caught the attention of investigators: *harmonious learning, fusion,* and
contagion notions. These three types, as will be shown, reflect the scientists'
unease to conceptualize both the static (structural) and dynamic (processual)
aspects of development at the same time. Of course, thinkers who are somewhat versed in the history of physics may argue that those two sides of
phenomena cannot, in principle, be described concurrently. However, what
may be true for microparticle physics in its relative simplicity, need not be
true in the case of highly complex developmental phenomena.

The "harmonious learning" notion can be seen in any sociogenetic account
which relies heavily on the socialization or enculturation perspectives as those
that have been popular in cultural anthropology (e.g., Cohen, 1971, Mead,
1963, Spindler, 1974). Here the social world provides the necessary information for the developing person, whose role is merely to learn and to become
an adequately functioning member of the given society (or culture as viewed
as an ethnic group). The learning process can be seen as "harmonious" in the
sense that the learner, over time, accepts the society's ways, and does not
alter the status quo of those in the process of learning (see also Van Geert,
1988). It is assumed that society provides the developing person (who is
viewed as a "novice") with a "socially shared" corpus of information, which is
uniform, non-contradictory within itself, and hence all-encompassing as it
"shapes" the novice in an inescapable way. This notion emphasizes structure
(first of the social information, and later, after learning has taken place, of the
person's intra-psychological functions), but leaves the complexities of the
transposition of the structure from the social to the personal worlds up to the
explanatory power (or its lack) of the label "learning" (and of the traditional
learning theories in psychology). The social basis for these notions seems to
be the history of education in Europe, which since the Middle Ages has
emphasized the one-sided transfer of knowledge from the teacher to the
student, albeit recognizing that this process can be a lengthy one.

The "fusion" notions can be seen to solve the sociogenetic problem by way
of positing a non-structured unification of the "personal" and "social" facets of
development, which may lead to synthesis of novelty (e.g., Boodin, 1913) or
to "appropriation" of the social information by the person (Lave, 1988;
Rogoff, 1990; Valsiner, 1991). The fusion-based perspective overemphasizes
the dynamic (processual) aspect of sociogenesis, and attempts to eliminate the
structural order of both the "social" and "personal" worlds. Its social roots

seem to be firmly in the history of the physical sciences, or at least in psychologists' interpretations of these sciences.

Finally, the notions that attempt to integrate both the structural and dynamic facets of sociogenesis belong to the category of "contagion." This type borrows its metaphoric basis from the reasoning of the medical sciences about infectious diseases. Not surprisingly, in the 1980s and 1990s that are characterized by societal discourse about AIDS, building a model of sociogenesis on the transfer of the knowledge of viral infection and immunization mechanisms comes easily under the appropriate suggestions from the prevailing social discourse. However, infectious diseases have been known in medicine for a long time, and hence it is not surprising that the contagion notion of sociogenesis has been utilized long before our times. This parallel was drawn clearly in Vladimir Bekhterev's explanation of the role of social suggestions as *contagium psychicum*, in analogy with that of infectious diseases (*contagium vivum*, see Bekhterev, 1903, p. 5). Similar to the infection-carrying biological microorganisms, the psychological infection is carried by words, gestures, and other aspects of social interaction. The recipient of this "infection" can of course actively fight against it, can neutralize the infection, and can make oneself immune to the given kind of contagion (see also the surfacing of the contagion idea in Cavalli-Sforza et al, 1982, p. 26). The recipient here is an active participant in the process of *contagium psychicum*, rather than merely a person who takes over the social suggestions as pre-givens, or learns the "right" ways of being in the culture.

Description of the Sociogenetic Process: An Explanation of Its Outcomes

What constitutes "explanation" in the social sciences is far from being clear. Most of the research traditions in psychology have been built on the assumption that the study of outcomes (i.e., already emerged results of some generative process, like personal finished products, test scores, etc.) can provide sufficient basis for inference about the mechanisms that generate those outcomes (Lightfoot & Folds-Bennett, 1992). However, that epistemological strategy equals setting up the cart to pull the horse, even if it is in line with the collective-cultural suggestions of the occidental societies (see Kojima, 1988, p. 243). In case of any developmental phenomenon, the refusal to study the actual process of development and to concentrate on the analysis of mere outcomes of development equals giving up the only possibility science has to unveil the mechanisms of development.

Therefore, in the case of sociogenesis, the realistic epistemological strategy would be to attempt to use the description of the process mechanisms as an explanation of the outcomes (Valsiner, 1987). However, the elaboration of this standpoint turns out to be complicated, as it requires the building of an explicit theoretical scheme of the process of sociogenesis which possesses sufficient generality to fit all the variety of specific encounters of the person with his/her social world. It has to account for not only the episiodes of *maximum social relatedness* of the developing person (such as hypnotic states, see Janet, 1925; or trance, Hughes, 1991), but also for periods of *seemingly total independence* of the person from all the social world around him. A sociogenetic theory must be sufficiently general so as to explain the emergence of personal autonomy and individuality.

Any scheme of sufficient generality is a hostage to the underlying assumptions that are axiomatically taken by its constructor. The main issue that underlies the question of sociogenesis is which assumptions about culture transmission are made by the investigator of sociogenesis.

Unidirectional and Bidirectional Cultural Transmission Models

The main reason for the poverty of our theorizing about sociogenesis can be seen in the prevailing unidirectional notion of culture transmission or socialization (Valsiner, 1989a, chap. 3; also see Wertsch, 1991, pp. 71-73). This view renders the recipient of the cultural transmission or socialization passive in his acceptance (or failure of it: a "miss" or an "error" of the transmission) of the cultural messages. The latter are de facto viewed as fixed and immutable entities, which are either accepted by the receiver as such, or (in case of their incomplete acceptance) an "error of transmission" is assumed to have taken place. Any change *in* the message itself that could be produced by the receiver remains beyond the explanatory power of the unidirectional culture transmission model, other than by attribution of "error" status to it (Valsiner, 1988).

The unidirectional transmission model fits with the nature of technological systems, where the information to be transmitted is fixed, closed to development, and where the accuracy of transmission of the *given* message is a desired goal. In contrast, development of any kind and level (biological, psychological, sociological) is an open-systemic phenomenon in which novelty is constantly in the process of being created (Valsiner, 1987, 1989a, 1991). Hence, the unidirectional culture transmission model is an artifact of uncritical transfer of ideas from the non-developmental to developmental domains of reality.

Although the unidirectional model is non-developmental in its implications, its use in psychology is widespread. Its implicit acceptance can be seen in case of the "harmonious learning" type of notions of sociogenesis (see above). To explain socio*genesis* on the basis of the unidirectional culture transmission model and through the explanatory use of learning, enculturation, or socialization concepts is inconsistent with the phenomena of sociogenesis (i.e., social construction of novel psychological phenomena in the intra- and inter-individual psychological domains).

In contrast to the unidirectional culture transmission model, its counterpart, the bidirectional culture transmission model, is free from a number of non-developmental implications (see also Valsiner, 1989a chap. 3). This model is based on the premise that all participants in the cultural transmission process are actively transforming the cultural messages: the communicator actively assembles a message of a certain unique form, and the receiver (equally actively) analyzes the message, and re-assembles the "incoming cultural information" in a personally novel form in the mind. This view of cultural transmission entails the construction of novelty *both* during encoding and decoding of the cultural messages. In some sense, the "message" as such never exists in any "given" form, as it is reconstructed by the encoder (who may start with a certain goal in mind, but may shift it while creating the message), and by the decoder in a similar manner. As the roles of the encoder and decoder are constantly being changed into each other, cultural transmission involves transformation of culture in real time, by all participants in the social discourse.

The bidirectional model of cultural transmission makes it possible to take an open-ended perspective to the sociogenetic process, which is appropriate if we are interested in the construction of novelty. It allows our conceptualizations of sociogenesis to become explicitly developmental. Of course, the construction of novelty in human development is based on the familiarity (see also Rheingold, 1985). In development, the socially available cultural input to the developing person sets up the pool of resources for the person's constructive activities, the actual outcome of which cannot be predicted before they have taken place.

In a certain respect, it can be said that the unidirectional model of culture transmission constitutes a special case of the bidirectional model, namely, the case in which the active role of the receiver of the cultural messages is at its minimum. In that case, the receiver's ways of active involvement in the reception process are reduced to the minimum (and hence can be viewed as the "passive reception" takes place). Wertsch (1991, pp. 78-79), following Bakhtin, captures that inclusiveness of the unidirectional culture transmission view in the wider co-constructionist ("dialogic") view by emphasizing the contrast between "authoritative" and "internally persuasive" discourses. However, the minimization of active reception process (in case of receiving "authoritative" texts) can itself be viewed as an active reception strategy (or meta-strategy, i.e., decision to refrain from active analysis and synthesis of the incoming message). In sum, it could be argued, in contrast with much of the history of psychology and anthropology of socialization, that the cultural transmission process is always a bidirectional constructive process.

Theoretical Foundations: Jean Piaget, William Stern, and Lev Vygotsky

The bidirectional cultural transmission model is rooted in a number of inventions in developmental psychology, among which the seminal work of Jean Piaget is most outstanding. Piaget is probably one of the most actively misinterpreted thinkers in the developmental psychology of the 20th century, as he is given credit (as well as criticism) for that part of his contributions (stage descriptions) that merely constitute a background for his developmental ideas (Chapman, 1988a). From the viewpoint of the bidirectional culture transmission model, the main contribution of Piaget was his move to axiomatically assume the active nature of the child's knowledge construction within his surroundings:

> We apply the term "genetic epistemology" to this study of the way in which the subject constructs and organizes his knowledge during his historical development (ontogenetic and sociogenetic). Genetic epistemology presupposes a psychological analysis, but it necessarily leads to an epistemological study treating the great problems of the theory of knowledge. In fact, the study of the construction of a structure of knowledge teaches us something of the nature of this structure, that is, of its epistemological mechanism: whether the structure has been derived from experience or has been constructed deductively; whether it derives from language alone (and thus remains purely analytic) or is synthetic and supposes operations or actions. (Piaget, 1965, p. 31)

Piaget's constructivist perspective on personal and social knowledge creation emerged under the conditions of his avoidance of his primary work obligations, while employed by T. Simon in his psychometric laboratory (see Piaget, 1952, p. 244). Aside from mere abandonment of his work tasks, Piaget of course followed the more general theoretical leads of Henri Bergson (1911) and James Mark Baldwin (1906, 1908, 1911). In parallel, the developing personalistic epistemology of William Stern (1938) deserves to be reinstated as one of the bases for considering the active/constructive role of the person in the course of cultural transmission (see Kreppner, 1992 in press; Werner, 1938). Of course, it remains the case that the notion of bidirectional cultural transmission owes most to the synthesizing mind of Lev Vygotsky (Van der Veer & Valsiner, 1991).

Differently from the major tendencies in our modern psychological discourse, which emphasizes the differences between Piaget and Vygotsky (as well as manages to overlook Stern's contributions), here we concentrate on the similarities of the perspectives of these three thinkers. All of them assume the person's active process of relating to his environment, and the construction of knowledge as an outcome of that process. The cultural messages that surround a developing person (the person's "lived-through" world; see Kreppner, 1992 in press), are acted upon by the person, whose assimilative/accommodative processes (see Piaget, 1971, pp. 138-213) transform the semiotically encoded information from/about the world into internalized personal knowledge. The latter takes the form of systems of "personal sense" (i.e., the personal cognitive/affective counterpart of "meanings" in the society), as Paulhan (1928) and Vygotsky (1934, or 1987) have pointed out. In other terms, person's active encounters with the world transform "collective-cultural" meanings into "personal-cultural" systems of sense (Valsiner, 1989a).

This distinction between "collective" and "personal" cultures is merely a heuristic device to remind ourselves that the person, in one's personal uniqueness, is always related to the cultural meaningful world through the process of constant internalization and externalization. Both the internalization and externalization processes are constructive. Under conditions of multi-faceted social suggestions of various kinds (emanating from different sources, often following different goals and thus being highly divergent), the person constructs cultural novelty in the form of personal sense, which becomes externalized and thus enters the process of communication with other persons as a part of the social suggestions system. The constructive and innovative nature of the internalization processes has been recognized (albeit not always explicitly) by the major sociogenetic theorists of this century (see Lawrence & Valsiner, 1992 in press).

The Co-constructive Viewpoint

The bidirectional cultural transmission model as the axiomatic basis for understanding sociogenesis has clearly defined implications for the kind of model that we are trying to construct. First, sociogenesis is a process that is characterized by *joint construction* (or co-construction) of the psychological system of the developing person by him/herself, and the goal-oriented "social others" who provide the person with the social suggestions (Valsiner, 1988, 1992a, 1992b). This process is dynamically goals oriented (as well as goal-constructing, or *teleogenetic*), so that any participant in it can set up, try to attain, and re-place (or merely abandon) previously set goals. The multiplicity of goals, as well as their varied generality and temporal extension (see Kindermann & Valsiner, 1989, pp. 31-33) leave one with the clear impression that the co-constructive process is highly variable and unpredictable, exactly as a consequence of the teleogenetic nature of the process. At any moment in the ongoing transaction, any participant can, at an instant if necessary, change his or her goal orientation, or strategies of conduct, thus leading the whole co-construction process to take a previously unexpected and unpredictable direction (see Winegar, 1988). Under conditions of episodic convergence of the participants' goal orientations, the phenomena of construction of "group norms" can be observed, as in the classic studies by Muzafer Sherif (Sherif, 1935, 1936, 1937). However, under conditions of divergence of participants' goal orientations the phenomena of co-construction become highly diffuse and seemingly disorganized (or chaotic), within which it is only the relative personal consistency over time that could be discernible. Our detection of personal consistency in social contexts emerges when the social co-construction process is in some diffuse state, in which case the persons' externalizations over time can be observed to have relative consistency and person-addressable detectability (see also Oliver, 1965). The detectability of personal psychological externalizations is a result of differentiation of the person-environment relationships.

Within developmental psychology, the emphasis on differentiation (and its reverse process, de-differentiation) of structure has played a prominent role most of the time (Janet, 1926; Piaget, 1971; Werner, 1957). Differentiation entails the notion of *hierarchical integration* of the developing new structural entities. These hierarchical orders can be of different kinds (ranging from "strict" hierarchies, within which the transitivity of relations between parts is upheld, to the "loose" hierarchies that are characterized by intransitivity and ill-defined nature of some of the constituent parts). Most social relationships within which co-construction takes place are hierarchical in their nature. That joint construction entails asymmetry of power (i.e., the "experts" of the culture, or the parental generation, is dominant over the "novices" in the set-up of their environments in toto), but no determination of the outcome by the dominant partner of the co-construction process. Cases of relative symmetry in interpersonal relationships constitute a special case of the asymmetric systemic relationships. This recognition of asymmetric power relationships between persons does not entail the passivity of one of the partners. The "novice" not only can, but will defy many of the suggestions, use them to construct one's own novel action patterns, and go beyond the state of the surrounding collective culture at every moment. This is in line with Baldwin's notion of "persistent imitation" (Baldwin, 1892), Royce's ideas of "social opposition" (Royce, 1894), and Vygotsky's notion of play (Vygotsky, 1933/1976).

The co-constructive role of the participants in any social encounter has obviously been well known in the pertinent research literature for a very long time (e.g., Bartlett, 1920a; Simmel, 1906). By observing his subjects in the context of a very ordinary activity—retelling stories—Bartlett observed how individual persons reconstruct their knowledge, guided both by their collective and personal cultures:

> ...reproductions...bring into operation various specific tendencies towards dramatisation, condensation, rationalisation, and so on; but at the same time they make it clear that the function of those tendencies, and also the moment at which they come into play, are determined in part by differences in the character of the material employed. Take one point only: material giving rise to pleasing affective tone is likely to be reproduced, and at the same time to be exaggerated. But whether any given material *does* produce such affective accompaniment depends very largely upon its relations to the customs and beliefs prevalent in the community to which the subjects belong. (920b, p. 290)

The active person creates his/her own novel version of a folk story, self description, account of an event, or any other narrative, but on the basis of the range of expectations and meanings present in the "collective culture." By way of producing novelty, individuals participate also in the reconstruction of the collective culture.

Finally, all development of knowledge in science involves the active scientist as a co-constructor of new knowledge, together with her "social others" as well as cultural context. Again, Piaget has captured that unity of the active person and the surrounding world in sufficiently generic terms:

> If one considers the subject as an assemblage of ready-made structures, one forgets that the subject does not exist in a given form once and for all time. *The subject is none other than the assemblage of the actions which he exercises on the objects, and these actions are unceasingly transformed in accordance with the objects and modify the subject.* To set out from the object independently of the actions of the subject is to assume an empiricistic or positivistic perspective which forgets that the object is attained only by successive approximations. *The whole history of the sciences shows that objectivity is not a starting datum, but is constructed and acquired by a continuous and laborious effort.* These successive approximations relate to the actions of the subject in his conquest and reconstruction of the object. (1977, pp. 30-31, emphases in italics added)

Thus, the co-constructionist perspective builds upon a number of established traditions in biology and psychology, all of which have shared the common goal of understanding development. It overcomes artificially constructed controversies in special disciplines (e.g., the specific view of incompatability of Piaget's and Vygotsky's perspectives, which has been generalized well beyond the proportions of the original dispute: that about the "egocentric" speech). However, by recognizing both the person's individual-psychological *active role* and their *mutual interdependence*, the co-constructionist perspective leads to a need for further theoretical and methodological elaboration.

Elaboration of the Co-Constructionist Model

The elaboration of the co-constructivist perspective here makes use of the "contagion" metaphor as outlined above. Let us start from the obvious fact that the developing person is constantly surrounded by social suggestions from the "collective culture" (i.e., a combination of "personal cultures" of each and every other person whose externalizations reach the environment of the child, either directly or indirectly). These social suggestions are the cultural encoded messages that surround the developing child. The forms into which these messages are encoded are highly heterogeneous, ranging from the usual airwave transmission of acoustic and visual information to external forms and colors of objects, haptic and tactile, or olfactory experiences of the child, and to specific emotiogenic episodes in which the child is a participant-observer (see Rogoff, 1990). In other terms, the developing child *cannot avoid* the contact with the collective culturally organized world, even if the child may be in a position to avoid *some specific* environmental contexts (organized collective culturally) some of the times. In other terms, the collective culture guarantees a wide but inescapable field of access to the cultural meaning systems, *encoded with high redundancy* in the everyday world of the child. The process of bidirectional culture transmission, exactly as it includes uncertainty due to the person's active co-constructor's role in it, entails a *massive overstimulation* of the developing person by a high variety of collective culturally similar (but never the same) suggestions (see Valsiner, 1989a, 1989b). Given the unpredictability of the outcomes of the sociogenetic process that involves active and constructive individuals, the best possible strategy to attain the collective-cultural goals is to provide a highly redundant heterogeneous cultural environment to the developing persons. The specific mechanisms for that effort to guide the sociogenetic process is to make the encounter with collective-cultural suggestions *unavoidable* in the course of the lives of the individuals. The latter are not always attuned to the social suggestions (see Janet, 1925, chap. 6), and may at times actively undermine the expected "effects" of these suggestions. However, by saturating the persons' life-worlds with the myriad of social suggestions all oriented in a similar direction, the collective-cultural objectives can be expected to be upheld.

This encoded collective cultural "message field" serves as the input to the developing person who is an "active agent within his enviroment" (Basov, 1931; see also Basov, 1991). Even if the externally located myriad of social suggestions can be considered in terms of "cultural viruses" that are always ready to "attack" the "target organism," the *definitive conditions* under which the "target" person handles these suggestions are those of the personal psychological structure that has developed into its present state ("personal culture" at the given time and context). At any moment in a person's present life-world, he acts upon the cultural world and not necessarily with full eagerness to appropriate it! The previous experiences of the person that has participated in the construction of the "personal culture" at the given time have also involved the internalization/externalization processes in the past. Previous contacts with the cultural world have helped the person to prepare himself for the present similar encounter (or, in our parallel to the viral infection terminology, have worked out "personal-cultural antibodies" in the psychological structure). Thus, the developing person can at any time be "immune" to the surrounding social suggestions by way of using a variety of strategies: *ignoring, neutralizing, trivializing* (distancing oneself from), *dismissing, resisting, rejecting*, or any other way. However, these strategies are the presentday outgrowths from the person's past experiences with the social suggestions, and these strategies make it possible for the developing person to construct one's "personal culture" in the future in ways that can differ cardinally from the "shared expectations" of the "collective culture." All present encounters with the socio-cultural worlds are steps in the co-construction of the future individuality of the person (see Cole, 1992; Valsiner, 1993 in press). As a result, the "personal culture" becomes transformed in novel directions, never before observed in the psychological phenomena of the person. By externalizing the results of the internal transformation the social suggestion is communicated further to other persons, whose handling of the suggestion is of similar active and multidirectional (resist or accept into the personal culture) kind.

The present view has a fundamental implication for theory and methodology of the co-constructivist research: the notion of "person" survives in this context of theoretical discourse (rather than vanishes in the middle of social rhetorics, or inclusion in action contexts, see Valsiner, 1991). This does not constitute "dualism," but rather a construction of a differentiated view of reality. The sociogenetic perspective is itself a result of the cultural-historical development of the image of the person as separated from the social context, but who remains clearly interdependent with that context. Without that conceptual separation, the very question of the origins (traditionally phrased in terms of exclusive separation of the two components, e.g., social *or* individual) of the psychological functions of individuals could not have arisen. Once the question has been raised, it is answered by the sociogenetic thinkers by using the strategy of inclusive separation: accepting both social *and* individual origins. Thus, individual persons are constituted (onto*genetically*) by their social life course, but at any given moment (onto*logically*) they display their individual psychological worlds (personal cultures) in their conduct. The sociogenetic thinkers thus overcome the person/society dualism by recognizing it as a result of systemic interactions between person and society.

The co-constructionist acceptance of the "dualism" between person and society merely indicates the ways (mechanisms) through which personal psychological worlds are being socially co-constructed in the course of an individual's life course. It does *not* claim that at any present state of a person's development all of his (or her) intimately personal feelings and thinking is a mere repetition of externally present social discourse as that exists. Instead, the co-constructionist perspective assumes that persons go beyond their surrounding "collective cultural" worlds by way of constructing their unique "personal cultures," and thus are at any given moment personally relatively autonomous (or "independently dependent," see Winegar, Renninger & Valsiner, 1989) in respect of their immediate social worlds. The "dualism" of person and society is resolved within the sociogenetic theoretical perspective by way of claiming common ontogenetic interdependence, leading to differentiation of the person from (and by way of) its social world. In other terms, the sociogenetic perspective solves this problem of dualism by *inclusive separation* of the person from the social world (see Valsiner, 1987, 1991), and by specifying the systemic mechanisms of development that maintain the interdependence between thus separated parts of the interactive system.

Appropriation by Internalization/Externalization

In contemporary discussions on sociogenetic mechanisms, the question of internalization (and its counterpart, externalization) is often replaced by talk about "appropriation" of culture (Doise, 1985, p. 104; Rogoff, 1990, pp. 193-197; Shore, 1991). This is a logical consequence of the dominance of "fusion" or "blending" metaphors of cultural transmission that tend to negate structural differentiation of the person and the environment (Valsiner, 1991). Reduction of the psychological functioning of a person to social rhetorics (Shotter, 1990), texts (Gergen, 1988) or situated activity contexts (Lave, 1988) is a solution to psychological research problems that solves them by eliminating them. In this respect, socio-cultural reduction of the person to the role of a mere reflection of the highly heterogeneous social world is not different from its opposing other extreme position of biological or physiological reductionism, which leads to the elimination of psychological phenomena.

Isomorphism cannot be assumed to be present between the personal and social worlds: hence the need to separate (inclusively, instead of exclusively) the personal culture from the collective culture, and explain the person's constructions of the former *on the basis of* the latter. The notion of appropriation is a descriptive term which (from the socio-cultural perspective) reflects the actual processes of internalization/externalization that are responsible for the individual construction of personal cultures. The central role in that process belongs to the active person who relates to the constantly uncertain life-world of one's own (see also arguments about internalization by Diaz,

Neal & Amaya-Williams, 1990). The role of the active person can be observed in the handling of "dialogicality" of the process of personal-cultural construction. Mikhail Bakhtin has expressed this notion (see also Wertsch, 1991, p. 59) quite eloquently:

> The word in language is half someone else's. *It becomes "one's own" only when the speaker populates it with his own intention,* his own accent, when he appropriates the word, adapting it to his own semantic and expressive intention. Prior to this moment of appropriation, the word does not exist in a neutral and impersonal language...but rather it exists in other people's mouths, in other people's concrete contexts, *serving other people's intentions*: it is from there that one must take the word, and make it one's own. (Bakhtin, 1981, pp. 293-294, emphases in italics added)

The emphases added to this quote express my intention that is added to the message: to point to the active role attributed to the person who is appropriating a word. The person creates "hybrid constructions" (see Wertsch, 1991, p. 59) on the basis of different "voices" by way of internalizing of these "voices," changing (transforming) them in the process, and externalizing these constructed new messages, now filled with the person's own intentions (as intermediate "products" of the constantly continuous sociogenetic process). Furthermore, the person can construct a new "voice" on the basis of previously existing ones, or exist in the middle of a cacophony of an ill-defined (but yet influential) "chorus" of voices. These are a few implications of the socio-cultural theoretical perspective for sociogenetic theory.

In the process of co-construction, different participating partners of a "dialogue" (e.g., the "voices" of *decontextualized rationality* and *contextualized representation* that become involved with each other in the mind; see Wertsch, 1990, pp. 120-122) create conditions for further distancing of the person from the social context (e.g., Sigel & Cocking, 1977). However, the creation of conditions (or, for a situation of *goodness-of-misfit,* see Valsiner & Cairns, 1992 in press) in and by itself is not sufficient for explaining actual development. On the basis of these conditions, the co-constructive person creates novel forms of personal culture, by way of synthesis (rather than through mere choice of one option over another). If the main point that was emphasized by Vygotsky is to be advanced further, the question of intrapsychological synthesis of the personal culture needs to be explicated in the sociogenetic theory (Van der Veer & Valsiner, 1991).

From the perspective of human development, appropriation of the collective culture is in reality the process of construction of the personal cultures, through internalization and externalization as mutually linked parallel processes (see also John-Steiner & Tatter, 1983; Obeyesekere, 1990 chap. 1; Semin, 1989; Werner & Kaplan, 1984, chap. 19). The general form of that process is that of structural transformation, as specified both by Piaget (1971) and Vygotsky (Emerson, 1983; Wertsch & Stone, 1985). However, the dynamic and necessarily uncertain nature of sociogenesis can be easily overlooked if the new structuralist ethos starts to build strictly deterministic formal models.

"Bounded Indeterminacy" and Co-construction in Sociogenesis

It is argued here that construction of novel forms in the sociogenetic process follows the principle of "bounded indeterminacy" (see Valsiner, 1987; for criticism see Van Oers, 1988). By way of using the notion of *constraint* as a mechanism that enables construction of novelty (Winegar, 1988; Winegar et al., 1989), developing human beings are constructing themselves with the help of both external (action) and internal (self-processes) regulation via constraining. The self-constraining of the person is a semiotic process; it takes the form of coordination sense structures (i.e., a component of the personal culture) with those of meanings ("collective culture"), and results in a *range of possible novel senses,* which can emerge in principle at the next time moment. The subset of that range, which becomes actualized while the person moves onto the next time moment serves as the set of intra-psychological constraints for further construction of the range of possibilities for understanding the life events that the person creates within the given environment. The constant semiotic self-constraining process is the personal-cultural mechanism for constructive handling of the "heteroglossia" of different "voices" (Wertsch, 1991) as the person at any present time is constructing the future (Valsiner, 1993 in press). Under the myriad of social suggestions from many sources, the developing person is co-constructing one's personally unique life course, and assembling new "voices" for both intra-psychological and inter-personal "dialogues."

The co-constructionist viewpoint is consistent in its emphasis on multi-linearity of development (Valsiner, 1989a). The construction of a person's life course entails the potentiality for many life courses, out of which the person's unique and idiosyncratic one is jointly constructed. At each bifurcation point in one's life course, the person negotiates with one's self-constraints and others' constraining suggestions for a solution for the next step "into the future," thus actualizing only some of the many possibilities. The ways of "self-immunization" in respect to others' social suggestions (e.g., by ignoring, neutralizing, dismissing, rejecting, etc.) constitute the selective tools of the active person; the strategies for combining different suggestions and creating novel ones are the root for novelty construction. Developmental progress can be described retrospectively in relation to a previous state of reference (see Chapman, 1988b), while the actual sociogenetic process involves the construction of a future life course in the present.

The bifurcational nature of the sociogenetic process makes it possible for the persons to be flexible in their relations with their cultural surroundings, demonstrate phenomena that are traditionally attributed to the category of "free will," and be inconsistent within themselves (in comparison with their past). There is available a multiplicity of active co-construction strategies for handling the social suggestions by other persons (i.e. their externalizations of their personal cultures) and by the collective culturally pre-organized environmental structure. The social communication process that starts from the assumption of shared understanding (Rommetveit, 1979), moves toward overcoming the mutual non-understanding (Robinson, 1988), the result of which is joint construction of novel understanding.

Major Methodological Challenges

The co-constructionist perspective creates a number of difficult methodological problems for empirical research. These problems are inherent in the developmental perspective as such, and since the co-constructionist perspective constitutes the most explicit developmental perspective in contemporary social sciences, it is not surprising that those issues cannot be bypassed.

Traditionally, the psychology has been oriented towards describing psychological phenomena, the form of which has already emerged in the course of development. It has tried to superimpose upon the highly fluid phenomena of development categorical systems that are pre-structured by the investigators (by some "metacontract"; see Elbers, 1986) and hence remain blind to "surprises" that the co-constructionist nature of development brings with it (see Valsiner, 1992, in press). As was argued above, the person's encounter with the social world is necessarily ill-defined, as the social world is heterogeneous, and the person can apply multiple strategies to the handling of that world.

It is therefore obvious that the methodological imperatives of traditional psychology do not fit the goals of making sense of the sociogenetic process. Therefore, the developmental perspective implies that the developing person be observed in the process of moving from "chaotic" or "fluid" (and hence categorically difficult to describe) phenomena to the emergence of clear form. It is exactly the unclassifiable phenomena we observe in child development or any human "dialogical" encounter with others or with one's own self that may need to be the target of co-constructionist analysis, yet at our present time, these phenomena are consistently being overlooked and eliminated from the research process (see Figure 1).

As is evident from Figure 1, the actual process of development takes place at the time period (time units 10–19) when the form of the developing phenomenon is *no longer* what it used to be (time units 1–9), while it is *not yet* what it ends up being in the future (time units 20–31). For any observer of the developing form, the "crisis period" of development, which entails the elimination of the previous form and synthesis of the new one, constitutes a great challenge. Not only cannot the emerging novel form be detected by matching it with a new strict form-template, but also the given observer may strongly disagree with any other observer as to the nature of the fluid phenomena under investigation.

This rather formalistic example can be elaborated on the basis of filling in the notions described in Figure 1 with material from Wertsch's Bakhtinian emphasis on the "dialogicality" of multiple "voices." If in time units 1–7 we can think of co-presence and oppositional relationship of three well-defined "voices," and at 8–9 see the disintegration of that structure, then in the time units 10–19 we can see the "dialogicality" become highly fuzzy, and the detection of separable and clearly defined "voices" almost impossible. Following that period of "voice turmoil," the developing system turns to a new structure of two "voices" and their relation. The period of development that is most relevant for the emergence of novelty is that when the structure of "voices" cannot be exactly determined. The reality of developmentally important processes seems to play some "hide-and-seek" game with the conscientious and determined developmental scientist. This example leads us to a general methodological paradox: *if development takes place at times of de-differentiation of the previous forms and during the emergence of the novel ones, then its observation in terms of static categorization may lead the investigator to overlook exactly the phenomena that he is most interested in.* The whole methodological instrumentarium of researchers is in need of reformulation, in order to have at least some hopes of access to the processes of development. It is clearly the "developmental crises" periods that need to be scrutinized in depth, with the retention of the temporal order in the data. Otherwise, the microgenetic research strategy is the appropriate one for research, despite the fact that it has been forgotten in contemporary psychology (Catán, 1986; Siegler & Crowley, 1991).

A similar issue arises in the hermeneutic process of knowledge construction in experimenter ↔ subject relationships, where it may be the moments of sudden mutual divergence of communication where the relevant phenomena are discovered (see Hermans, 1991; Hermans & Bonarius, 1991a, 1991b). The person who takes the role of a "subject" in the research process is constantly creating novelty on the basis of the previous state of relationship with the world. However, our methodological rules often remain blind to the developmental openness of the subject under study (although at other periods in psychology's history this was not the case; see Danziger, 1990).

Our methodological complications demonstrate that the sociogenetic process does not stop at the beginning of a research encounter (even if the researchers might find it convenient to pretend that it does), but continues all through the research process. One is again reminded by Piaget's adequate description of objectivity in science (quoted above).

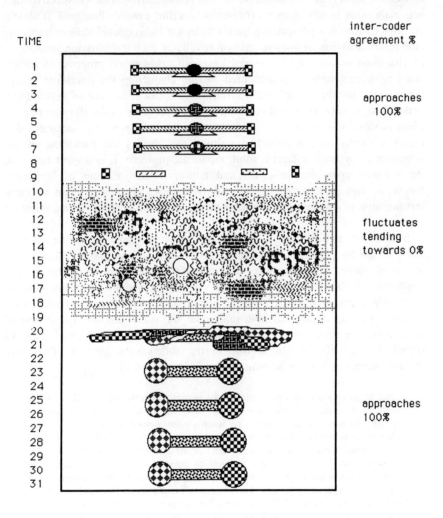

FIGURE 1. Periods of "crises" as loci of emergence of new form.

General Conclusions: Co-constructive Sociogenesis

Any theory of sociogenesis must explain inconsistency of persons by way of consistent theory of a general kind. The co-constructionist perspective that was elaborated in this chapter constitutes an effort towards that goal. It should be obvious that this perspective builds upon the bidirectional culture transmission model that entails construction of novelty at each transmission junction.

The main reason social sciences have not made much progress in understanding sociogenesis was attributed in this chapter to the uncritical acceptance of the uni-directional culture transmission model in most of psychology, anthropology, education, and sociology. When progress in the development of ideas is slow, the reason can be some meta-theoretic semiotic constraint that exists presently in the collective culture, and guides the reasoning of the scientists away from adequate solutions to the problem. It is argued here that the reliance upon the uni-directional notion of transmission of "finished" messages has constituted such constraint—the assumption that cultural transmission is similar to information transmission in technical communication systems.

In contrast, the process of sociogenesis was presented as a case of joint construction by persons of different relationships to one another, and to the world at large. Understanding this co-construction depends upon further synthesis of the ideas of a number of developmental theorists—Piaget, Vygotsky, Stern, and Wertsch—all of whom have been fascinated by the ways in which persons develop as both individual and social entities. The course of co-constructive sociogenesis is filled with nonlinearities and chaotic states, all of which may play a central role in the sociogenetic process. Thus, our theories need to take into account the basic "world view":

> ...that in the course of normal development a person repeatedly surpasses the previous limits of his capacities. But in so doing, especially in his capacity for handling episodes of interpersonal relations, he learns—when viewed closely—not by linear addition or progression, but by irregular reorganizations or transformations of these relationships. While the qualitative character of these reorganizations is more or less recognized by the gestalt theories in terms of individual perception, it needs to be stressed that changes of interpersonal competence restructure existent relationships in the world of interacting persons. The adolescent who finally revolts and beats up his father may have increased his autonomy, but in doing so has...transformed his self. And because that self is as much the product of others' activity as of his own, they too have transformed their appraisal, not only of his powers, but of the whole network of relationships in which they are enmeshed. (Foote, 1957, p. 40)

Mechanisms of sociogenesis create both social and personal phenomena in parallel and allow for the creation of the wonderful worlds of our intimate psyches, which can never be fully shared by other human beings, but which

can be externalized in the process of efforts to create interpersonal understanding, a goal that is so usual, necessary, and often so complicated in our
individual life-worlds.

Note

An early version of parts of this chapter was presented at the workshop
Mechanisms of Sociogenesis, at Rijksuniversiteit Utrecht, December 13–14,
1990. A number of the ideas expressed here were also part of an invited
presentation at the Australian Conference on Developmental Psychology,
Perth, Western Australia, in July 1990.

References

Ananiev, B.G. (1930), Sociogenetic method in the study of human behavior. In A.B.
   Zalkind (ed.), *Psikhonevrologicheskie nauki v SSSR*. (pp. 29-33). Moscow-
   Leningrad: Gosudarstvennoie Meditsinskoe Izdatel'stvo.
Bakhtin, M. (1981), *The dialogic imagination*. Austin: University of Texas Press.
Baldwin, J.M. (1892), *Suggestion and will*. International Congress of Experimental
   Psychology. Second Session (pp. 49-54). London: Williams & Norgate.
Baldwin, J.M. (1895), *Mental development in the child and the race*. New York:
   MacMillan.
Baldwin, J.M. (1902), *Social and ethical interpretations in mental development*. New
   York: MacMillan.
Baldwin, J.M. (1906), *Thought and things, or genetic logic. Vol. 1. Functional logic,
   or genetic theory of knowledge*. London: Swan Sonnenschein.
Baldwin, J.M. (1908), *Thought and things, or genetic logic. Vol. 2. Experimental
   logic, or genetic theory of thought*. London: Swan Sonnenschein.
Baldwin, J.M. (1911), *Thought and things, or genetic logic. Vol. 3. Interest and art*.
   London: Allen.
Baldwin, J.M. (1930), James Mark Baldwin. In C. Murchison (ed.), *A history of
   psychology in autobiography*. Vol. 1. (pp. 1-30). New York: Russell & Russell.
Bartlett, F.C. (1920a), Some experiments on the reproduction of folkstories. *Folk-Lore*,
   31, 30-47.
Bartlett, F.C. (1920b), Psychology in relation to the popular story. *Folk-Lore*, 31,
   264-293.
Basov, M. (1931), *Obshchie osnovy pedologii*. Moscow-Leningrad: Gosudarst vennoe
   Izdatel'stvo.
Basov, M. (1991), The organization of processes of behavior. In J. Valsiner & R. Van
   der Veer (eds.), Structuring of conduct in activity settings: The forgotten contribu-
   tions of Mikhail Basov. Part 1. *Soviet Psychology*, 29, 5, 14-83.
Bateson, G. (1972), Metalogue: What is an instinct? In G. Bateson, *Steps to an
   ecology of mind*. (pp. 38-58). New York: Ballantine Books.

Bekhterev, V.M. (1903), *Suggestion and its role in the social life.* 2nd ed. St. Peters burg: K.L. Rikker.

Bergson, H. (1911), *Creative evolution.* New York: Henry Holt & Co.

Boodin, J.E. (1913), The existence of social minds. *American Journal of Sociology,* 19, 1, 1-47.

Cairns, R.B. (1979), *Social development.* San Francisco: W.H. Freeman.

Cairns, R.B. (1985), *Sociogenesis and aggression: A modern perspective on the ontogeny and phylogeny of violence.* Unpublished Manuscript.

Cairns, R.B. (1992 in press), The making of a developmental science: The contributions and intellectual heritage of James Mark Baldwin. *Developmental Psychology.*

Catán, L. (1986), The dynamic display of process: Historical development and contemporary uses of the microgenetic method. *Human Development,* 29, 252-263.

Cavalli-Sforza, L.L., Feldman, M.W., Chen, K.H., & Dornbusch, S.M. (1982), Theory and observation in cultural transmission. *Science,* 218, 19-27.

Chapman, M. (1988a), *Constructive evolution.* Cambridge: Cambridge University Press.

Chapman, M. (1988b), Contextuality and directionality of cognitive development. *Human Development,* 31, 92-106.

Cohen, Y.A. (1971), The shaping of men's minds: adaptations to imperatives of culture. In M.L. Wax, S. Diamond & F.O. Gearing (eds.), *Anthropological perspectives on education.* (pp. 19-50). New York: Basic Books.

Cole, M. (1992), Context, modularity and the cultural constitution of development. In L.T. Winegar & J. Valsiner (eds.), Children's development within social context. Vol 2. *Research and methodology.* Hillsdale, NJ: Erlbaum.

Danziger, K. (1990), *Constructing the subject.* Cambridge: Cambridge University Press.

Diaz, R.M., Neal, C.J., & Amaya-Williams, M. (1990), The social origins of self-regulation. In L.C. Moll (ed.), *Vygotsky and education* (pp. 127-154). Cambridge: Cambridge University Press.

Doise, W. (1985), On the social development of the intellect. In V.L. Shulman, L.C.R. Restaino-Baumann, & L. Butler (eds.), *The future of Piagetian theory: Neo-Piagetians* (pp. 99-121). New York: Plenum.

Elbers, E. (1986), Interaction and instruction in the conservation experiment. *European Journal of Psychology of Education,* 1, 1, 77-89.

Emerson, C. (1983), Bakhtin and Vygotsky on internalization of language. *Quarterly Newsletter of the Laboratory of Comparative Human Cognition,* 5, 1, 9-12.

Foote, N.N. (1957), Concept and method in the study of human development. In M. Sherif & M.O. Wilson (eds.), *Emerging problems in social psychology.* Series III (pp. 29-53). Norman, OK: University Book Exchange.

Gergen, K. (1988), If persons are texts. In S.B. Messer, L.A. Sass, & R.L. Woolfolk (eds.), *Hermeneutics and psychological theory.* (pp. 28-51). New Brunswick, NJ: Rutgers University Press.

Gergen, K. (1991), *The communal creation of meaning.* Paper presented at the Jean Piaget Society meeting, Philadelphia, PA.

Hermans, H.J.M. (1991), The person as co-investigator in self-research: valuation theory. *European Journal of Personality*, 5, 217-234.

Hermans, H.J.M., Bonarius, H. (1991a), The person as co-investigator in personality research. *European Journal of Personality*, 5, 199-216.

Hermans, H.J.M., Bonarius, H. (1991b), Static laws in a dynamic psychology? *European Journal of Personality*, 5, 245-247.

Hughes, D.J. (1991), Blending with another: an analysis of trance channeling in the United States. *Ethos*, 19, 2, 161-184.

Janet, P. (1925), *Psychological healing*. New York: MacMillan.

Janet, P. (1926), *De l'angoisse a l'extase*. Paris: Félix Alcan.

Janet, P. (1930), Pierre Janet. In C. Murchison (Ed.), *A history of psychology in autobiography*. Vol. 1 (pp. 123-133). Worcester, MA: Clark University Press.

John-Steiner, V., & Tatter, P. (1983), An interactionist model of language development. In B. Bain (Ed.), *The sociogenesis of language and human conduct* (pp. 79-97). New York: Plenum.

Kindermann, T., & Valsiner, J. (1989), Research strategies in culture-inclusive developmental psychology. In J. Valsiner (ed.), *Child development in cultural context* (pp. 13-50). Toronto: Hogrefe & Huber.

Kojima, H. (1988), The role of belief-value systems related to child-rearing and education: The case of early modern to modern Japan. In D. Sinha & H.S. Kao (eds.), *Social values and development* (pp. 227-253). New Delhi: Sage.

Kozulin, A. (1990), *Vygotsky's psychology: A biography of ideas*. Cambridge, MA: Harvard University Press.

Kreppner, K. (1992 in press). William L. Stern. *Developmental Psychology*.

Lave, J. (1988), *Cognition in practice*. Cambridge: Cambridge University Press.

Lawrence, J.A., & Valsiner, J. (1992 in press), Social determinacy of human development: An analysis of the conceptual roots of the internalization process. *Human Development*.

Lightfoot, C., & Folds-Bennett, T. (1992), Description and explanation in developmental research: separate agendas. In J. Asendorpf & J. Valsiner (Eds.), *Stability and change in development: A study of methodological reasoning* (pp. 207-228). Newbury Park, CA: Sage.

Marková, I. (1987), On the interaction of opposites in psychological processes. *Journal for the Theory of Social Behaviour*, 17, 279-299.

Marková, I. (1990a), The development of self-consciousness: Baldwin, Mead, and Vygotsky, In J.E. Faulconer & R.N. Williams (eds.), *Reconsidering psychology: Perspectives from Continental philosophy* (pp. 151-174). Pittsburgh, PA: Duquesne University Press.

Marková, I. (1990b), On three principles of human social development. In G. Butter worth & P. Bryant (eds.), *Causes of development* (pp. 186-211). Hillsdale, NJ: Erlbaum.

Mead, G.H. (1903), The definition of the psychical. *Decennial Publications of the University of Chicago, 3* (Ser. 1), 77-112.

Mead, G.H. (1910), What social objects must psychology presuppose? *Journal of Psychology*, 7, 174-180.

Mead, G.H. (1934), *Mind, self, and society*. Chicago: University of Chicago Press.

Mead, M. (1963), Socialization and enculturation. *Current Anthropology,* 4, 2, 184-188.

Obeyesekere, G. (1990), *The work of culture: symbolic transformation in psychoanalysis and anthropology.* Chicago: University of Chicago Press.

Oliver, S.C. (1965), Individuality, freedom of choice, and cultural flexibility of the Kamba. *American Anthropologist,* 67, 421-428.

Paulhan, F. (1928), Qu'est-ce que le sens des mots. *Journal de Psychologie,* 25, 289-329.

Piaget, J. (1952), Jean Piaget. In E.G. Boring, H. Werner, H.S. Langfeld & R.M. Yerkes (eds.), *A history of psychology in autobiography.* Vol 4 (pp. 237-256). Worcester, Ma.: Clark University Press.

Piaget, J. (1965), Psychology and philosophy. In B.B. Wolman & E. Nagel (eds.), *Scientific psychology: Principles and approaches* (pp. 28-43.). New York: Basic Books.

Piaget, J. (1971), *Biology and knowledge.* Chicago: University of Chicago Press.

Piaget, J. (1977), The role of action in the development of thinking. In W.E. Overton & J. McGallagher (eds.), Knowledge and development. Vol. 1. *Advances in research and theory* (pp. 17-42). New York: Plenum.

Rheingold, H.R. (1985), Development as the acquisition of familiarity. *Annual Review of Psychology,* 36, 1-17.

Robinson, J.A. (1988), "What we've got here is a failure to communicate": The cultural context of meaning. In J. Valsiner (ed.), *Child development within culturally structured environments.* Vol. 2. *Social co-construction and environmental guidance of development* (pp. 137-198). Norwood, NJ: Ablex.

Rogoff, B. (1990), *Apprenticeship in thinking.* New York: Oxford University Press.

Rommetveit, R. (1979), On common codes and dynamic residuals in human communication. In R. Rommetveit & R. Blakar (eds.), *Studies of language, thought and verbal communication* (pp. 163-175). London: Academic Press.

Royce, J. (1894), The imitative functions, and their place in human nature. *Century Magazine,* 26, 137-145.

Semin, G. (1989), On genetic social psychology: A rejoinder to Doise. *European Journal of Social Psychology,* 19, 401-405.

Sherif, M. (1935), A study of some social factors in perception. *Archives of Psychology,* No. 187, 1-60.

Sherif, M. (1936), *The psychology of social norms.* New York: Harper & Brothers.

Sherif, M. (1937), An experimental approach to the study of attitudes. *Sociometry,* 1, 1-2, 90-98.

Shore, B. (1991), Twice-born, once conceived: meaning construction and cultural cognition. *American Anthropologist,* 93, 1, 9-27.

Shotter, J. (1990), *Knowing of the third kind.* Utrecht: ISOR.

Siegler, R.S., & Crowley, K. (1991), The microgenetic method: A direct means for studying cognitive development. *American Psychologist,* 46, 6,606-620.

Sigel, I.E., & Cocking, R.R. (1977), Cognition and communication: a dialectic paradigm for development. In M. Lewis & L.A. Rosenblum (eds.), *Interaction, conversation, and the development of language* (pp. 207-226). New York: Wiley.

Simmel, G. (1906), The sociology of secrecy and of secret societies. *American Journal of Sociology,* 11, 4, 441-498.

Spindler, G.D. (1974), The transmission of culture. In G.D. Spindler (ed.), *Education and cultural process* (pp. 279-310). New York: Holt, Rinehardt & Winston.

Stern, W. (1938), *General Psychology From the Personalist Standpoint.* New York: Macmillan.

Valsiner. J. (1987), *Culture and the development of children's action.* Chichester: Wiley.

Valsiner, J. (1988), Ontogeny of co-construction of culture within socially organized environmental settings. In J. Valsiner (ed.), *Child Development within Culturally Structured Environments. Vol. 2. Social Co-construction and Environmental Guidance of Development.* (pp. 283-297). Norwood, NJ: Ablex.

Valsiner, J. (1989a), *Human development and culture.* Lexington, MA: D.C. Heath.

Valsiner, J. (1989b), Collective coordination of progressive empowerment. In L.T. Winegar (ed.), *Social interaction and the development of children's understanding* (pp. 7-20). Norwood, NJ: Ablex.

Valsiner, J. (1991), Building theoretical bridges over a lagoon of everyday events. *Human Development,* 34, 307-315.

Valsiner, J. (1992a), Introduction: Social co-construction of psychological development from a comparative-cultural perspective. In J. Valsiner (ed.), *Child development within culturally structured environments. Vol. 3. Comparative-cultural and constructivist perspectives.* Norwood, NJ: Ablex.

Valsiner, J. (1992b),. Epilogue: Comparative-cultural co-constructionism and its discontents. In J. Valsiner (ed.), *Child development within culturally structured environments. Vol. 3. Comparative-cultural and constructivist perspectives.* Norwood, NJ: Ablex.

Valsiner, J. (1992c), Social organization of cognitive development: internalization and externalization of constraint systems. In A. Demetriou and E. Efklides (eds.), *The modern theories of cognitive development go to school.* London: Routledge & Kegan Paul.

Valsiner, J. (1993 in press), Making of the future: temporality and the constructive nature of human development. In G. Turkewitz & D. Devenney (eds.), *Timing as initial condition of development.* Hillsdale, NJ: Erlbaum.

Valsiner, J., & Cairns, R.B. (1992 in press), Theoretical perspectives on conflict and development. In C.U. Shantz & W.W. Hartup (eds.), *Conflict in child and adolescent development.* Cambridge: Cambridge University Press.

Valsiner, J., & Van der Veer, R. (1988), On the social nature of human cognition: An analysis of the shared intellectual roots of George Herbert Mead and Lev Vygotsky. *Journal for the Theory of Social Behavior,* 18, 117-135.

Van der Veer, R., & Valsiner, J. (1988), Lev Vygotsky and Pierre Janet: On the origin of the concept of sociogenesis. *Developmental Review,* 8, 52-65.

Van der Veer, R., & Valsiner, J. (1991), *Understanding Vygotsky: A quest for synthesis.* Oxford: Basil Blackwell.

Van der Veer, R., & Valsiner, J. (1992 in press), Sociogenetic perspectives in the work of Pierre Janet. *Storia e Critica della Psicologia.*

Van Geert, P. (1988). The concept of transition in developmental theories. In W.J. Baker, L.P. Mos, H.V. Rappard & H.J. Stam (eds.), *Recent trends in theoretical psychology.* (pp. 225-235). New York: Springer.

Van Oers, B. (1988), Activity, semiotics and the development of children. *Comenius,* No. 32, pp. 398-406.

Vygotsky, L.S. (1934), *Thinking and speech.* Moscow-Leningrad: Gosudarstvennoe Sotsialno-eknomicheskoe Izdatel'stvo.

Vygotsky, L.S. (1933/1976), Play and its role in the mental development of the child. In J. Bruner, A. Jolly & K. Sylva (eds.), *Play* (pp.537-554). Harmondsworth: Penguin.

Vygotsky, L.S. (1987), *The collected works of L.S. Vygotsky. Vol. 1: Problems of general psychology.* New York: Plenum.

Werner, H. (1938), William Stern's personalistics and psychology of personality. *Character and Personality,* 7, 109-125.

Werner, H. (1957), The concept of development from a comparative and organismic point of view. In D.B. Harris (ed.), *The concept of development* (pp. 125-147). Minneapolis: University of Minnesota Press.

Werner, H., & Kaplan, B. (1984), *Symbol formation.* Hillsdale: Erlbaum.

Wertsch, J.V. (1990), The voice of rationality in a sociocultural approach to mind. In L.C. Moll (ed.), *Vygotsky and education* (pp. 111-126). Cambridge: Cambridge University Press.

Wertsch, J.V. (1991), *Voices in the mind.* Cambridge, MA: Harvard University Press.

Wertsch, J.V., & Stone, C.A. (1985), The concept of internalization in Vygotsky's account of the genesis of higher mental functions. In J.V. Wertsch (ed.), *Culture, communication, and cognition: Vygotskian perspectives.* (pp. 162-179). Cambridge: Cambridge University Press.

Winegar, L.T. (1988), Children's emerging understanding of social events: co-construction and social process. In J. Valsiner (ed.), *Child development within culturally structured environments. Vol. 2. Social co-construction and environmental guidance of development* (pp. 3-27). Norwood, NJ: Ablex.

Winegar, L.T., Renninger, K.A., & Valsiner, J. (1989), Dependent-inde-pendence in adult-child relationships. In D.A. Kramer & M.J. Bopp (eds.), *Transformation in clinical and developmental psychology* (pp. 157-168). New York: Springer.

Part 2

New Conceptual Approaches

4. The Sociogenesis of Processes of Sociogenesis, and the Sociogenesis of Their Study

John Shotter

"Man has, as it were, become a kind of prosthetic god. When he puts on all his auxiliary organs he is truly magnificent; but these organs have not grown on him and they still give him trouble at times." (Freud 1962, pp. 38-39)

A Metamethodological Prelude: Beyond Epistemology

Very generally problems to do with sociogenesis are to do with the development of our relations to our surroundings. And these problems are connected with those to do with the relation—some would say, the contest—between objectivism and relativism, or that between realism and social constructionism: the problem of finding some basis somewhere to which to appeal in warranting one's claims to be offering knowledge of at least some kind of worth to others. Knowledge is thought to be of worth to others if it is knowledge of circumstances or states of affairs "outside" of oneself, rather than being merely knowledge of one's own, "inner," personal desires or opinions.

In the past, attempts to solve this problem have treated it both as a singular problem and as a philosophical problem, as involving that branch of philosophy known as epistemology. As if once the epistemological problem was solved, the problem of our relation to our surroundings would also be solved. In line with certain remarks of Wittgenstein (1953)—that essentially, there are countless ways in which we might relate our thought to speech, and our speech to the world, countless ways in which what Vygotsky (1986) calls "the interfunctional relations" between "higher psychological functions" might be formulated—I want to argue that, rather than functioning mechanically and systematically, our mental processes reflect in their functioning essentially the same ethical and political considerations influencing transactions between people, out in the world. Our feeling in the past, that the problem should be treated merely an epistemological problem, represented, as Rorty (1980, p. 61) puts it, the "triumph of the quest for certainty over the quest for reason."

The desire for a theory of knowledge is a desire for constraint—a desire to find "foundations" to which one might cling, frameworks beyond which one must not stray, objects which impose themselves, representations which cannot be gainsaid. (Rorty, 1980, p. 315)

While Rorty succeeds in deflating philosophy's claims to hegemony in this area, however, what is missing from his account is any discussion of how thought and speech and thought and social practices interconnect. He stops short of taking seriously his own insight: to wit, that what we call thought is nothing more and nothing less than sets of historically locatable social practices. Or, to put the matter in Wittgenstein's (1981, no. 656) terms, if we try to characterize the "foundations" of language we will fail, because "language is variously rooted; it has roots, not a single root." This opens up the problem of the relation between thought and speech, thought and social practices to other, more "empirical" forms of investigation, for it means that rather than being of a "mechanical" kind, "interfunctional" relations, such as those between language and thought, become a matter of human choice and argumentation; they become contested. That is what I mean to explore.

Before I say anything further about the general tenor of my approach to this problem, I must point out the unusual way in which I shall formulate it (a way which, I think, is in fact in line with Vygotsky's approach to these issues). In beginning reflective thought about the nature of the world, we have a choice: either to think of it as based in invariances (fixed things) and to treat change as problematic, or, to think of it as in flux (as consisting in activities) and to treat the attainment of stability as a problem. I take this second view; thus central to all that follows is a vision of the world, and of our knowledge of it, as *both* consisting in *activities* of various kinds. Indeed, in line with William James' (James, 1950) image of mental activity within individuals as a flowing stream of activity, containing an array of swirls, and eddies, and vortices, I assume an ontology for the world at large as consisting in an array of "loci of formative or creative activity," or an "ecology of interdependent agencies." Where a part of what it is to say that an entity is an agency, is to say that within the particular region or moment of reality it occupies, it can make *at least some* events occur, that is, exert its formative power, independently of events that occur "outside" of that region or moment.

Within such a view, however, "things do not settle or endure out of their natural state" (Vico, 1968, para. 134). A stable social practice has to be sustained in existence by various "regulatory devices" of a social kind. It is only by the continual administration of such constraints that social orders are sustained in existence, but it is precisely these administrative procedures that are being continually contested.

This has at least two important implications for how we should proceed in our investigations:

1. In the formulation of agencies I offered above, within the particular region or moment they occupy they can make at least some events occur. Here the formulation "at least some" is necessary, because between the centers of such loci are zones of activity within which it is uncertain as to which of the loci the activity "belongs." These "zones of uncertainty" are zones of

contest and struggle. Speaking of social activity in this way means that it is true from a reflective, *retrospective* view of things we can say (as Rorty, 1989, for instance, does), that there is nothing "beneath" socialization, or prior to history, which is definatory of the human being, and that "making" goes all the way down. But *prospectively* and practically, from the view at the point of communication, it is not true. There, each agency is, so to speak, conditioned or constrained in what it can "make" by what it "finds" other agencies around it to be doing, or to have done; not only must it give them a "say" too, but it must "listen" to what they have said or are saying as well. Thus at this less global level, what I want to say, is that "making" and "finding" are intertwined all the way down and all the way back. So although overall I want to present what *in theory* may look like a thoroughgoing socio-historical constructionism, at a more regional, momentary level, it has, as we shall see, what *in practice* might be called a contingently realist aspect to it.

2. The other implication has to do with the fact that when we talk of the various "sites" in social life within which such contests occur, when we talk of "society," "the individual," "the person," "the citizen," "civil society," etc., we all too often assume that we all know perfectly well what the "it" is that is represented by the concepts we are arguing about. We find it difficult to accept that "political objects" such as these are not "there" in some primordial naturalistic sense; that talk "about" them only comes to "make sense" as their character is developed within a discourse. But to claim that discourses work to produce rather than simply to reflect the objects to which the words uttered within them seem to refer, is still make a claim with an unclear meaning. We still unconsciously assume (like Humpty-Dumpty) that when we use a word, it means what we want it to mean, nothing more, nothing less. Nowhere is this more apparent than in our talk about talk, in which we assume that words are *surrogates* (Harris, 1980) which STAND IN[1] for the things in our world, and that communication is a process of *telementation* (Harris, 1981), in which we put our ideas INTO words in order to SEND them to the minds of others. It is these unrecognized image schematisms, implicit in almost all our talk about talk that, as Reddy (1979) points out, lead us to expect "success without effort" as the norm in communication rather than its opposite. We fail to realize that unless effort is expended in the negotiation of meanings, we mostly fail properly to communicate. The fact is, said Wittgenstein (1953, no. 13), that "when we say: 'Every word on language signifies something' we have so far said *nothing* whatsoever, unless we have explained exactly *what* distinction we wish to make."..."Our talk gets its meaning from the rest of our proceedings," (Wittgenstein, 1969, no. 229).

The Problem of "Interfunctional Relations":
Their Nonmechanical Nature

If we turn now to Vygotsky's approach to these problems, we can see how congenial his formulation of the problem of development is to our post-Rorty, antifoundationalist stance, that is, a stance antagonistic to the project of formulating one-way systems of dependencies "rooted" in indubitable, self-evident, first principles. For, right at the beginning of *Thought and Language* (Vygotsky, 1986, p. 1), he formulated the problem of development as to do with the changing of "interfunctional relations," especially of the relations between thought and language. He claimed then (i.e., in 1934) that "inter-functional relations in general have not as yet received the attention they merit." This was because, he claimed, "the unity of consciousness and the interrelation of all psychological relations [was/is] accepted by all....It was taken for granted that the relation between two given functions never varied; that perception, for example, was always connected in an ideal way with attention, memory with perception, thought with memory" (pp. 1-2). Yet, as he goes on to say, "all that is known about psychic development indicates that its very essence lies in the change of the interfunctional nature of conscious-ness" (p. 2).

We can link what Vygotsky says here with what Wittgenstein discovered when he returned again to the problem of the link between language and thought, which he felt he had solved in the *Tractatus*. There, he made such claims as: "We make to ourselves pictures of facts" (T:2.1), and "The picture is a model of reality" (T:2.12). Further, such a model is "linked with reality" (T:2.1511) by being "like a scale applied to reality" (T:2.1512), and so on. But what *is* the character of the "link" or the "hook up" between phenomena and their representations? What counts as *appropriateness* here? Furthermore, here is a central weakness. For the trouble is, as Wittgenstein says in the *Tractatus*: "The picture...cannot represent its form of representation..." How can we get to know its form then? Well, the model itself "*shows it forth*," he says (T:2.172, my emphasis); thus, to the extent that its *form* is *shown* in its structure, its correspondence to reality is something which one must "just see." However, as Lewis Carroll realized (in the tale of Achilles and the Tortoise), we cannot be cognitively (or physically) coerced, through irrefut-able reasoning, to accept such claims. In other words, as Wittgenstein real-ized, the fact is, as he put it later in his book, *On Certainty*: "...the idea of 'agreement with reality' does not have any clear application" (1969, no.215). Thus, if this is the case, if saying something *about* the world is *not* a matter of "picturing" or "parallelling" the structure of the world in the structure of our statements, how can we link our use of language to our circumstances in such a way as to be able to say something *about* them? What is the use to which we can put our words? The answer he gives is this:

> There are *countless* kinds: countless different kinds of use of what we call "symbols",
> "words", "sentences". And this multiplicity is not something fixed, given once for all;
> but types of language, new language-games, as we say, come into existence, and others
> become obsolete and get forgotten... (1953, no. 23)

There are in actual fact, he is claiming, an indefinite number of ways in which the connection between an utterance and its circumstances is, or can be, literally, made and our claims to knowledge justified or warranted. The "logical" form used in a picturing relation to our supposed reality, is simply one among many other ways of formulating claims to knowledge about one's circumstances. Others, such as narrative, metonymic, or even ironic forms are possible also. Indeed, he says: "It is interesting to compare the multiplicity of the tools in language and of the way they are used..., with what logicians have said about the structure of language. (Including the author of the *Tractatus-Logico-Philosophicus*.)" (1953, no. 23). The trouble is, in science as in logic (as also in psychology), because we mistakenly "*compare* the use of words with games and calculi which have fixed rules..." (1953, no. 81), we always think that words *must* have stable, unequivocal, already determined *meanings*. But in the openness of ordinary everyday life, in comparison with the closed world of logic, this is precisely *not* the case. Indeed, in ordinary conversation, it is the *novel* use of *fixed* forms—like the carpenter's novel use of his or her standard tools—which leads to a result appropriate to the unique circumstances in hand.

In line with Wittgenstein's remarks, that essentially there are countless ways in which we might relate thought to language, and language to thought; countless ways in which interfunctional relations might be formulated, I want to suggest that, rather than functioning mechanically and systematically, our mental processes reflect in their functioning essentially the same ethical and rhetorical considerations influencing transactions between people, out in the world. If this is true, then it has implications for us in attempting to theorize this relation. For, if the relation between (a person's) speech and its understanding (by another) is anything like the relation between thought and speech (within an individual), then an understanding too is something that is not preformed, but it is something that is "successively developed" (and checked) in a back-and-forth process over time.

People's linguistic task cannot be in any way like that depicted in Saussure's (1960, pp. 11-12) classic, paradigmatic account of the communicative situation, in which an immaterial idea or concept in the mind of one person (a speaker or writer) is *sent* into the mind of another, essentially similar person (but now in the role of a listener or reader), by the use of material signs such as vibrations in the air or ink marks on paper (see Reddy, 1979). It must be much more like Vygotsky's process of "instruction," in which a person of one kind "makes" something known to another of a (usually very) different kind (e.g., an expert to a layperson, an adult to a child). But how might this process work?

Theory in the Investigation of Made but Contested Phenomena

It is this issue that I want to explore further, for it opens up a whole new micro-social sphere of study to do with the countless different processes which in the past have been covered by special, *general* terms, such as "assimilation," "accommodation, and "equilibration" in Piagetian psychology.

The trouble with general principles is that they are only ever understood in terms of a whole set of *ceteris paribus* (all things being equal) clauses. But these render "rationally invisible" all the daily, so-called idiosyncratic details of how we actually conduct our scientific (and daily) affairs: How in detail we actually conduct our investigations, how we "write up" our results, how we "adjust" what we do to the institutional and social demands upon us. These so-called "social" and "personal" aspects of the process, these small "divergences," "accidental differences," "approximations," "anomalies," are left out of account. In other words, science's account of its own conduct hides its own sociogenesis from view. Only if a whole new approach is fashioned, is it possible to understand the nature of the abstractly described "equilibratory" processes of "joint action," in which practice is adjusted to theory, and theory to practice. Only by taking into account these "local and particular" details, while at the same time making use of "perspicacious presentations" (Wittgenstein), or "exemplary models" (Foucault), is it possible to *show* the relations involved in the socio-historical production of theoretically accountable human activity.

Here again Vygotsky gives us some cues. After talking about the problem of interfunctional relations, he goes on to describe *two* methods for the analysis of complex psychological wholes or activities:

1. In analyzing an activity into its *elements* the "inner" (or intentional) connectivity between all the elements is lost: "The living union of sound and meaning we call the word is broken up into two parts, which are assumed to be held together merely by mechanical associative connections" (1986, p.5), external to the elements themselves. Now someone else who worried at this problem in the same way was John Dewey, who said of this same problem in relation to the reflex arc concept, the following:

> Instead of interpreting the character of sensation, idea and action from their place and function in the sensori motor circuit, we still incline to interpret the latter from our preconceived and preformulated ideas of rigid distinctions between sensations, thought,

and acts. The sensory stimulus is one thing, the central activity, standing for the idea, is another thing, and the motor discharge, standing for the act, is a third. As a result, the reflex arc is not a comprehensive, or organic unity, but a patch work of disjoined parts, a mechanical conjunction of unallied processes. (Dewey, 1948/1896, p. 361)

An activity draws its meaning from its "place" or "position" within a more overall activity within which its plays a part. In other words, mental (as opposed to physical) processes possess *intentionality*; there seems to be a principle of "inner," meaningful connectivity at work, which is ignored when mental activities are analyzed into elements.

2. This leads me to a mention of the second method of analysis Vygotsky described, the one he preferred: Instead of analysis into elements, he talked of analysis into *units*, where by units he talked of *word meanings*. What Vygotsky means by this is, I think, obscure. He seems, via Sapir (1921/1972), to have accepted a Saussurian notion of language almost totally as being a *system* of arbitrary signs functioning as symbols for concepts, in which communication is the *conveying* of an idea from the inside of one head to the inside of another (I'm following the Kozulin translation here). "The higher, specifically human forms of psychological communication are possible," he says, "because man's reflection of reality is carried out in generalized concepts" (1986, p.8).

Now I do not want here to follow Vygotsky's notion of *word meaning* as the relevant unit any further, but I do want to take the idea of unit analysis as such a step further, for I think it provides us with a hint that we shall find useful later. Elsewhere, Vygotsky (1978, p. 8), provides us, I think, with an important methodological suggestion, when, in discussing the relevance of Marx's *theory-method* for an understanding of developmental processes, he says:

> The whole of *Capital* is written according to the following method: Marx analyses a single living "cell" of capitalist society—for example the nature of value. Within this cell he discovers the structure of the entire system and all its economic institutions....Anyone who could discover what a "psychological" cell is—the mechanism producing even a single response—would find the key to psychology as a whole.

It is this idea—put instead, perhaps, in terms of *exemplars, paradigms,* or *perspicacious concrete examples*—which I think we shall find important.

To reinforce my claim here, let me remind you of my basic assumption in all of this: that whatever invariances there are in the world, they are ones that we ourselves, using ways and means of own devising, bring into, and sustain in existence. Thus, of necessity, my approach must be the reverse of our usual (analytic) manner of proceeding: I will not be offering and then be attempting to prove true, any theories or characterizations, laws or principles, or mechanisms of sociogenesis. I cannot. For that *implicitly* would be not only be to assume already existing orders of dependency in the world, but also, to assume that what only recently has come into existence can, in its historically developed final form, be extended indefinitely backwards, to explain its own formation. But all this is only to repeat in other words Vygotsky's views stated above.

In line with the hint he gives us, then, rather than discussing theory, I will adopt a more empirical approach, that is, I will explore "accounts" of *possible* kinds of influence that might be at work in the "shaping" of the development of our activities at a very early stage, before any stabilities have been established within them. For (in my view), what later is properly called "the theory" of a phenomenon is a consequence of a whole social, not a prior principle underlying its existence. The term "theory" only makes sense as such when set against, but also in among, particular, already stabilized, cultural practices, within which there has been a period of "equilibration" of both theory to practice, and practice to theory.

This suggests that there are thus, at least two forms of sociogenesis involved here, to do with the two different directions of equilibration, so to speak, in which social practices are established (although I will mention a third, even more basic, non-equilibratory form of sociogenesis later).

Two Forms of Sociogenesis

One form is from the side of the equilibration of practice to theory, so to speak, and has to do with the way in an effective theory-practice relation slowly emerges, and is finally established. As Ludwik Fleck (1979) shows in his historical account of the development of the Wasserman reaction, once the practice is established and working well, we tend to project back into it a *clear* origin and an *orderly* course of development, which it did not in fact have. As Fleck says, "if after years we were to look back upon a field we have worked in, we could no longer see or understand the difficulties present in that creative work."

> The actual course of development becomes rationalized and schematized. We project the results into our intentions; but could it be any different? We can no longer express the previously incomplete thoughts with these now finished concepts.
>
> Cognition modifies the knower so as to adapt him harmoniously to his acquired knowledge. The situation ensures harmony within the dominant view about the origin of knowledge. Whence arises the "I came, I saw, I conquered" epistemology, possibly supplemented by a mystical epistemology of intuition. (Fleck, 1979, pp. 86-87).

From within such systems, a certain *statement* seems to represent "a self-evident reality which, in turn, conditions our further acts of cognition. There emerges a closed, harmonious system within which the logical origin of individual elements can no longer be traced." (Fleck, 1979, p. 37) Yet, as Fleck shows, to understand the sociogenesis of a (finally effective) process, it is the actual nature (not its distorted nature from within the now finished system) of both its origin *and* the surroundings occasioning its growth that we must grasp. For it is these that function as both the "seed" and the "soil," so to speak, which gives the final system its *style*—where a *Denkstil* can be thought of as a generative "proto-idea" (metaphor, image) along with a set of strategies for eliminating anomalies (Bloor, 1976) in the regulation of its development.[2]

The other form of sociogenesis works more from the other side, the side of the equilibration of theory to practice. For sometimes effective practices are simply set up *in practice*, and are then interpreted *later* as showing something fundamental about the nature of human nature. Thus, it is a mistake to attribute their development to general forces, rather than to look into the particular, practical details involved. Hence, about his earlier attempts to understand the workings of power, Foucault (1979) comments that "What was lacking [there] was this problem of the 'discursive regime', of the effects of power peculiar to the play of *statements*. I confused this too much with systematicity, theoretical form, or something like a paradigm" (my emphasis, p. 113). He realized that he had to investigate the constitution and meaning of singular events, outside of an overall framework of interpretation, because the *form* of a "form of life" is a *consequence* not a *cause* of its production. Hence Foucault's later concern with the description of particular, new and "exemplary" practices, productive of new forms of social relation and subjectivity, evidenced below:

> Were I to fix the date of completion of the carceral system, I would not choose 1810 and the penal code, nor even 1844, when the law laying down the principle of cellular internment was passed; I might not even choose 1838, when books on prison reform... were published. The date I would choose would be January 22, 1840, the date of the official opening of Mettray....Why Mettray? Because it is the disciplinary form at its most extreme, the model in which are concentrated all the coercive technologies of behaviour.[3] (Foucault, 1979).

What Foucault is attempting to do here, in choosing an *exemplary model*, is to show how a new "social space," so to speak, is created in which both a certain form of subjectivity, *and* an associated form of objectivity are created together, a "time-space" which is created, not by individuals, but seemingly by (a transformation) social practices themselves—a problem to which we must return.

My purpose in mentioning both Fleck's cognitive, "thought-style" (*Denkstil*) approach and Foucault's more practical, "genealogical" approach—and one should notice, by the way, that Fleck is concerned with the sociogenesis of scientific knowledge, while Foucault is concerned with planned (not spontaneous) developments in everyday life—is to introduce a new, nontheoretical approach to the task of analyzing the "equilibratory" processes to do with relating theory to practice, and practice to theory. We need at least these two approaches.

A Third Form of Sociogenesis: Sensory Topics

However, we should not assume that social life at large has a homogeneous ontology, that it is always and everywhere the same. Elsewhere (Shotter, 1984, 1990), I have talked of it as consisting of something like an *ecology* of partially interdependent moments and regions of formative activity. While new forms may be *deliberately* created as transformations of those already existing with certain regions and moments—and this is where the two approaches already mentioned are, I think, relevant—other forms may be created *spontaneously* within the chaotic *zones* between two relatively well formed activities, the zones within which they "rub up against one another," so to speak[4]—and this is where the third approach I mentioned is, I think, needed.

In the past (Shotter, 1984), I have explored this phenomenon in abstract terms, under the heading of "joint action." Now, I no longer feel it is appropriate to invent general, abstract processes—such as "equilibration," or "joint action"—and to hold "them," as mysterious agents, responsible for the adjustment which takes place; it is just this move which, to repeat, works to hide all the actual, socio-political processes of importance.[5] A better approach involves what might be called a *poetics* of relational forms—I mean, in line with Vygotsky's idea of a "cell" which contains in its concrete constitution *the structure* of the entire set of significant relational forms involved, something which will function as an analytic paradigm. Such a paradigm is supplied, I think, by Vico in his *New Science* in his discussion of the coming into existence of what he calls "sensory topics." But before I turn to his account, I must mention two "correctives" to our thought, two "conceits" we must cure ourselves of if we are to see the point of his poetic example.

One is "the conceit of nations": we cannot get our beginnings from "within" a culture (nation), for they lie "outside" at least its *normal* forms of reality. Within a culture, they will thought to be *extraordinary*. The second is that as trained scholars, we are not in a good position to study the problem of the origins of human society. The opposite of the case. Thus we need to undo a good deal of our training, to see the extraordinary as the source of the ordinary. Indeed, Vico says, we must reckon as if there were no books in the world, and grasp the nature of the extraordinary stance it requires if we are to take it seriously. But what does it mean to take this maxim of Vico's seriously? Vygotsky (1986) puts it well when he says that "in learning to write the child must disengage himself from the *sensory aspect* of speech and replace words by images of words" (p.181, my emphasis). It is this sensory or sensuous aspect of speech which is so difficult for us now, as literate people, to recognize and to describe; it is, however, this sensuous aspect of speech which will be our main concern below.

This, then, is the force of Vico's correctives: If we are to grasp the nature of the beginnings of language, and reckon as if there were no books in the world, it is the (for us) extraordinary nature of oral, pre-literate, non-conceptual, non-logical forms of communication that we must understand. We must grasp the nature of a form of communication which consists, not in a sequential occurrence of events or things, not in a series of products or of component meanings, but which "subsists" in the continuous flow of sensuous, "moving" activity between people.

In such an unbroken flow of responsivity, in which at first, as Vico puts it, "each new sensation cancels the last one" (para. 703), how do people manage to create and establish within the flow of experience between them a "place" (*topos*), an "is," within the flux of sensation that can be "found again"? How is a recognizably distinct, but socially shared *feeling* about one's circumstances, to which all those involved can later return, formed? For without the possibility of referring to something recognizable as familiar, individuals would live, as Mead (1934, p. 351) puts it, "in an undifferentiated now..," responsive like animals only to immediate and proximate influences. Without the metaphor of written texts and of meanings as static images (representations) to help us, how might we imagine the nature of people's first mental activity? While modern theories of knowledge begin with something present to the mind (e.g., Descartes begins with self-evidently true, clear, and simple innate ideas) Vico begins by asking how it is that the mind comes to have anything present to it at all (Verene, 1981).

And it is precisely to this question that Vico claims to have an answer, indeed, it is the master key of his science. "We find," he says,

> that the principle of these origins both of languages and of letters lies in the fact that the early gentile people, by a demonstrated *necessity* of nature, were poets who spoke in poetic characters. This discovery, which is the master key of this Science, has cost us the persistent research of almost all our literary life, because with our civilized natures we moderns cannot at all imagine and can understand only by great toil the poetic nature of these first men. (para.34, my emphasis)

But to understand what he means here by saying that the early people were, by necessity, poets (where the word *poet* is from the Greek *poietes*, meaning one who makes, a maker, an artificer), we must divide the process of making into two parts: the first, to do with the forming of a *sensory topic*, and the second, with the forming of an *imaginary universal*, which, from a "rooting" in it, "lends" the topic a determinate form. We shall find the resources we need in characterizing both in the following paradigm example.

In paras. 379-391 of the *New Science*, Vico analyzes what he calls the "civil history" of the saying that it was "From Jove that the muse began." Taking it seriously, he suggests that fear of thunder indeed functioned to give rise to both the first sensory topic and imaginative universal. For, as everyone runs to shelter from the thunder, all in a state of fear, an opportunity exists for them to realize that it is the *same thing* that they all fear; and a look or a gesture will communicate this. What we might call a "moment of common reference" exists between them. What "inner mechanisms" might be making such a realization possible is not Vico's concern here; his concern is with the "outer" social conditions. And here it is the fear shared in common that provides the first fixed reference point that people can "find again" within themselves and know that others "feel the same way."

For this kind of fear, this fear of thunder, is not an ordinary fear of an immediately present dangerous event to with one can respond in an effective manner. There is no immediate practical response available to them in response to thunder. It is "not a fear awakened in men by other men, but fear awakened in men by themselves" (para. 382). Their fear is of a kind which seems to point *beyond* the thunder. When people hear it, they become confused and disoriented, they move furtively and with concern for each other; the thunder's presence is the *unspoken* explanation of their actions. And often, "when men are ignorant of the natural causes producing things, and cannot explain them by analogy," says Vico (axiom, para. 180), "they attribute their own nature to them" (see epigraph quote). Thus at this point:

> The first theological poets created the first divine fable, the greatest they ever created: that of Jove, king and father of men and gods, in the act of hurling the lightning bolt; an image so popular, disturbing and instructive that its creators themselves believed in it, and feared, revered and worshipped it in frightful religions....They believed that Jove commanded by signs, that such signs were real words, and that nature was the language of Jove. The science of this language the gentiles believed to be divination. (para. 379)

And it was by learning to read the auspices (natural "signs") that one could learn how, ahead of time, to conform oneself to Nature's (Jove's) requirements.

But the fable of Jove, the imaginary universal, lent form to, and was rooted in, the prior establishing of a *sensory topic*, a sensuous totality linking thunder with the shared fears at the limits of one's being and with recognizing the existence of similar feelings in others because of shared bodily activities. It is created, not out of a heterogeneous amalgam of events, but *within* a developed and developing totality of relations between people.

> The first founders of humanity applied themselves to a sensory topic, by which they
> brought together those properties or qualities or relations of individuals and species
> which were so to speak concrete, and from these created their poetic genera. (para.495)

The sensory topic from which the image of Jove originated, is thus a "topos," a "place" in which it is possible to "re-feel" *everything* which is present at those times when "Jove" is active. And, as such feelings are slowly transformed into more external symbolic forms, the inarticulate *feelings* remain as the "standards" against which the more explicit forms may be judged as to whether they are adequate characterizations or not.

Sensory topics are the primordial places, the *loci*, constituting the background basis of the mentality of a people. They make up its common sense, its *sensus communis*. Without a common sense, there is no basis in which to "root" the formation of any imaginative universals. Yet, such a common sense is in no way *systematic*. It is, says Heider (1958, p. 2), "unformulated and only vaguely conceived." "It embraces the most heterogeneous kinds of knowledge in a very incoherent and confused state," says Schutz (1964, p. 72). It is "immethodical," says Geertz (1983, p. 90), i.e., it caters both to the inconsistencies and diversity of life; it is "shamelessly and unapologetically ad hoc. It comes in epigrams, proverbs, *obiter dicta*, jokes, anecdotes *contes morals*—a clatter of gnomic utterances—not in formalized doctrines, axiomatized theories, or architectonic dogmas." Yet strangely, as Geertz goes on to say, for all its disorder, such knowledge has "accessibleness" as another of its major qualities. Indeed, as Vico points out, it is first in *practical* activities that people must create (by ingenuity/*ingengno*) the meaningful links between what is demanded in a situation, and what is available (by way of resources)[6]—a meaning must be "lent" to the sensing of one's surroundings.

What Vico outlines above then, is a poetic image in terms of which one might understand the *mute*, extraordinary, common-sense basis for an articulate language, where such a basis constitutes the unsystematized, primordial contents of the human mind, its basic paradigms or prototypes. And as Wittgenstein (1953) says about the functioning of such a paradigm or prototype: "In the language-game it is not something that is represented, but it is a means of representation...something with which comparison is made" (no. 50). They are the feelings or intuitions against which the adequacy of concepts may be judged.

Time and the Generative Potentials in a Relational Field

Thus, within a sensory topic, within an identifiable "place" in the flow of sensuous activity between people, are "brought together [all] those properties or qualities or relations of individuals and species which were so to speak concrete," upon which a poetic genera, an imaginative universal, may be based. These first anchor points are to do, not with "seeing" in common, but with "feeling" in common, with the giving or lending of a shared significance to shared feelings in an already shared circumstance.

How might we imagine the nature of such "common places"? Could we call them structures? What does it mean to say that they contain (are a locus of) generative potentials?

We are helped here, I think, by Prigogine's (1980; Prigogine & Stengers, 1984) account of the dynamic stabilities (I shall call them *loci*) occurring in processes of flow. They are created and maintained (by being continually reproduced) within the continuous but turbulent, structurizing processes at the boundaries between two kinds of flowing activity, processes which seem to be closely related to living processes. They have some quite extraordinary characteristics, not least, in the nature of their inner complexity and their continual generation of novelty. Their extraordinary nature stems, Prigogine claims, from an emphasis upon what in the past has been ignored: namely, *time*. Upon reappraising the role of time we find that our "belief in the "simplicity" of the microscopic [the 'building block'] level now belongs to the past," he says (Prigogine, 1980, p. xv). In the new, time-space:

> The elementary particles that we know [which above I have called loci of activity: JS] are complex objects that can be produced and decay. If there is simplicity somewhere in physics and chemistry [and in other fields of study], it is not in microscopic models. It lies more in idealized macroscopic representations. (p. xiii, my additions)

It is the temporal nature of the component activities constituting such loci, and the fact that they are always on the way to becoming other than what they already are, which accounts for their continual novelty.

The growth of such loci (their emergence out of chaos and their sustenance within their chaotic surroundings) is an irreducible aspect of their temporal nature. It cannot be parceled out and added in later when convenient. Thus it makes no sense to talk of such loci as being constructed piece-by-piece and then set in motion; they cannot be made up of parts (if that is still an appropriate term), themselves devoid of temporality, i.e., out of previously *unrelated* parts. In their emergence, they grow from simple into richly structured loci in such a way that their "parts" at any one moment in time owe, not just their character, but their very existence both to each other, *and* to their relation with their parts at some earlier point in time. In other words, the "history" of their relations is just as important as their "logic"—if, that is, it still makes sense to talk in these terms, when both modes of description require representation within the coherent forms of order thought intelligible within a culture (cf. Vico's "conceits").

Thus, no matter how remarkable the "static" geometrical structure (the structure at an instant) of such flowing processes may appear to be, they cannot properly be called *structures* at all. For strictly, any genuinely spatial structure contemplated at a given moment is *complete*, i.e., all its parts are given at once, simultaneously, whereas, the temporally developing loci of which we are speaking are always *incomplete*. There is always more to come within such loci; they are intrinsically creative in the following sense: Rather than static unities-of-homogeneity (made up of similar building blocks), Prigogine calls the stabilities within a flow, unities-of-heterogeneity, for, they can only be seen as (dynamic) unities if their regions are at every moment *different*, in some sense, from what they were at a previous moment (else they would appear as "frozen"). But in what sense? The difference cannot be a change in configuration, else the stability would not remain recognizable as the same stability (as having the same form) from one moment to the next. There must be an irreducible *qualitative* difference between its successive phases for it to be recognizable as a stability within a flow; each phase must be novel in some respect by contrast with the phase preceding it—a novelty that is expressed in its capacity to retain its unity in relation to a whole range of unpredictable changes in its surroundings.

Thus, in relational terms, what we have here is a unity in which its phases and aspects are not related to each other as *separable*, existentially identifiable component parts, but are related only as *sensibly* distinct and distinguishable[7] aspects of the same flowing totality. Each loci is a region of structurizing activity (an agency?), within which a diffuse, dynamic unity is continually, creatively sustained by the (disorderly) exchanges at its boundaries, exchanges between it and the other activities surrounding it, which depend in their turn upon dynamic exchanges at greater and lesser levels, and so on.

Thus, in the now *time-full* world introduced by Prigogine, the idea of building up a complex structure by constructing it out of simple parts ("building blocks," "elementary particles," etc.) must be relinquished. If we are to talk of a "sensory topic" as a "human construction," then as a construction it cannot be similar to a building, or a mechanism, or to any structure put together out of previously unrelated parts. Whatever its "elementary components" are, we can feel sure that they are in some sense relational, i.e., they exist only as sensibly distinct, *novel* moments within an otherwise flowing totality. In other words, there is no point in thinking of relational fields and the nature of their "generative potentials" as systematically ordered "things," they are loci of activity. Although they have no specifiable *form*, they can be specified by their *formative* powers. Elsewhere (Shotter, 1984), I have characterized their nature as having an "already specified further-specifiability," i.e., they give rise to a particular *style* of continuous unforeseeable originality.

This aspect of loci of activity suggests to us another fundamental change we must make in our thinking: While in classical modes of explanation, we focus upon the repetition of identical *forms*, in relational terms, every event occurs within a context of previous events to which they are related. Thus it is not in an event's repetition but in its *novelty* that its significance (function) should be sought.

Conclusions

I have analyzed here then, not any mechanisms of sociogenesis, nor any *theories* of sociogenic processes, but a number of *paradigms*: concrete poetic exemplars rich enough to act as creative sources of both questions and answers. The necessity to do this was occasioned by the fact that when we paid the attention to interfunctional relations that they merited, we realized that what in the past we had taken for granted as invariable, was in fact highly variable. Indeed, attention to the actual, empirical details of such transactions revealed a complex but uncertain process of testing and checking, of negotiating the form of the relationship in terms of a whole great range of, essentially, *political* and *ethical* issues—to do with productive (formative) and negative (causal) powers, with entitlements, judgments, matters of care and concern, etc., for, in our social lives together, we all have a part to play in *a major corporate responsibility*: that of maintaining in existence the communicative "currency," so to speak, in terms of which we conduct all our social transactions. It is this fact: that our ways and means of "making sense" to (and with) one another have not been given us as a "natural" endowment, nor do they simply of themselves endure; what is possible between us is what we (or our predecessors) have "made" possible. And which we are concerned both to maintain, but also to modify to our own circumstances.

References

Bloor, D. (1976), *Knowledge and Social Imagery*. London: Routledge and Kegan Paul.

Dewey, J. (1948/1896), The concept of the reflex arc. In W. Dennis (ed.), *Readings in the History of Psychology*. New York: Appleton-Century-Crofts.

Fleck, L. (1979), *The Genesis and Development of a Scientific Pact*. Chicago: Chicago University Press.

Foucault, M. (1972), *The Archaeology of Knowledge*. A.M. Sheridan (trs.), London: Tavistock.

Foucault, M. (1979), *Discipline and Punishment: The Birth of the Prison*. A.M. Sheridan (trs.), Harmondsworth: Penguin Books.

Freud, S. (1961), *Civilization and Its Discontents*. New York: W.W. Norton and Co.

Geertz, C. (1983), *Local Knowledge: Further Essays in Interpretative Anthropology.* New York: Basic Books.

Gleick, J. (1987), *Chaos: Making a New Science.* London: Cardinal.

Harris, R. (1980), *Language-makers.* London: Duckworth.

Harris, R. (1981), *The Language Myth.* London: Duckworth.

Heider, F. (1958), *The Psychology of Interpersonal Relations.* New York: Wiley.

James, W. (1950), *The Principles of Psychology, Vol. I.* New York: Dover.

Lakoff, G. and Johnson, M. (1980), *Metaphors We Live By.* Chicago: University of Chicago Press.

McGuire, W.J. (1973), The yin and yang of progress in social psychology. *Journal of Personality and Social Psychology,* 26, 446-456.

Mead, G.H. (1934), *Mind, Self and Society.* Chicago: University of Chicago Press.

Prigogine, I. (1980), *From Being to Becoming: Time and Complexity in the Physical Sciences.* San Francisco: Freeman.

Prigogine, I. and Stengers, I. (1984), *Order out of Chaos: Man's New Dialogue with Nature.* New York: Batam Books.

Reddy, M. (1979), The conduit metaphor. A. Ortony (ed.). *Metaphor and Thought.* London: Cambridge University Press.

Rorty, R. (1980), *Philosophy and the Mirror of Nature.* Oxford: Blackwell.

Rorty, R. (1989), *Contingency, Irony and Solidarity.* Cambridge: Cambridge University Press.

Sapir, E. (1972), *Language: An Introduction to the Study of Speech.* New York: Harcourt Brace, orig. pub. 1921.

Saussure, F. de (1960), *Course in General Linguistics* C. Bally, A. Sechehaye (eds). London: Peter Owen.

Schutz, A. (1964), *Collected Papers II: Studies in Social Theory.* The Hague: Martinus Nijhoff.

Shotter, J. (1980), Action, joint action, and intentionality. M. Brenner (ed.). *The Structure of Action.* Oxford: Blackwell.

Shotter, J. (1984), *Social Accountability and Selfhood.* Oxford: Blackwell.

Shotter, J. (1990), *Knowing of the Third Kind: Essays on Rhetoric, Psychology and the Culture of Everyday Social Life.* Utrecht: ISOR.

Verene, D.P. (1981), *Vico's Science of the Imagination.* Ithaca: Cornell Univ. Press.

Vico, G. (1948), *The New Science of Giambattista Vico.* T.G. Bergin and M.H. Fisch (ed. and trs.), Ithaca, NY: Cornell University Press.

Vygotsky, L.S. (1978), *Mind in Society: The Development of Higher Psychological Processes.* M. Cole, V. John-Steiner, S. Scribner, E. Souberman (eds.) Cambridge, MA: Harvard University Press.

Vygotsky, L.S. (1986), *Thought and Language.* Translation newly revised by Alex Kozulin. Cambridge, MA: MIT Press.

Vygotsky, L.S. (1987), Thinking and speech. In *The Collected Works of L.S. Vygotsky: Vol. 1.* R.W. Rieber and A.S. Carton (eds.), N. Minick (trs.). New York: Plenum.

Wittgenstein, L. (1953), *Philosophical Investigations.* Oxford: Blackwell.

Wittgenstein, L. (1969), *On Certainty.* Oxford: Blackwell.

Wittgenstein, L. (1981), *Zettel,* (2nd Ed). G.E.M. Anscombe and G.H.V. Wright (eds). Oxford: Blackwell.

Notes

1. I have used the useful uppercase way of indexing metaphors introduced by Lakoff and Johnson (1980).

2. Elsewhere (Shotter, 1984), I have suggested that what it is for formative activities to have a certain *style* is for them to have "already specified, further self-specifiability."

3. And he continues: "In it were to be found 'cloister, prison, school, regiment'. The small, highly hierarchized groups, into which the inmates were divided, followed simultaneously five models....This superimposition of different models makes it possible to indicate, in its specific features, the function of 'training'.... Where Mettray was especially exemplary was in the specificity that it recognized in this operation of training....It was the first training college in pure discipline: the 'penitentiary' was not simply a project which sought its justification in 'humanity' or its foundations in a 'science', but a technique that was learned, transmitted, and which obeyed general norms....It was the emergence or rather the institutional specification, the baptism as it were, of a new type of supervision—both knowledge and power—over individuals who resisted disciplinary normalization....But the supervision of normality was firmly encased in a medicine or a psychiatry that provided it with a sort of 'scientificity'; it was supported by a judicial apparatus which, directly or indirectly, gave it legal justification."

4. The influence of motifs from so-called "Chaos Theory" are apparent here (Gleick, 1987).

5. Now it is not that these processes of "adjustment" have not been noted in the past. Indeed, McQuire (1973) has noted that what a psychological experiment may test "is not whether [a] hypothesis is true but rather whether the experiment is sufficiently ingenious stage manager to produce in the laboratory conditions which demonstrate that an obviously true hypothesis is correct" (p. 449). Or, as Smedslund (1984) says about the supposed experimental testing of obviously true hypotheses: "This possibility of reinterpreting pseudoempirical studies as involving the testing of procedures is universally present" (p. 249). In each case, however, what is underestimated is the difficulty of the process of "linking" or "hooking up" theory to practice. They both fail to take account of the fact that in our everyday social life together, we do not find it easy to relate ourselves to each other in ways which are *both* intelligible (and legitimate), *and* which also are appropriate to *"our"* (unique) circumstances; and the fact that on occasions at least, we none the less do succeed in doing so.

6. Vico saw also the conceit of scholars as due to their detachment from the necessities of life. Indeed, in his history they came last on the tree of knowledge: "First (were) the woods, then cultivated fields and huts, next little houses and villages, thence cities, finally academies and philosophers: this is the order of all progress from the first origins." (Vico, 1948, para.22)

7. Where by the term *sensibly distinct*, I mean that each aspect is not perceived as a distinct, momentary whole, but that each aspect is nonetheless distinguishable from every other to the extent that its coming into existence can be sensed, i.e., its emergence makes a sensuous difference.

5. Iconology and Imagination: Explorations in Sociogenetic Economies

Chris Sinha

Introduction

This paper is both about human cognition, its origin and development; and about prevailing notions of cognition and rationality, their origin and history. What I shall propose, more speculatively than argumentatively, is that to understand the linkage between these two genetic processes is one way to understand, or to give content to, the concept of sociogenesis. The linkage in question is both reflexive (it involves the relationship between thought, and thought about thought), and productive (it involves processes which make possible new kinds of thought). I shall further propose that the "site," or "space," which these linking sociogenetic processes inhabit and populate is what I shall refer to, following Castoriadis (1987), as the *social imaginary*. My starting point is the observation that the cognitive sciences find themselves today in a situation of crisis. The established, or "classical," paradigm of cognitivism is under attack on many fronts, ranging from its account of cognitive processing mechanisms, to its underlying "objectivist" philosophy. Cognitivism is (very summarily) the view that human mental processes can be characterized in terms of the manipulation of a set of discrete, arbitrary physical tokens, by a set of explicitly statable algorithmic rules operating upon those tokens. While I do not wish to rehearse here every one of the manifold criticisms of cognitivism that have been advanced in the last decade or so, it is possible to summarize some of their principal features under the following four major themes: I address these issues at length in Sinha (1988); see also, amongst many others, Marková (1982), Bruner (1990), and Plunkett and Sinha (1991).

The cognitivist paradigm, because of its overriding concern for formalization, is unable to comprehend the crucial role of context (social, communicative, ecological) in human cognitive processes.

The cognitivist paradigm is unable to provide an adequate account of human epigenetic development, and remains locked in an outmoded and sterile opposition between nativism and environmentalism. The cognitivist paradigm employs serial-symbolic computational processing models which fail to capture the dynamic and contextually sensitive properties of human cognition and perception. Alternative (parallel distributed processing) computational architectures are superior in respect of both their capacity to model human cognition, and their neurobiological plausibility.

The cognitivist paradigm is built upon an outdated metaphysics of the (individual) mind as a "mirror of nature" (Rorty, 1980), of knowledge as an objective mapping of a mind-independent reality, and of rationality as a disembodied set of algorithmic procedures divorced both from human biological and cultural incarnation, and from imaginative structures of human understanding.

My focus here is upon the last of these themes, which is in some ways the most general one, but which at the same time raises a very specific set of issues concerning the concepts of reason, representation, figuration, and imagination.

The first aim of this paper is not so much to explore "from within" what Johnson (1987) calls the "crisis in the [objectivist] theory of meaning," with its attendant consequences for the cognitive sciences, as it is to pose the question: What sociogenetic mechanisms and processes may have been responsible for the predominance of the objectivist view of meaning and rationality in the classical Western theory of mind?

My second aim in this paper is to show that not only modern cognitivism, but also Freudian and Piagetian developmental psychologies, are structured around a fundamental opposition between (incorporeal) reason and (corporeal) imagination, in which the former is posited as a "higher" evolutionary stage than the latter. Finally, I wish briefly to address the question of how we might better understand the complex interrelations between the ontogenesis and sociogenesis of cognitive processes. Obviously, all this is an ambitious undertaking, and I can only attempt a preliminary exploration of the issues in this paper.

Iconology and Imagination

In recent, well-known books, Mark Johnson (1987) and George Lakoff (1987) argue that objectivism is an inadequate basis for theories of human language, meaning, and cognition. For our current purposes, we can gloss "objectivism" as encompassing a number of well-known doctrines of meaning and rationality, such as truth-based logical semantics, the correspondence theory of truth, the "classical" theory of categorization (see below), the presumed primacy of univocal, literal meaning in language, the peripheral status of metaphoric meaning, and so forth. As Johnson and Lakoff remark, there is nothing about such theories which requires them to address the specific, biologically and culturally embodied dimensions of human experience. Indeed, in the guise of "machine functionalism," the view that reason and meaning are disembodied and transcendent has acquired an almost self-evident status in cognitivist philosophy of mind.

For cognitivism, the relation of reference between symbol and world is either sidelined (methodological solipsism) or is regarded as a technical issue to be solved by a truth-based logical semantics. At the heart of the cognitivist account is the "idea," common to both rationalist and empiricist philosophies, which in the course of the centuries has been progressively purged of its original imagistic and picture-like characteristics or connotations. In modern cognitivism, an idea is essentially an argument of which something can be predicated in the "language of thought" (Fodor, 1976).

The alternative, "New Romantic" account advanced by Johnson (1987) and Lakoff (1987) sees "ideas" as being more like images. The categories employed in human cognition and language are like images in that they are not "clear and distinct," but have "fuzzy" boundaries; and they are not atomic primitives, but have internal structure, though not one of a "compositional" nature. Ideas, or concepts, in the New Romantic account, are also articulated in "idealized cognitive models" of an image-schematic nature, and image-schematic structures are derived from bodily experience: thought is embodied.

The New Romantic account does not conceive of the link from symbol to world as being governed by truth conditions, but as being a function of experience and its embodiment, in biological organisms and human cultures. There is a continuity between meaning in the broad sense of "being in" or "having" a world, and linguistic meaning as a special case. All meaning, including linguistic meaning, is situated in recurrent patterns of bodily experience, and the imaginative projections of these experiential patterns across different domains of understanding.

In identifying, or aligning, the imagination with the corporeal, Lakoff and Johnson are following a long line in Western thought. However, while the dominant tradition, from Plato onwards, has counterposed the "merely" sensible and sensuous (to which the imagination is seen to belong) to the logos, New Romanticism not only reverses the traditionally lowly valuation placed upon the imagination; it also emphasizes the involvement of the bodily and the imagistic in processes of reasoning, language, and discourse. The body and the icon, long banished from the domain of the rational, are postulated in the work of Johnson, Lakoff, and others (e.g., Langacker, 1987) to play a crucial role in human cognitive processes. How, and why, did they become excluded in the first place?

"Iconology" is a term which was introduced by the art critic Erwin Panofsky (1939), who distinguished it from the more traditional "iconography," or classification of religious and artistic images. W.J.T. Mitchell (1986) writes:

> If Panofsky separated iconology from iconography by differentiating the interpretation
> of the total symbolic horizon of an image from the cataloguing of particular symbolic
> motifs, my aim here is to further generalize the interpretive ambitions of iconology by
> asking it to consider the idea of the image as such. (Mitchell, 1986, p. 2)

Iconology, then, in Mitchell's interpretation, is the study, not just of images, but of the idea of the image: of its relations to its cognates—imagery, imagination, figure—and to its other—text, discourse, word. And, as Mitchell makes clear, this "idea" (remembering that for generations of philosophers, following Aristotle, an idea was itself a mental image) is far from being "clear and distinct." Rather, it is "essentially contested"; it has been, through-out recorded history, a focus and a site of political, social, religious, and intellectual conflict, of a struggle between iconophilia (idolatry) and icono-phobia (iconoclasm). Iconology, then, is about both the relationship between image and text, and about the different discourses through which this relation-ship has been thought and contested. So much (for the time being) for iconology, what about "sociogenetic economies"? Here I have availed myself of a notion which has found wide currency in French structuralist and post-structuralist approaches to linguistics and psychoanalysis, but whose most explicit formulation is to be found in Jean-Joseph Goux (1990). The "intu-ition" underlying the notion was expressed in the early part of the twentieth century by the anthropologist Marcel Mauss, who proposed that "exchange is the common denominator of a large number of apparently heterogeneous social activities" (Goux, 1990: 2). By the 1960's it was becoming almost a commonplace to suggest that a unification (in terms both of delineating the conceptual field, and of understanding the historical conditions for the emergence) of the human sciences might be provided by a generalized notion of exchange, since "the semiotic, economic and psychoanalytic horizons all emphasized the question of substitution and its correlative, value" (Goux, 1990, p. 2).

Yet, as many critics were to point out, the analogy between linguistic communication, monetary exchange, and the symbolic structures proposed by psychoanalysis (especially in its Lacanian variant) may be nothing more than an analogy, and a misleading one at that. That Saussure (1966) employed economic and monetary metaphors in formulating the principles of structural linguistics, is perhaps nothing more than an instance of a "new" science borrowing the terminology of an already established one, for heuristic and didactic purposes. That Lacan (1966) chose a linguistically based exposition of the "symbolic economy" of the unconscious, may be accounted for by reference to the exhaustion and anachronism of the standard "hydraulic" metaphors. And "exchange," considered as an economic-anthropological category, is so far from homogeneous in its membership that the inevitable question arises as to whether the very concept is not a universalistic projection (or fetish?) of the generalized commodity form of the advanced capitalistic mode of production. In short, there are good reasons to doubt that the concept of "exchange" is capable of revealing any more than superficial commonalities between the different human sciences.

Here, though, Goux takes another tack. Instead of "exchange," he posits a notion which is both more "abstract" and more "historicist" (that is to say, a socially and historically emergent concept): the concept of the general equivalent. This, following Aristotle, he glosses as a standard "which, by making things commensurable, renders it possible to make them equal" (Goux, 1990, p. 3). The "discovery" or "invention" of the general equivalent (or generalized concept of exchange and exchangeability) first occurred, probably, in Ancient Greece—Goux's work coincides, here and elsewhere, with the ideas of the philosopher Alfred Sohn-Rethel (1978), a parallel which I have not the space here to pursue further—and inaugurated a "fundamental configuration" of symbolic practices and value-economies which has persisted and reached its most developed expression in our present societies. This fundamental configuration Goux summarizes thus:

> the accession of the father to the rank of privileged subject, controlling the conflict of identification; the elevation of the phallus to the place of centralized standard of objects of drive...the privileged position of language as a phonic signifier potentially equivalent to all other signifiers through the operation of verbal expression—all these appear to be promotions of a general equivalent. In each case, a hierarchy is instituted between an excluded, idealized element and the other elements, which measure their value in it. In short...the Father becomes the general equivalent of [psychoanalytic] subjects, Language the general equivalent of signs, and the Phallus the general equivalent of [psychoanalytic] objects, in a way that is structurally and genetically homologous to the accession of a unique element (let us say Gold, for the sake of simplicity) to the rank of the general equivalent of products. Thus, what had previously been analyzed separately as phallocentrism (Freud, Lacan), as logocentrism (Derrida), and as the rule of exchange by the monetary medium (Marx), [can be seen as] part of a unified process. (Goux, 1990, p. 4).

Goux adds that there is no question here of asserting any particular causal priority (e.g., of "base" over "superstructure"); and that the historical emergence of this "fundamental configuration" (the rule of the general equivalent, as we might say), is also identifiable as the historical condition for the birth of philosophy "as we know it"—that is, the problematic of equivalence and its logic, as this finds its expression in the "idea of the idea" (an abstraction of identity from perceptible difference) and the law of the excluded middle. Here and below I am extending Goux's argument, or at least using a slightly different vocabulary from his. At this point, we must ask: what precisely is the nature of the equivalence relationship which is constituted between any two terms, the privileged and the non-privileged, that which is the measure of value and that which is measured or equalized? The answer, surely, is that the relationship is symbolic, in the sense that it is the totality of such equivalences The term "equivalences" refers in this context to all possible symbolic (classificatory, metaphoric, metonymic) identifications in all possible societies, which make up the "symbolic order" of any given society, and which finds its expression both in the language and in the institutions of that society.

However, as Castoriadis (1987) makes clear, the realm of the symbolic is not, either in the individual or in the society, one which exists *sui generis* or autonomously: every symbol presupposes an imaginary relationship between the symbol and that which is symbolized; and conversely, the realm of the imaginary (in the life of both societies and individuals) finds its expression in and through symbolization. As Castoriadis (1987: 127) puts it:

> the imaginary has to use the symbolic...to pass from the virtual to anything more than this ... But, conversely, symbolism too presupposes an imaginary capacity. For it presupposes the capacity to see in a thing what it is not, to see it other than it is...to the extent that the imaginary ultimately stems from the originary faculty of positing or presenting oneself with things and relations which do not exist...we shall speak of a final or radical imaginary as the common root of the actual imaginary and of the symbolic. This is, finally, the elementary and irreducible capacity of evoking images.

Johnson (1987), as we have seen, emphasizes the constitutive role of the imaginary (and the corporeal) in the cognitive processes of individuals. He stresses, as does Lakoff (1987), that the interpretation of the meanings conveyed or expressed by the symbolic system of natural language depends upon metaphoric projections and identifications which find their "root" meaning in human bodily experience and in the "radical imaginary," the capacity to evoke and deploy imagery. Such meanings are intersubjectively shared, inasmuch as individual language users share a common, embodied, human predicament or "being-in-the-world." But the social dimension of the imaginary (including its role in language and cognition) extends beyond this "inter-corporeality" (Merleau-Ponty, 1964). As Castoriadis argues, underlying the symbolic order of any given society, and "grounding" its system of social significations, is an order or "pattern," which he refers to as the social imaginary, and which he speaks of as providing "the conditions for the representability of everything that the society can give to itself." Castoriadis continues:

> These patterns do not themselves exist in the form of a representation one could, as a result of analyses, put one's finger on. One cannot talk in this case of "images," however vague and indefinite the sense ascribed to this term. God is perhaps, for each of the faithful, an "image"...but God, as an imaginary social signification, is neither the "sum," nor the "common part," nor the "average" of these images; it is rather their condition of possibility and what makes these images, images "of God"...The imaginary social significations do not exist strictly speaking in the mode of representation;

they are of another nature, for which it is of no use to seek an analogy in the other spheres of our experience. Compared to individual imaginary significations, they are infinitely larger than a phantasy (the pattern underlying the Jewish, Greek or Western "image of the world" is of infinite extension) and they have no precise place of existence (if indeed the individual unconscious can be called a precise place of existence.) They can be grasped only indirectly and obliquely...as the invisible cement holding together this endless collection of real, rational and symbolic odds and ends that constitute every society, and as the principle that selects and shapes the bits and pieces that will be accepted there. (Castoriadis, 1987, p. 143)

Employing Castoriadis' notion of the social imaginary, we can now say that what, with Goux (1990), we identified as the rule of the general equivalent, as a general ordering principle manifesting itself in the sphere of symbolic economies, can be seen as having its roots in the re-structuring of the social imaginary itself, in such a way that the "space" of the latter is made to conform to an omnipresent "image" of rationality—a rationality that is, as Castoriadis (1987, p. 156) points out, in its decontextualized self-sufficiency, a second-order imaginary. In this respect, one can speak of the colonization of the social imaginary by the logos, such that imagination (radical, figurative, and social) becomes a kind of repressed other, haunting reason's construction of the world in its own image.

Metonymy, Writing, and the General Equivalent

The thesis that I shall, speculatively, advance in this section is twofold: (1) that what Lakoff (1987) identifies as the "classical" theory of categorization—a thing either belongs or does not belong, without residue, to a particular category—has as its historical (sociogenetic) condition of existence the emergence, in a complex of sociogenetic economies, of the rule of the general equivalent, and (2) that a major role in this sociogenetic process was played by the invention of the phonetic alphabet. Before proceeding further, however, I want briefly to address the concept of "sociogenesis" itself.

As I employ it, this concept implies some sort of relationship between individual human development (ontogenesis), and the historical, socio-cultural circumstances in which individual human development occurs, and has occurred. In this context, we can refer, in the first place, to the issue of the socio-historical conditions of emergence of the discourses in which human cognition and its iconology are given shape and substance as an "object" of philosophy and science. Thus, in a following section, I shall examine theories of human psychological development, with respect to their implicit or explicit iconologies (their stance in iconological matters). There is, however, more to it than this, and I shall also try to step down a level, from the meta-discourse of iconology, to ask (in the final section) the question: in what way can we adequately understand the development, in human beings, of conceptualization as a psycho-social activity, and the role of both the radical imaginary and the social imaginary in this activity?

These two questions can be linked by posing a third question, which is the focus of this section: What is (or was, and is) the sociogenetic process which gave rise to the conceptualization of thought itself in terms of abstract, decontextualized general equivalence?

The difficulty with this question lies in the fact that it crosses the two different levels of possible analysis which are referred to above. Goux's analysis of the rule of the general equivalent attempts to show how it is that socially circulating representations (of language, of political economy, of the psyche) have some common point of genetic origin, historically locatable and traceable in the webs of discourses reaching down through the centuries. But we might go further, and suggest that the sociogenetic mechanism which (for example) elevates the phallus to the signifier (in the realm of the social imaginary) of the object of power/desire, is the very same mechanism which constitutes not only the subject of psychoanalytic discourse, but also actual, individual subjects.

The rule of the general equivalent is, if this is so, a sociogenetic mechanism whose effectivity is at the level both of the description and of the thing described. It is inscribed in our discourses, and also in that which the discourse purports to delineate. Psychoanalytic discourse is the appropriate discourse for a phallocentrically constituted subject; its "ideal" structure mirrors the sociogenetic mechanisms which place the subject in a specific (patriarchally determined) relationship to power and desire.

The same point can, of course, be made in relation to the "mysterious" commodity-form, as analyzed by Marx; it is both an imaginary (ideal) abstraction, and a sociogenetic process of production of real social relations. And the same point can also be made in relation to that mysterious notion introduced by Saussure of the "arbitrariness" of the sign: was it meant as a methodological principle, or as a real characterization of a relation between two imaginary terms (signified and signifier), which, on Saussure's own account, cannot exist without each other?

These mysteries of reflexivity and level of discourse are especially recalcitrant in the case of thought (cognition) and its sociogenesis. For, as I have said, it is easiest to think of the rule of the general equivalent as constituting, in Western thought, the "idea of the idea": the representation of the representation of the essence which is unchanged despite the flux of appearance. And this is, in itself, a challenging and bold thesis. But what if we were to make the thesis bolder still? What if we were to hypothesize that this very same sociogenetic mechanism (or complex of mechanisms) constituted or made possible thought itself, not just philosophy (thought about thought), but the thought which is philosophy's object?

What if what we call (developed) human cognition is a product of a sociogenetic mechanism (the rule of the general equivalent), that is mediated by ontogenetic processes, and whose entry into human culture can be dated to around about the fifth century BC in the Ionian peninsula (and maybe elsewhere, at around the same time)? What if this "developed" human cognition is not a universal of either biology or of culture, but a specific socio-historical acquisition? If this is so, it might help to explain why the "crisis" of the rule of the general equivalent is nowhere so acutely manifest and so laden with implications as in the sciences of cognition itself.

If, however, we are to think of a sociogenetic mechanism (such as the rule of the general equivalent) as having effects at different levels which are at the same time somehow reciprocally linked, we need some reflexive conceptual apparatus, and a vocabulary in which to express it. To attempt an expansion of this: only a certain kind of "thought" can permit a certain kind of "thought about thought," and that "thought about thought" constitutes the thought thought-about as that kind of thought, and both the thought thought-about and the thought about it are brought into existence by the self-same sociogenetic process.

To make this point more concrete, let us examine the thesis advanced by Goux (1990). This is, essentially, that the originary, and still operative, "fundamental configuration" of what we might call the "Western political economy of the social imaginary" is constituted by a constellation of institutions and their associated ideologies: namely, patriarchy, monotheism, monetary exchange, and logocentrism. Now, the problem with this formulation, as it is, is that it leaves unstated the problem of the cognitive dimension of logocentrism, by which term I mean simply the notion of a decontextualised, linguistified, and univocal notion of "meaning" as residing in word and text (see also Wertsch, 1991).

Goux (1990) does, indeed, specify the sociogenetic relationships which bind together patriarchy, monotheism, the mediation of commodity exchange by money, and Mosaic and Protestant iconoclasm (the latter being, of course, linked with logocentrism), and I shall return to these relationships in the following section, in which I shall analyze the iconoclastic presuppositions to be found in the developmental psychologies of Freud and Piaget. Yet these relationships are best seen in terms of the mutual motivation of the different components of the constellation by each other, rather than in terms of specific sociogenetic (generative) processes permitting the historical emergence of any particular one of them. Since my concern here is (primarily) with cognition, and the iconology of "thought about thought," it is upon logocentrism that I wish to focus.

Specifically, I wish to bring into play another social institution and social practice, and suggest that it played a crucial role in making possible a logocentric stance to meaning and rationality as univocal, determinate and decontextualized. That institution and practice, I suggest, was phonetic-alphabetic writing, and my proposal is that this institution and practice made possible new ways of conceiving of categorization, in terms of an opposition between "essence" and "appearance" and in terms of the law of the excluded middle. In short, I am proposing that the invention of the phonetic alphabet was the primary cognitive sociogenetic mechanism making possible the "classical" theory of categorization, and thus in introducing the cognitive prerequisites for the "capture" of the Western social imaginary by the rule of the general equivalent.

As should be clear from the foregoing, I am not suggesting that any single mechanism was solely responsible for the sociogenetic institution of the rule of the general equivalent, which cannot have been a single "event," and which should also in any case be thought of in terms of tendencies and relative dominances, rather than as some absolutely all-governing principle. Rather, what I want to examine here is the role played by the invention of the phonetic alphabet in constituting one of the conditions of possibility—through notational externalization—of an operative and conscious concept of generalized equivalence, with specific cognitive and meta-cognitive properties and consequences.

It is important to note here that it is a particular kind or mode of writing (phonetic-alphabetic), rather than writing "in general," that I am proposing as being implicated in the sociogenesis of the concept of generalized equivalence. However, I shall first very briefly discuss the role of writing in general, in both cognitive and monetary economies.

First, Olson (1977), Scribner and Cole (1981), and others have drawn attention to the possibility that literacy, in certain particular socio-functional contexts, may induce cognitive effects at the level of metalinguistic and metacognitive processes. These effects may be seen as the inducement of a shift towards "decontextualized" or "abstract" thinking. What I shall suggest is something similar, but with a focus on the congruence between a particular cognitive figural process, and the figurative bias underlying abstract logical reasoning. This bias, as Rotman (1978) and Walkerdine (1988) have pointed out with respect to mathematical and other kinds of formal reasoning, is metonymic in character.

The advantage of this specification is that it recognises that "abstraction" and the "theoretical attitude" are realized, or made manifest, in both the metaphoric and the metonymic dimensions of language and representation (Sinha, 1988). The studies of Olson (1977), Cole (1981), and others have tended to see the issue of "abstraction" as one involving semantic and propositional content: that is, as a process whereby semantic content becomes decontextualized along a metaphoric dimension. In contrast, I shall focus here upon the metonymic ("part-whole" or "container-contained") figure, without commitment as to whether writing in general, or alphabetic writing in particular, also induces a kind of textual-semantic "abstract cognitive attitude"; of the kind conveyed by Olson's notion of a historic shift, attributable to Protestantism and the rise of mercantile capitalism, from a notion of "meaning as mediated by authority," to a notion of "meaning as solely residing in the text." I shall, however, have something to say about the sociogenetic mechanism whereby alphabetic writing potentiates a notion of abstract or formal truth, which is of course intimately connected with the notion of decontextualized propositional or cognitive content. The further exploration of the interactions between metonymic and metaphoric modes of "abstraction," and its relation to writing, lies beyond the scope of this paper.

Second, there is no question that graphic notation has its roots very far back in human prehistory, perhaps as far or even farther back than language itself (Harris, 1986). It is also clear that, from the very first, graphic notations of language, that is, writing, played a significant role in ordering and regulating economic transactions, of tribute, trade, and so forth, and in economic activity (e.g., stock-taking and accountancy) in general. The invention of the phonetic alphabet quite definitely post-dates the general use of writing for recording economic information, and I do not wish to suggest that its effects on economic systems (e.g., the emergence of commodity exchange and monetary systems) were direct. Rather, it is more plausible to see the emergence of monetary value-equivalence (monetary token-equivalence), and the emergence of the phonetic alphabet, involving graphic token-equivalence, as being mutually reinforcing processes in the sociogenesis of the rule of the general equivalent.

Having said that, let me now turn to the specific role of phonetic-alphabetic writing in the externalization of the notion of generalized equivalence, and the way that this "frames" meaning and value in such a way that the classical, abstract "concept of the concept" becomes possible. I shall start by distinguishing between three general classes of metonymy, or "container-contained" relations, namely: Category–Member, Substance–Sample, and Type–Token. I want to emphasize that these relations do not map in any straightforward way onto each other, even though each of them does imply some kind of equivalence. Thus, all members of a category are equivalent, inasmuch as they may be named by the term for the category. However, as Lakoff (1987) and others have pointed out, this does not mean that all category members are equivalent in their "goodness," "centrality" or "typicality." Category membership is (in natural languages) both vague, and contestable or negotiable in its boundaries. Similarly, samples of a substance exemplify the substance, and are equivalent in that respect, but some samples may be better, purer, and more "representative" than others. Finally, tokens which instantiate some value are all equivalently tokens of that value (be it a monetary or a semiotic value), but their empirical or perceptible form may vary: the phonetic realization of phonemes being a crucial and well-known case, but we may think also of coins, notes, and so forth.

Thus, all these three metonymic relations involve some kind of equivalence relation obtained between the elements comprising that which is "contained," and a "container." The "container" can be seen as precisely the "abstraction" that "represents" and constitutes the contained as being equivalent in some way. Yet the relations are different: a member of a category is not a sample, since a category is not a substance, and vice-versa. The type-token relationship does, it is true, share properties of each of the other relations. A type can be thought of as a category with an infinite (potential) membership; and tokens may be thought of as sampling either a concrete substance (as in gold coinage) or an abstract substance, as for example the "content" level of Hjelmslev's version of structuralist linguistics (Hjelmslev, 1953).

At the same time, the type-token relation exemplifies most clearly the notion of "abstract equivalence," an equivalence which is governed by a value which is "beyond" the phenomenal form of the token. This value is imaginary (it is constituted in and as representation); but it has real effects in constituting and structuring the real, and the perception of the real. Value, as constituted in type-token relations, is constituted in and through the social imaginary.

The category-member and the sample-substance relationships also exemplify (or embody) the social imaginary, since categorization is, in a sense, the world as it is structured and composed for any given language and culture. And categorization processes also impose themselves on, and are also partly shaped by, the "substances" which make up the natural (and "spiritual" or "mental") worlds. These two metonymic relations, and their interplay, govern to a large degree the experienced world of any given culture.

I would maintain, however, that a large body of research supports the conclusion that categorization, while being highly culturally variable, is not arbitrary: it is partly determined by properties both of the natural world and of the psychophysiology of human perception. In their ecological situatedness, categorization processes (including those governing conceptions of substance) are socio-natural in character; they are Janus-faced, facing both nature and culture, and embodying the co-articulation of nature and culture in specific cultural settings.

The type-token relationship is different. In categorization, "substance" partially lends form to its representation: the category member is an instantiation of a category which is, as it were, "marked," or informed, by the properties of its most representative members. In contrast, in the type-token relationship the substance is a realization of the abstract form: the token, as "substance," is informed by the purely abstract type. Of course, it is also the case that types do not emerge arbitrarily. Phonemic systems of languages find their conditions of possibility in the physiology of the human vocal tract. But this shows only that types can also be considered as categories, subject to the same kind of socio-naturalistic double determination as any other category. What concerns me here is not the type considered as a category, but the type-token relation as such, which is different from the category-member relation, while depending for its operation upon it. The type-token relation is signification in its "purest" form, and though it is material in both its effects and its structure, it is irreducible to any naturalistic plane (and this irreducibility is constitutive, of course, of precisely the difference between phonology, which is part of linguistics, and phonetics, which is part of the natural sciences.) We can add here, too, that although the type-token relationship depends upon categorization processes, it is also the case that the manifestation of categorization in human language depends upon the type-token relationship. Without language, which operates as a system of types, there can be no linguistic categorization and no linguistic semantics, no metaphor and no cultural meaning.

It is for this reason that I wish to suggest that the type-token relationship is crucial for an understanding of the concept of abstract, general equivalence, and how it came to achieve the status of a dominant structuring principle in the social imaginary. My proposal is that the invention of the phonetic alphabet, which externalized in a notational system the type-token relationship, made it possible to consider equivalence as an abstract and general "rule." That is to say, whereas before the phonetic alphabet, the type-token relation was merely immanent in signification and its products, the phonetic alphabet makes this relationship manifest and graspable as a principle with diverse and powerful applications. And this principle is precisely the principle of abstract general equivalence, or the concept of the concept.

The new departure made possible by the phonetic alphabet is the externalization in notation of the mediation of meaning by abstraction (sometimes referred to in terms of the "double articulation of language" and the "arbitrariness of the sign.") And, once made manifest, the notion of abstract general equivalence can itself be generalized, over language and over concepts of mind and reality, yielding a radical restructuring of the social imaginary.

The mode of this generalization, I suggest, consists, in the first instance, of the transposition of the concept of general equivalence to the two other metonymic relations which I described above. This transposition yields a transformation of the governing relations between "container" and "contained," such that the "container," rather than being a sign or representation which signifies a "place" for the generality of its "contents," becomes rather a function defining an extensional set. Through this transformation, the (initially distinct) category-member and substance-sample relation become co-articulated and mutually definitive, in the form of the following "abstract" relationships: set–member of set and concept (essence)–instance of a concept. The co-articulation of these relationships yields the fundamental equivalence mapping which is presupposed by a truth-valued (bivalent) logic: [set] =

members and predicate [arguments], where the first notation expresses an extensional and the second notation expresses an intensional logical semantics. To put it another way, the co-ordination of the transformed metonymic relations stipulates that a category is defined as an extensional set, each of whose members instantiates a property expressible as an intensional predicate. This co-ordination constructs and defines the "abstract objectivist" notion of truth. Without exploring the issue further in this paper, I should like to remark that the recent attempts to use "natural kind terms" as paradigmatic of meaning (e.g., Kripke, 1980) represents an attempt to resolve the current "crisis" in the abstract-objectivist theory of meaning (Johnson, 1987) by formulating the substance-sample relation as "foundational"; while Lakoff's (1987) and Johnson's (1987) "experiential realism" represents a critique of any such intensionalist or essentialist arguments.

In summary of this section, I have suggested that the semiotic transformation of metonymic relations, in terms of a concept of general equivalence, derived, via its externalization in the phonetic alphabet, from the type-token relation as "pure signification." This, I suggest, was a specific sociogenetic mechanism enabling the re-constitution of "thought about thought" within an abstract-objectivist, or logocentric, framework. This sociogenetic transformation also constituted a radical restructuring of the social imaginary, by virtue of which the rule of the general equivalent was constructed as extensible over the entire domain of the social, and by means of which, also, its figurative-imaginative "origin" was "repressed" and re-constituted as the other of language, law, and logic.

Iconology and Developmental Theory

In this section I examine the iconological presuppositions, or stances, of the most influential "modern" developmental psychological theories: those of Freud and Piaget. This examination will reveal a striking degree of unanimity: developmental psychology, since its inception, has been unrelentingly icono-clastic and logocentric. The concept of a developmental or genetic psychology had, as many commentators have pointed out, its principal roots in evolutionary and socio-biological theories (Sulloway, 1979). The evolutionary biological matrix within which developmental psychology took shape was also, from the very beginning, intertwined with the notion of a depth psychology, in which semiotic and iconological transformations mediate between "primitive" and "civilized" psychic layers. The linkage between evolutionary depth, and iconological depth, is expressed in Freudian psychoanalysis in the distinction between "latent" and "manifest" mental content. For the greater part of both the nineteenth and the twentieth centuries, the dominant theory of representation in experimental psychology was associationism. In an associationist framework, there is no principled difference between the "verbal" and the "imagistic" aspects of thought: they are conceived of as simply different kinds of presentation of the same atomistic content. The mechanism of thought—the association of ideas—operates on this content indifferently to its particular mode of presentation in consciousness, and that which remains unconscious is a kind of shadow, which parallels those trains of associations that for one or another reason do break through the threshold of consciousness.

Disputes about the possibility of, for example, "imageless thought," did not involve any important departure, on either side, from this model, since what is held to be at question is not whether images and words are essentially different "kinds," but whether the one can be present to consciousness without the other.

Freud's theory of dreams and the unconscious differs profoundly from any such assumption that image and word are merely alternative modes of presentation of an identical content. When a psychoanalyst like Lacan (1966) maintains that the unconscious is "structured like a language," this cannot mean that the latent content of the unconscious somehow obeys a syntax which is akin to that of a natural language, for Freud emphasized continually that the unconscious does not know logic, or time, or syntactic ordering. It is not so much the unconscious itself that is structured like a language, as the operations by means of which unconscious contents, forced into self-dissimulation by censorships and prohibitions, are articulated and ordered as signifiers at the level of manifest content-the dreamwork and the processes of symptom formation.

The world of the dream may also violate logic and time, but it does so in ways that can be understood as having a "logic" that is its own (condensation/metaphor, displacement/metonymy.) The world of the dream is a partially logicized representative of another world, the actual unconscious, which is entirely other to the logos. The unconscious is not a set of propositions awaiting transformation by the dreamwork, nor even a set of propositions lacking temporal, modal or other inflection or qualification. Nothing like a proposition "exists" in the unconscious, and for this reason it is even misleading to speak of unconscious desires, for desire is (or can be formulated as) a propositional attitude, and human desires are engendered in language as much as in the unconscious "investments" (in a pre-symbolic "economy") that power them.

What then is the content of the unconscious? Freud speaks of *Trieb* (drive, pulsion), but drives must have an object, and the "place" of this object is the imagination. The unconscious is the realm of the imaginary, of fantasy, and of the body imagined. And it is here that Goux's remarkable analysis of Freud's text on Michelangelo's statue of Moses becomes relevant. Freud, he says, "was unable to interpret the Moses completely without analyzing analysis, that is, without analyzing the cultural presuppositions of his discovery and, somewhere along the line, denouncing, perhaps we had better say, 'disclosing,' the roots of psychoanalysis in Judaism" (Goux, 1990, p. 144); and specifically in the link "between the Judaic prohibition against worshipping images and the prohibition against incest with the mother" (Goux, 1990, p. 137). Goux continues:

> What Moses condemns when he castigates the idolaters is actually, in a historical perspective, the cult of female, maternal deities, and the fertile incest rites accompanying this cult. The law given to the Jewish people by Moses...is first of all a radical prohibition not only against incest itself but against any incest with the mother in the imaginary...With his written law, Moses institutes a blindness with regard to image, imagination and phantasy—all of which are associated with sensuality and love for the mother. Thus he brings to completion the exodus from Egypt—not merely out of the land that bears this name but also out of the inner Egypt, the land of sphinxes, tombs, and hieroglyphics, land of the imagination and of its invasive icons...From this perspective, we might say that Freud's psychoanalysis constitutes a second exodus from Egypt, for it proclaims that image and phantasy are delusion and that behind the seductive draperies of the imaginary, an enduring symbolic structure homologous to a language must be discovered. Psychoanalysis seeks not to interpret the image with another image but to dissolve it, to reduce it, to repress its welling forth by translating it into language. (Goux, 1990, p. 138-139)

But there is something strange here. For, as I have already said, we cannot seriously maintain that "beyond" the manifest level of "dream-content"—the "Egypt" to which we can travel in our imagination—is a language. No, "beyond" that is only the unconscious, another Egypt, which is governed by an imagination (not a law) that precedes "subjection in" language and submission to the patriarchal law. The only sense in which a language, or anything like it, lies "beyond" the imaginary is the sense in which the journey from latent to manifest content can be described as a kind of translation, subject to certain modes of quasi-linguistic operations, whose dynamics can be understood only on condition that certain prohibitions have themselves taken seat in the unconscious. And this condition, the condition of repression, is also the precondition for psychoanalyis itself, the double condition which makes it possible for Goux to speak, apparently so strangely, of psychoanalysis itself "repressing" the imaginary, by repressing its own condition for existence as Freud's "science of the talking cure."

What then is repressed? Not just the imaginary, perhaps not even the imaginary as such, because despite Freud's deep suspicion of it, he of course recognizes it as a place or topos, while seeking to subject it to language, in practice as well as in theory. What is repressed is rather the recognition that the imaginary is the other, not just to language, but also to the law of the father: it is the place of the mother. As Goux says, in Judaism,

The prohibition against figural representation amounts to a violent, radical rejection of the maternal. The Jewish tradition thus develops as a systematic exclusion of all metaphysical images of the mother. Conversely, the corollary of this rejection is the importance attributed to the letter, to writing, to alphabetic signifiers. Moses' scribes cannot use hieroglyphics without breaking the law. Rid of its iconic dimension, the symbolic will tend to be reduced to the articulation of scriptural strokes. The utter extirpation of the prolific imaginary, in favor of the agency of the letter, effected by those who followed in Freud's footsteps, is without doubt fully in keeping with this violent devaluation of the imaginary by a writing that decrees law and name, beginning with Mosaic iconoclasm. (Goux, 1990, p. 145)

Let me now attempt a summary of the above. Freudian psychoanalysis is a depth psychology in which the imaginary is a topos, which is other to language: images do not accompany words or constitute a complementary mode of presentation of the same content as that expressed in language, but are representatives of a deeper, more "primitive" layer of the psyche. The imaginary does not ground language, but subverts it, and must be checked by rendering it in and subordinating it to language. Psychoanalytic theory is fundamentally iconoclastic, and this iconoclasm is sociogenetically related to the rejection, expulsion, and repression of the maternal and the material. The devaluation of the image of the mother, and of sensuous materiality, is coupled with the domination of patriarchal law and language as representatives of both spirituality and reason.

The subject of psychoanalysis (both the actual, individual subject/patient and the topic or topos) is thus constituted not only in language, but also against the imaginary, from whose bondage science must release him/her/it. This emancipation (or exodus) is simultaneously a recognition of, and subjection to, the law, which must (on pain of neurosis or of the loss of one's identity) be inscribed or introjected in the structures of the Unconscious itself, as operations which simultaneously enable repression and render that which is repressed intelligible. Freudian psychoanalysis is a rationalization (in every sense, including the psychoanalytic one) of a sociogenetic process of the production of a specific type of subjectivity, in specific historical circumstances.

Furthermore, the iconoclasm of psychoanalysis mirrors the iconoclasm accompanying the "exodus" from the land of the glyph to the land of the alphabet. According to Harris (1986), "the modern consensus view [of the origin of alphabetic writing] favours the North Semitic alphabet as the earliest known form and dates its appearance to the first half of the second millenium BC" (p. 31). Alphabetic writing, then, may have been not only a cognitive technology favoring and permitting the elaboration of an abstract-objectivist notion of truth, coupled with the concept of the concept, but also a means of preserving a written record whose form of expression, in being stripped of iconicity, makes it uniquely appropriate for the revelation of the one truth of the One God in a sacred text.

Alphabetic writing was, if this speculative, sociogenetic story has any validity, the cognitive-mechanical link between two different aspects of the notion of univocal meaning, which has played such a central role in Western thought: meaning as logically connected to truth conditions on single sentences, and meaning as authoritatively inhering in textually-connected, written sentences. The alphabet represents the binding together of the different strands of sociogenetic process—patriarchy, monotheism, the monetary economy, and writing—eventuating in the rule of the general equivalent; and the elevation of a logocentric, abstract-objectivist reason to a position of dominance and exclusion over and against Imagination. As we have seen, the opposition between reason and imagination (the latter seen as primitive, dangerous, unruly, and feminine) is enshrined in the theory and practice of Freudian psychoanalysis. I want now to suggest that the same iconoclasm is also to be discerned in the developmental theory of Jean Piaget, albeit in a different manner.

In Piaget's work we encounter what seems at first sight a paradox: although Piaget is dismissive of, and accords an essentially conservative (non-progressive) role to imagination and to what he terms figurative thought, he does not, as we might then expect, valorize language over figuration. On the contrary, both language and figurative thought are considered to be instances of a unitary "semiotic function," which can be understood as that dimension of cognition that comes into being with the advent of mental representation. Representation is a literally ambivalent (double-valued) concept in Piagetian theory. First, it denotes the ability to mentally evoke absent realities, that is to say, imagination. Second, it denotes symbolization, by which Piaget understood not a relation between a sign and a simple object, but a relation between a (figurative) signifier and a schema; and a schema, while having a figurative (indexical/iconic) component, is principally defined by (or grounded in) actions and (later) operations. Now, representation, for Piaget, is certainly a crucial aspect of human cognition, its advent being co-terminous with the acquisition of full object permanence, and constituting what Piaget terms (echoing, no doubt consciously, Kant's phraseology) a "Copernican revolution" in the thought of the child. However, although representation is for Piaget a necessary condition for the development from pre-operational to operational thought, it is neither in itself a sufficient condition, nor the principal cause and motor of that development. This latter role is fulfilled by action, and the co-ordination of actions through their government by operative structures. These structures lie "beyond" figuration, and constitute the conditions of possibility for the "logicization" of representation.

In the structure of Piaget's theory of representation, we can discern striking similarities to the structure of psychoanalytic theory. Piaget's theory, like

Freud's, is a "depth" psychology, in which the "manifest" content of representation (figuration and symbolization) stands in a relation of rule-governed (language-like) dependence to a deeper structure which is not language but which can only be rendered in a language-like, symbolic notation. This deep structure, for Piaget, is the logos in its purified form, stripped of the figurative and imagistic contaminations of actual, natural languages.

Natural languages, for Piaget, are doubly removed from the "operative" locus of pure reason: first, in that they depend upon sensible figures (the signifiers), and second in that these signifiers, being genetically related to the imagination, are mediated by the imagination in their relation to the operative structures. For this reason, natural languages can only imperfectly reflect and approximate to the "ideal" notation of a logical language (a notation that Piaget variously sought in the work of "Bourbaki," in the propositional calculus, and in the theory of groups). In virtue of this imperfection and contamination, natural languages cannot be accorded more than a peripheral role in the developmental unfolding of the Logos immanent in the relation between the epistemic subject and the real-rational world that it constructs.

The quest for an ideal, logical, universal language is, of course, a familiar trope of Western philosophy, from Leibniz through to logical positivism. But I want to suggest that it is also one manifestation of an equally deep-seated iconoclasm which can be traced back at least as far as the Protestant (and especially English Puritan) concern to expunge rhetoric and "fanciful" imagery from scientific and scholarly discourse. Piaget was, as is evident from his early writings, a thinker with a deeply religious view of the mission of science and philosophy, a view suffused with an idealistic and humanist Protestantism: not so much a harsh, predestinarian Calvinism, as a vision of the harmonious and dialectical unfolding of a nature which is ultimately and immanently identified with reason.

Yet, like Freud with Judaism, Piaget inherited from his own intellectual and religious background a profound iconoclasm, an iconoclasm that extended to language itself, which he saw as an imperfect vessel of reason. And, like Freud, Piaget can be seen as the constructor of a psychology from which the Mother, and desire for the Mother, has been expelled—not just literally, in Piaget's neglect of emotion and of the early socio-communicative environment of the infant, but also metaphorically, in his mistrust and neglect of the sensuous materiality of both representation, and the reality that representation informs (see Sinha, 1988, on the notion of the "materiality of representation"). Piaget's patriarchal, masculinist, Apollonian psychology is based upon a denial and a refusal (itself a characteristically Protestant theme) of mediation; his epistemic subject unfolds in monadic self-sufficiency towards a rationality immanent in, and guaranteed by, a law that is beyond imagination. For Piaget, as for Freud, this "beyond" of imagination is also "above," commanding imagination and engraving its authority within it.

In summary, Freud and Piaget both view the imagination as being other to rationality: the imaginary is identified with primitivity, with the (desire for the) maternal and the feminine, and with egocentrism, and rationality is identified with the reality principle, with the law of the father, and with operational thinking. What I have elsewhere (Sinha, 1988) called the "phylo-cultural complex," the mapping of notions of childhood and primitivity onto each other within an evolutionary framework, can in many respects be read as the principle theoretical expression of an iconoclasm that has marked developmental theory since its inception.

Ontogenesis and the Social Imaginary

Hans Furth (1990) has recently attempted to achieve a synthesis of Freudian and Piagetian developmental theories by employing Castoriadis' notions of the radical and the social imaginary. My comments on Furth may reflect some misreadings of his position, in part due to the condensed and allusive nature of his paper, and in part due to constraints on the length of this paper. He identifies the ontogenesis of the radical imaginary with the emergence, at around 2 years of age, of the capacity for symbolic ("pretend") play and mental imagery.

Cognitively (and following Piaget), this capacity is due to the emergence of a representational ability, predicated upon the differentiation of the object from specific sensorimotor action structures. Affectively (and following Freud), this same capacity involves a libidinal investment in the object, dissociated from any biologically-given reproductive function.

> These two ruptures in biological adaptation form the indispensable core elements of the radical imaginary and explain why adaptation is an inadequate conception for the open-ended constructiveness of human psychology...This constructive power requires the logical comprehension of the separated object and ... the motivational freedom of a libido that is not instinctually tied to its biological purpose. From this perspective, the meaning of an image (or of pretending) is the mental object to which the child's libido is attached: "want-my-object," where object stands for "my world, my society." (Furth, 1990, p. 208-209).

Like Castoriadis, Furth (1990) sees the radical imaginary as the source of the social imaginary, inasmuch as the cognitive-affective significations that constitute the play of radical imagination are social significations: the ultimate object of imaginary desire and knowledge is the social world or surround that lends meaning to the child's actions, even as the child's imagination projects personal meaning onto the world. The dialectic of development involves a mutually informing and co-constructive relationship between the radical imaginary (the source of intellectual and social transformation), and the specific, historically given social significations (or symbolic order) that constrain the field of play of the radical imaginary.

> The radical imaginary, as a particular developmental creation, is peculiar to the one individual, while as a particular historical creation, it is peculiar to the particular society. In the first case we see society within the individual, in the second the individual within society. (Furth, 1990, p. 212)

It would seem, then, that Furth is departing from the iconoclasm that I have argued to be central to both Piagetian and Freudian developmental theories, and that, like Lakoff and Johnson, he is arguing that the imagination should be seen as being at the core of human mental life. However, Furth explicitly reintroduces a logocentric and iconoclastic dimension to his theory, in his discussion of the child's development from the age of about 7 years (that is, the age period characterized by Piaget in terms of "concrete operations," and by Freud in terms of "latency"). Furth writes: "children must first construct a play reality before awareness of social, logical and physical constraints leads them to make the adult distinction between pretend and serious...around age 7, at which time the play reality of children is safely conserved in their 'unconscious'." (p. 207). The telling notion of "safe repression" recurs in Furth's text:

> After [7 years], logical operations reach a critical closure...Faced then with the internal demands of conscious logic and the external pressures of social reality, children by this time have completed the psychological repression of their pretend world....In the early years serious learning is secondary and is in fact constantly distorted in the service of the child's imaginary. But after its safe repression and unconscious conservation, learning and cooperation take on an increasingly serious, nonplayful character...having more or less willingly repressed their imaginary worlds, [children] are open to the impact of the "real" social world...progress in logical and societal understanding in the few years following age 7 is truly phenomenal and easily observable in all cultures. (Furth, 1990, p. 210-211)

Given my previous discussion of the sociogenesis of the rule of the general equivalent, it is natural to read Furth's theoretical approach as involving a translation of the processes which I have designated as a historical transformation of the structure of the social imaginary, onto the timescale of ontogenetic development (at least within Western cultures). Just as (I have proposed) the imagination is positioned by logocentric, univocal reason as an excluded and repressed other, so within the (Western) individual (Furth proposes), the radical imaginary is "safely" repressed as an "indelible core of human society and each person within it" (1990, p. 210) Behind all adult achievements are unconscious forces which have been gathered and structured in childhood. Because "These forces are pregnant with what is considered the best [creative imagination, etc.] as well the worst [ambivalence, frustration, delusion, etc.],"

(1990, p. 212) their "safe" socio-psychological repression is a necessary condition for the constructive growth of the social individual.

There are two sets of critical remarks that I wish to address to Furth's developmental theory. The first set concerns his apparent obliviousness to the culture-specific nature of his developmental story, as well as to the recent demonstrations by cognitive scientists such as Johnson and Lakoff of the continuing centrality, into Western adult mental life, of imaginative structures of understanding. Gustav Jahoda, in his critical commentary appended to Furth's article, notes that "the picture drawn by Furth of the life of the young child...is EurAmerico-centric" (p. 215). Furth's account, far from abandoning the traditional iconoclasm of developmental theory, merely repeats its central presupposition: Imagination represents, once again, a "primitive" stage which must be simultaneously abandoned and (unconsciously) preserved, in the growth towards mature reason. Logic, and awareness of its objectivizing constraint, are equated with both social stability and psychic health.

In this respect, Furth's account is a normative generalization of Western views of the relations between reason and imagination, over all places and times. This is not to deny that this normative account does indeed express the "truth" of our own social practices of the education and socialization of children, inasmuch as these practices are themselves expressive and reproductive of the symbolic order and social imaginary of modern Western society. Furthermore, inasmuch as this society "functions properly," Furth's account also expresses a "truth" of child development itself. Yet it is, at best, a half-truth; since it denies and excludes the constitutive, and not merely "motivating," role of embodiment and imagination in all human cognition, including Western human cognition. In a sense, because Furth wishes, on the one hand, to recognize the centrality of the imaginary in human development, and on the other hand, also to preserve the iconoclastic premises upon which Piaget and Freud erected their theories, his own text can be seen as a deeply ambivalent expression of the iconological crisis of the contemporary cognitive sciences.

This is not the place to attempt an alternative account of human cognitive, linguistic, and communicative development. There can be no doubt, however, that such an alternative account is both necessary and possible, and that its construction could contribute to both a theoretical and a practical emancipation of imaginative reason from the objectivist straitjacket of logocentric, univocal rationality that currently constrains it. Here, I will conclude with my second set of critical remarks to Furth's account.

Furth regards "repression" (that is, the repression of the imaginary) as being both a psychological and a social process. He remarks cryptically:

> Personal repression was described...in Freudian terms as the conservation of the radical imaginary in a person's psychological structure. But insofar as this becomes the struc-

ture to which adult society is presently assimilated, it is clear that social repression in the Marxian sense is already at work in that primary repression. Personal and social unconscious are in fact two sides of the same human situation. (1990, p. 212)

Furth goes on to reject the possibility of "a utopian social situation that would have no repression, no alienation nor false consciousness, even as there is no person without these characteristics" (1990, p. 212). No doubt this latter, as a generality, is true. No doubt, either, that it is a sentiment in tune with our time, when we have become chary of "utopias' as a result of historical experience of where attempts to realize them actually lead to.

The problem, though, is that Furth seems to locate the "danger" of utopias precisely where all iconoclasts have always seen danger: in the imagination, and (presumably) particularly in its destructive and aggressive aspect (perhaps here Furth is taking inspiration from Melanie Klein as well as from Freud). Yet it is arguable (and has often been argued) that the totalitarian nightmares that motivate Furth's rejection of the utopian imagination are grounded, not in the imaginary as such, but in the rationalisation (bureaucratic, logocentric, and univocal) of the social imaginary that so largely characterises modern, Western societies—and their "Utopian" dreams and nightmares.

If it is true (and I don't wish to quarrel with this) that reason is a bulwark of sanity against the (not, today, so imaginary) danger of a resurgence of "primitive," "blood-and-soil" ideologies of "imagined communities" (Anderson, 1991), it is also true that objectivist reason and its socio-technological concomitants have, while professing universality, systematically excluded, denied, and repressed the claims of human communities that "fail" to live up to its own image of what it is to be rational and civilized.

None of us, either, can fail to be aware of the danger in which the unremitting exploitation of the natural world places our, and other, species.

There is a temptation to say "rationality" is part of the problem, not the solution. We need not, however succumb to this temptation, if we are able to recognise that the problem with rationality lies not in its internal normative machinery, but in the exclusions that, in the guise of objectivism, it effects on the claims of imagination, community, embodiment, and, simply, reasonableness. That the sciences of cognition are, at last, awakening from their long dream of reason, putting, as Johnson (1987) puts it, the body back in the mind, may be an encouragement to believing that human reasonableness can yet make some headway on a larger, global scale. That isn't Utopia, but there must surely be a place in it for the utopian imagination.

References

Anderson, B. (1991), Imagined Communities. London: Verso.

Bruner, J.S. (1990), *Acts of Meaning*. Cambridge, MA: Harvard University Press.

Castoriadis, C. (1987), *The Imaginary Institution of Society*. Cambridge: Polity Press.

Fodor, J. (1976), *The Language of Thought*, Hassocks: Harvester Press.

Furth, H.G. (1990), The "radical imaginary" underlying social institutions: its developmental base. *Human Development* 33: 202-213.

Goux, J.J. (1990), *Symbolic Economies,* Ithaca, NY: Cornell University Press.

Harris, R. (1986), *The Origin of Writing,* London: Duckworth.

Hjelmslev, L. (1953), *Prolegomena to a Theory of Language*, Bloomington, IN: Indiana University Press.

Johnson, M. (1987), *The Body in the Mind: The Bodily Basis of Meaning, Imagination and Reason*. Chicago: Chicago University Press.

Kripke, S.A. (1980), *Naming and Necessity*. Oxford: Blackwell.

Lacan, J. (1966), *Ecrits*. Paris: Editions due Seuil.

Lacan, J. (1977), *Ecrits: A Selection*. London: Tavistock.

Lakoff, G. (1987), *Women, Fire and Dangerous Things: What Categories Reveal about the Mind*, Chicago: Chicago University Press.

Langacker, R. (1987), *Foundations of Cognitive Grammar, Vol. 1 Theoretical Prerequisites*. Stanford, CA: Stanford University Press.

Marková, I. (1982), *Paradigms, Thought and Language*. Chichester: Wiley.

Merleau-Ponty, M. (1964), *Signs*. Evanston, IL: Northwestern University Press.

Mitchell, W.J.T. (1986), *Iconology: Image, Text, Ideology*. Chicago: Chicago University Press.

Olson, D. (1977), From utterance to text: the bias of language in speech and writing. *Harvard Educational Review,* 47, 257-281.

Panofsky, E. (1939), *Studies in Iconology*. Oxford: Oxford University Press.

Plunkett, K. and Sinha, C. (1991), *Connectionism and Developmental Theory*. Aarhus: Psykologisk Skriftserie.

Rorty, R. (1980), *Philosophy and the Mirror of Nature*. Oxford: Blackwell.

Rotman, B. (1978), *Mathematics: An Essay in Semiotics*. Bristol: University of Bristol, Monograph.

Saussure, F. de (1966), *Course in General Linguistics*. New York: McGraw-Hill.

Scribner, S. and Cole, M. (1981), *The Psychological Consequences of Literacy*. Cambridge, MA: Harvard University Press.

Sinha, C. (1988), *Language and Representation: A Socio-naturalistic Approach to Human Development*. London: Harvester-Wheatsheaf.

Sohn-Rethel, A. (1978), *Intellectual and Manual Labour*. London: Routledge.

Sulloway, F. (1979), *Freud: Biologist of the Mind*. New York: Basic Books.

Walkerdine, V. (1988), *The Mastery of Reason*. London: Methuen.

Wertsch, J. (1991), *Voices of the Mind: A Socio-cultural Approach to Mediated Action*. London: Harvester-Wheatsheaf.

6. The Concept of Sociogenesis in Cultural-Historical Theory

René van der Veer

In 1924, American Congress passed the Immigration Restriction Act that specified quotas for the immigration of people from the southern and eastern European countries. This major political event was greatly influenced by the active lobbying of eugenicists who argued that the consistently low IQ scores obtained by immigrants from these countries reflected a biologically based intellectual inferiority (Gould, 1981; Lewontin, Rose, & Kamin, 1984; Kevles, 1985).

At approximately the same time in the Soviet Union, persons whose parents (had) belonged to the social class of the bourgeoisie were submitted to political examinations and purges. Because of their inappropriate social background, they were often deemed unfit to occupy important positions in society and dismissed, imprisoned, or executed (Graham, 1987; Van der Veer & Valsiner, 1991).

These political events in the USA and the USSR were facilitated by the dominance of two extreme views on human behavior and development that formed each other's perfect mirror image. Prominent American and British psychologists such as Spearman, Galton, and Burt defended a biological determinist view of human behavior and had no difficulty at all in providing politicians with arguments in favor of eugenic measures. In their view, the different average IQ scores obtained by different races, nationalities, or (sub)cultural groups were caused by their different biological makeup. Ultimately, as twin studies had allegedly proven beyond reasonable doubt, the explanation of human behavior was to be found in the genes. In contradistinction to these Anglo-Saxon researchers, their Soviet counterparts subscribed to a cultural determinist view of human behavior arguing that, ultimately, all cultural and mental phenomena were determined by the social class of the person, which in its turn was determined by economic factors, such as productive relations. The remnants of this view can still be felt in present-day Soviet psychological writings (cf. Van der Veer, 1990).

These two extreme views on the causal determinants of the human mind formed part of the historical context of Lev Vygotsky's attempt to formulate his own view of human development. It is the purpose of this paper to outline several aspects of Vygotsky's view of human mental development and to raise some questions for further reflection. It will be realized that such an analysis is not only of historical interest: a theoretically fully adequate view of human mental development is still lacking and the ghosts of biological and cultural determinism continue to roam among us (cf. Lewontin, et al., 1984).

That essentially biological and cultural determinist views of human development dominate the scientific debate within psychology up to the present day has recently been argued in an important book by Ratner (1991). The author argues that seemingly interactionist views, such as the one advocated by Piaget, are, in reality, heavily tilted towards the maturational, biologist side and do not take into account the concrete conditions of human life. Likewise, he criticizes learning theorists, such as Bandura, for their extreme environmentalism. The author points out the detrimental effects of these views in such areas as perception, emotions, and memory and forcefully argues the validity and potential fruitfulness of a Vygotskian, sociohistorical point of view in which human mental functioning is viewed as the result of the individuals' participation in concrete social interactions and their employment of cultural tools.

Some Key Ideas of Vygotsky's View

Vygotsky opposed the biological and cultural determinism of his time and explicitly acknowledged the role of both environment and genotype in child development. However, he resisted a simple interactionist model in which the trajectory of human development is viewed as the summative result of the influences of a stable environment plus a stable genotype. He explicitly argued that organism and environment both change during their continual interaction and emphasized the role of individual life histories. In his *Foundations of Paedology* (Vygotsky, 1935), for example, he argued that the concept of environment is, in itself, problematic as the same environment plays different roles in different age groups and for different individuals. The same environment is subjectively experienced and intellectually understood in different ways by children of different ages and varying backgrounds (Vygotsky, 1935, p. 60). Moreover, the environment is, like the child, far from stable, but in a continual flux, not in the least because the children themselves are actively changing their environments (Vygotsky, 1935, p. 68). With these observations Vygotsky pointed out that the concept of environment is relative to the individual or species we study and that organism and environment change in complex interactions (cf. Hinde, 1982, pp. 86-87). This view implied that a developmental state at a certain moment can never be decomposed into x percent genes plus y percent environment, as the order of events (determining the individual's life history) is crucial.

Vygotsky also surmised that higher psychological functions are less dependent on hereditary factors than lower ones and suggested that the role of heredity may change for certain mental properties as children grow older. These ideas seem to have been partly based on the longitudinal twin research carried out at the time in the Moscow Medical-Genetic Institute (Luria, 1936, 1937; Luria & Mirenova, 1936; Mirenova, 1932; Vygotsky, 1935, pp. 50-51). The results of this research have never been fully published, as its basic idea was at variance with the cultural determinist ideology. Incidentally, the idea of testing twins repeatedly for the same mental traits, that is, following a longitudinal design, seems to be relatively rare in contemporary twin studies.

Lower and Higher Psychological Functions

Vygotsky's suggestion that higher psychological functions are less dependent on hereditary factors than lower ones deserves our attention. It implies dividing psychological processes into those closer to the genotype (or less environment-dependent) and those further removed from the genotype (or more environment dependent). While such a distinction can never be clear-cut—as functions will vary on a continuum and depending on the environment in question—it shows that Vygotsky attempted to formulate the intricate interplay between genotype and environment in more concrete terms. In his view, children's cognitive development rested on the transformation of lower psychological functions in a process of mastering cultural knowledge and skills and resulting in what were called higher psychological functions.

The distinction between lower and higher psychological functions in its present form goes basically back to Wundt (cf. Danziger & Shermer, in press) and seems intuitively plausible. Lower functions are generally associated with psycho-physiological processes such as reaction time, GSR, etcetera, while processes such as thinking and problem solving belong to the higher functions. It is not altogether clear, however, why these quasi-physiological processes would be less dependent on the environment, nor did Vygotsky ever clearly and consistently explain until what age we may encounter lower psychological functions, or whether they may exist forever.

In Vygotsky's view, the lower psychological processes evolved during the biological evolution of the species (that is, they are innate), whereas higher psychological processes evolve through the mastering of cultural rules and scripts in the individual's life history. This view implied that the processes thought to be specific to the human species, such as language and thinking, presupposed the existence of a cultural heritage and the social other or *socius* in Baldwin's terms. Higher psychological functions do not unfold according to a pre-programmed developmental sequence, but are mastered in a process called sociogenesis.

The Idea of Sociogenesis

Of course, many psychologists and philosophers had proposed similar views of human development and Vygotsky was very well acquainted with their work. He had thoroughly studied the work of, among others, Baldwin, Durkheim, Freud, Janet, and Natorp, and often referred to them when formulating his own view of sociogenesis. Janet, in particular, had made several speculations about the social origin of several higher conducts that seemed quite attractive to Vygotsky. He agreed, for example, with Janet's speculation that the singular power of words over another person's or one's own behavior goes back to a period in the history of mankind when words were commands spoken by the chief of the tribe to rule his people (cf. Van der Veer & Valsiner, 1988, 1991). Having positively referred to Janet, he once summarized Janet's and his view of sociogenesis in the following way:

> That, which now is united in one person, and seems to us a unified holistic structure of complex higher inner psychological functions, was once in history composed of separate processes divided over individual persons. To put it simply, the *higher psychological functions evolve from collective social forms of behavior*....We might point to the central and leading role of the whole cultural development, whose fate cannot be confirmed more clearly than by that law of the transition from social to individual forms of behavior, that might also be called *the law of the sociogenesis* of the higher forms of behavior....Thus, *the structures of the higher psychic functions represent a copy of the collective social relations between persons.* (Vygotsky, 1931, pp. 483-485; emphasis added).

Thus, higher forms of behavior develop as the child starts internalizing social relations and attitudes. Janet (1928) had suggested that the child's personality basically develops with the internalization of important others' attitudes towards the child. Likewise, children's self-control was thought to be a verbal control, based on children's realization of the singular power words tend to have on others. In this view, then, the individual self does not exist originally but gradually evolves during childhood in a peculiar, roundabout way. While Vygotsky basically accepted that children's higher psychological processes evolve through the internalization of rules, scripts, knowledge, and attitudes provided by the social others, he tried to merge this conception with the (Marxist) idea of cultural tools, or instruments.

Instruments

The transmission of culture from one generation to another is a complex bidirectional process that proceeds in a variety of ways. It is possible with Vygotsky to conceive of culture as a conglomerate of cultural tools, but only at the risk of losing a large part of the meaning of the concept "culture." Several reasons led Vygotsky, who was one of the finest connoisseurs of European culture of his time (cf. Van der Veer & Valsiner, 1991), to narrow down the concept of culture in this way. Among other things, he was greatly impressed by Köhler's (1921) seminal research on chimpanzees using physical tools. Köhler's work served as an example of how higher animals and human beings might use tools in problem solving (cf. Van der Veer & Valsiner, 1991). Vygotsky also tried to link up with Engels' analysis of the role of labor in human anthropogeny. Finally, thinking of culture as consisting of tools or instruments seemed particularly apt for the study of cognitive human development (as compared to emotional, or affective development).

To Vygotsky the major cultural tools of human beings were verbal signs, or concepts. In his view they play a role in human behavior that is very similar to that of tools in the behavior of chimpanzees. However, in a whole series of investigations carried out by Vygotsky and his associates, it was attempted to prove the view that the use of these types of cultural instruments was preceded in ontogeny by a period in which children only use physical tools. Human cognitive skills would first be mediated by physical means, then by external speech, and, finally, by internal speech. We can see, then, that in this series of investigations, Vygotsky, rather than using the Janetian framework of the internalization of social attitudes and relations, used a "Marxist" framework of internalizing external cultural tools. Instead of emphasizing the social other or *socius*, as he did in the quotation given above, he now tended to concentrate on the mastering of cultural tools that form the embodiment of the knowledge acquired by a specific culture. It is seldom realized that this implied a conceptual shift that resulted in a different concept of sociogenesis. Moreover, the idea that cognitive skills should necessarily go through a phase of mediation by material means is probably unfortunate. A detailed discussion of Vygotsky's and Leont'ev's (1931, 1932) forbidden colors experiment will make this apparent (cf. Van der Veer, 1991 for further information and a replication of this study).

The Forbidden Colors Experiment: An Example

In Leont'ev's (1931, 1932) forbidden colors experiment, children and adults were presented a memory/attention task and provided with auxiliary means to aid performance. Leont'ev (and Vygotsky) wondered whether subjects of different ages would show different use of the instruments (colored cards) provided, whether this would be reflected in task performance (in terms of the number of mistakes made), and whether reliance on external instruments would gradually disappear as subjects grew older. The latter result would constitute an indirect argument in favor of the internalization hypothesis. Thirty subjects participated in the experiment of whom 7 of preschool age (5 to 6 years old), 15 of school age (seven children of 8 to 9 years old and 8 children of 10 to 13 years old), and 8 adults. No further information (e.g., SES, sex, ethnic background) about these subjects was provided.

The Nature of the Task

Leont'ev (1932, pp. 64-65) presented his subjects with three or four series of 18 questions, out of which 7 concerned the color of things. In each series the 2nd, 4th, 8th, 9th, 12th, 15th, and 17th question required a color answer. The other questions were either arbitrary (e.g., "Do you like reading?"), or in some way prepared the next color question. Thus, one of Leont'ev's questions was "Have you seen the sea?," which was immediately followed by the next question "What color is the sea?". The subjects were instructed to answer each question promptly and in one word, especially in the case of colors. The first series of 18 questions was presented without any additional limitations, that is, the subjects were free to answer whatever they liked. In the second series the actual rules of the game were explained: the subject should (1) not repeat the name of one and the same color within one series; and (2) avoid mentioning two specified "forbidden" colors. The third series differed from the second one insofar as the subject was now given a set of nine colored cards and told that these might help him to accomplish the task ("They must help you to win," Leont'ev, 1932, p. 64). A fourth series was only presented in cases where the subject did not show evidence of having found out how to use the cards, or did so only towards the end of the experiment. Apparently, before this fourth series, the subjects were told explicitly how to make use of the cards.

From Leont'ev's account it becomes clear that for the subjects the whole setting was that of a "game," which they could either lose or win. The experimenter tried to introduce a relaxed atmosphere and linked the questions together—by means of phrases such as "Tell me!," or "What do you think?"—to simulate a normal conversation-like situation. Also, because the experimental situation was very much like a traditional game played in Russian (and Dutch) families, it may be assumed that the subjects felt "at home" during the "game" and "played" at an optimal level.

The Nature of the Questions

Most of Leont'ev's questions were very simple and well within comprehension of his subjects. Examples of his questions were: "Can you draw?"; "Did you ever listen to music?"; "What color is the sea?"; "Do you like dogs?"; "Do you want to be big?," "What colors can leaves be?," etcetera. It should be remarked, however, that not all of the questions could be answered equally easily. To illustrate this, let us look at Leont'ev's second series where the forbidden colors were green and yellow. His 7 color questions were, respectively: (2) "What color is your shirt?"; (4) "What color are the railway-carriages?"; (8) "What color is the floor (generally)?"; (9) "and the walls?"; (12) "What color are lilacs?"; (15) "What color can leaves be?"; (17) "What is your favorite color?".

It is clear that some of these questions (e.g., 17 and, maybe, 15) leave considerable freedom to the subject, while others (e.g., 2 and 12) permit only one possible answer, unless the subject is prepared to give an untruthful, arbitrary answer (e.g., "Lilacs are red"). The rules of the game allow for such arbitrary answers, but it is quite likely that young subjects will find it very hard to give them. Unfortunately, Leont'ev said virtually nothing of this varying level of difficulty, mentioning only (Leont'ev, 1932, p. 65) that some questions were more "provocative of error" than others. We also do not know whether in the list given above, the second question was meant to provoke an error, that is, we do not know whether the experimenter deliberately selected some detail of the subject's clothes that had a "forbidden" color. We may conclude, then, that some questions were more difficult than others in the sense that they, if answered truthfully, required the mentioning of one of the forbidden colors. For other questions there were more degrees of freedom.

The Colored Cards

Leont'ev provided his subjects with nine colored cards of unknown size. His colors were black, white, red, blue, yellow, green, purple (lilac), brown, and gray. The "forbidden" colors he used were green, yellow (in the second series), blue, red (third series), black, and white (fourth series). The fact that each color was represented only once and that nine cards were available is of great significance for the strategies of card use that may be followed. Thus, quite a few children followed the simple strategy of turning first the two forbidden colors upside down and then, following each color question, successively mentioned one of the remaining color cards and turned it over. In this way they avoided mentioning both the forbidden colors and the repetition of any color. Having nine cards at one's disposal, this strategy can always be employed as there are exactly seven color questions in each series.

The fact that each color is represented only once in the set of colored cards as well as the fact that it contains all "forbidden" colors is, of course, also of significance. Interesting variations of the game and possibly other forms of card use would arise if this were not the case.

Forms of Card Use

Leont'ev (1932, p. 70) claimed that the various methods of using the cards could be reduced to two different forms. One strategy was to put the forbidden colors out of the range of vision, to exhibit the remainder, and—as the subject was answering the questions—to place the already named cards on one side. This approach was very similar to the one mentioned above, but there is one essential difference. In the strategy we described, the subject can "mechanically" read off the remaining colors, which puts virtually no demands on either memory or attention processes. The only thing the subject has to do properly is to turn over the colored cards after their use. In no way, thus, does he or she have to keep track of the colors already mentioned or even to remember the forbidden colors. In the first strategy mentioned by Leont'ev, the cards are not turned over; they are merely put out of sight, which makes this strategy presumably slightly more difficult to maintain. Leont'ev (1932, p. 70) regarded this method as "the least perfect" one, reasoning that the subjects often did not use the colored cards as a real mediating device, and only put the card aside *after* having given their answer. Putting aside the cards, then, was little more than the registering of the spontaneously given answers. Leont'ev (1932, p. 74) was inclined to interpret this strategy as a temporary phenomenon caused by the subjects' enchantment by the method: they were so impressed by the magic power of the cards that they used them irrespective of the questions asked. Such a "formalist" phase in the use of mediating devices was characteristic for both ontogeny and phylogeny. Leont'ev (1932, p. 74) speculated:

> Probably it is just this phase of the domination of external psychological mediums, through which the development of the higher instrumented, "significative" acts of behavior pass, that reveals itself in the history of the cultural development of humanity, in those numerous and extremely worked-out systems of external methods of behavior which compose a typical feature of primitive society.

Some pages before, Leont'ev (1932, pp. 69-70) had compared the same behavior—putting the forbidden colors out of sight—to the "way...an Australian or African savage might act in freeing himself from a dangerous man by destroying his image or symbol." Thus, the fascination with a specific elaborate method and the inability to see its limitations and real value would be characteristic of both children in a certain age period and of humanity in its "primitive" or "magic" period. For this reason, Leont'ev and Vygotsky (see Van der Veer & Valsiner, 1991) used to call children who used such a strategy—and children who showed no card use at all—"primitive" or "natural" as opposed to the "cultural" children who employed "more sophisticated" strategies.

In the second strategy discerned by Leont'ev, the cards remain in sight (the child may separate them into two rows or columns, for instance) and before each answer the child consults the available cards. In this case, then, the cards are used *before* the answer is given and the subjects' behavior can be called mediated in the real sense of the word. Undoubtedly, the second method is more difficult to follow as the cards used so far are now not simply ignored, but consulted. It is only after this consultation of both the forbidden color cards, the cards used, and the remaining cards that the subjects can give their answer. To Leont'ev this meant that the second strategy reflected a higher form of (mediated) thinking typical of a later stage of mental development.

The Number of Mistakes and Their Interpretation

The most important quantitative results of Leont'ev's experiment were formed by the number of incorrect answers to the color questions in the various age groups. Table 1 summarizes his data.

Two things seem immediately evident from this table. First, the number of incorrect answers (with or without cards) seems to diminish with age. Second, performance with colored cards (Series III/IV) seems better than performance without (Series II). It was the second fact that was theoretically the most interesting to Leont'ev, and a substantial part of his paper was devoted to its

TABLE 1. The average number of incorrect answers in relation to the availability and non-availibility of colored cards (after Leont'ev, 1932, p. 69)

Age	N (no. cards)	Series II (cards)	Series III/IV II–III/IV	Differences
5–6	7	3.9	3.6	0.3
8–9	7	3.3	1.5	1.8
10–13	8	3.1	0.3	2.8
22–27	8	1.4	0.6	0.8

interpretation. As can be seen, the youngest children made virtually the same number of mistakes (3.9 versus 3.6 out of 7 possible mistakes) in both card (Series III/IV) and non-card (II) series. For older children, however, the results were decidedly better for the card series (differences between Series II and III/IV of, respectively, 1.3 and 2.8). Finally, for adults the results were still in favor of the card series, but the advantage was considerably smaller (a difference between Series II and III/IV of only 0.8). Combining these results with his qualitative observations of the subjects' behavior and the answers they gave to his questions Leont'ev came to the following interpretation of his findings.

The youngest children (5–6 years old) gave incorrect answers to slightly more than half of the color questions and the difference between the series with and without cards was very small. Leont'ev explained that these children were very easily distracted from the task and did not discover, by themselves, how to use the cards. Even after the explicit instruction on how to use them that preceded Series IV (sometimes, also, the children were allowed to watch the card use of more able peers) the children remained unable to handle the cards (Leont'ev, 1932, p. 68). At best they superficially imitated the card use of others, but their whole behavior as well as their answers to questions asked by the experimenter demonstrated a complete lack of understanding of their function. In fact, Leont'ev observed several times that the colored cards actually hindered the correct performance of children as they were drawn to some cards and kept repeating their attractive colors. In general, then, the youngest children were unable to detect and/or understand the instrumental function of the colored cards. It can be concluded, therefore, that their answers were not mediated by the external stimuli provided, but formed an immediate reaction to the question or to some accidental part of the environment. Quite another picture can be observed in the case of the older children. These children showed a considerably better result in the series with cards (Series III/IV) than in that without (Series II). As can be seen in Table 1 the differences were, respectively, 1.8 and 2.8. Leont'ev suggested that this improvement from Series II to Series III/IV was due to the children's better understanding of the functions of the cards. The children were now increasingly capable of using the cards, often detecting their correct use spontaneously, that is, not needing the additional instruction or modeling and the extra Series IV. Leont'ev concluded that these children understood the instrumental function of the colored cards and that their thinking, thus, was mediated through external means.

The results of the adults were at first sight rather puzzling: while their number of mistakes was quite low, there was virtually no difference between the card and non-card series. At any rate, the difference between the performance in Series II and III/IV was considerably smaller (0.8) than the corresponding difference (1.8 or 2.8) for schoolchildren. In fact, the magnitude of the difference was rather similar to that of the preschool children. Moreover, observation pointed out that the adult subjects manipulated the colored cards far less than the schoolchildren did. It would seem, then, that the behavior of adults was as unmediated or "natural" as that of these youngest children. Leont'ev, however, did not at all believe in such a peculiar form of mental regression. Instead, he claimed that

> the second series of stimulation [that is, the colored cards] gets emancipated from primary external forms. What takes place is what we here call the process of "ingrowing" of the external means: the external sign turns into an internal one. (Leont'ev, 1932, p. 76)

Leont'ev argued, thus, that the behavior of adult subjects remains mediated, but that the mediation process shifts from external to internal means. He provided two arguments to substantiate his claim: First, he pointed out that the phenomenon of internalization of external means is a very general one as in the case of children who learn to do calculations by heart only after extensive training with paper and pencil calculations. It, therefore, seemed unlikely that the adults in the present task would suddenly relapse into "natural," unmediated behavior. Second, several of the adults did make use of the cards, but without manipulating them. Having spread out the cards, usually with the forbidden colors in a special position, they would fixate them after each color question and then give the correct answer. To Leont'ev this strategy formed a perfect illustration of the shift to internal means: while younger children have to remove the forbidden colors physically, the adults can carry out this operation "in their heads" using the cards only as a sort of reminder. The observed cases, therefore, demonstrated a mental operation that is halfway its internalization process.

This set of results was explained by Leont'ev in the following way: That the very young children did not display any spontaneous card use shows that children of this age do not understand the potential of cultural instruments and are still in their "pre-cultural" or "natural" period. Their performance on the task is, consequently, rather poor, and card and no-card conditions lead to equivalent results. That slightly older and older children do show improvement from no-card to card conditions proves that children of this age realize the power of the cultural instruments and are able to use them successfully. Finally, that adults show good performance in both the no-card and card condition, while at the same time relying far less on the cultural instruments provided, suggests that adults shift towards another form of mediated performance: rather than relying on external cultural instruments, such as colored cards, they rely on internal cultural instruments, such as words. In other words, what we witness in this experiment is a process of internalization.

On the Interpretation of the Forbidden Colors Task

A number of critical comments have been made concerning the nature and
methodology of the forbidden colors task and the interpretation of its results
(Adams, Sciortino-Brudzynski, Bjorn, & Tharp, 1987; Van der Veer, 1991).
For our present purpose it will suffice to say the following: First, to designate
children who do not use the colored cards provided as "pre-cultural," or
"natural" is rather misleading. It is, however, the logical result of Vygotsky's
narrowing down of the concept of culture. A child may be "natural" in
Vygotsky's and Leont'ev's (see Van der Veer & Valsiner, 1991) way of using
that word (that is, not making use of intricate cultural instruments), but
"cultural" in another, and far more normal, sense of that word (that is,
following all sorts of cultural models and having been molded by a specific
culture in many ways). Vygotsky's and Leont'ev's view is unfortunate as it
would imply that children up to 8 years old are somehow not really partaking
in their culture. It is also inconsistent with Vygotsky's claim in other places
(e.g., Vygotsky, 1984, p. 281) that children are social (and, thus, cultural)
from their birth. Secondly, to conclude from the increasing performance of
adults and their diminishing card use in a cross-sectional experiment that
adults increasingly rely on internal cultural means is an indirect proof of
internalization at best. Thirdly, it seems an unfortunate idea to suggest that
internalization always proceeds from the use of physical, material tools, such
as colored cards, to internal tool use. The idea of literal internalization loses
some of its plausibility in the case of colored cards (unless the children would
eat them, of course) and other physical, material means. What seems far more
plausible is to think of internalization as a process in which (meta)cognitive
skills are initially provided in the form of verbal assistance by more able
peers or adults, which are gradually internalized by the child (cf. Wertsch's
work on mother-child dialogues; Wertsch, 1980), or as a process of shifting
from some external cultural mediators (e.g., cards) towards *other* internal
cultural mediators (mostly words). Unfortunately, the forbidden colors
experiment and other similar experiments conducted by Vygotsky and his
associates were not suited for the study of this process.

Implications for a Concept of Sociogenesis

Vygotsky tried to integrate various views on the sociogenetic origin of
specifically human behavior in one comprehensive theory. In doing so he
made two conceptual distinctions that deserve additional thought: First, he
distinguished between lower psychological processes tied to the genotype of
the individual and higher psychological processes acquired during the indivi-

dual's life history. Such a distinction is conceptually tenable and fruitful as long as one doesn't think it possible to somehow partition out the biological and social-cultural aspects of human behavior. As Lewontin, Rose, and Kamin (1984, p. 282) have argued, "the biological and the social are neither separable, nor antithetical, nor alternatives, but complementary....All human phenomena are simultaneously social and biological, just as they are simultaneously chemical and physical" (cf. Ratner, 1991). Secondly, he distinguished "natural," or "pre-cultural," and "cultural" periods in the development of specific cognitive processes such as memory. This distinction was unfortunate as it either suggested that children up to a certain age do not form part of the culture they grow up in or implied a use of the concept of culture in the very restricted meaning of tool use. Both views are untenable and contrary to claims made by Vygotsky (1925/1987) in other places.

For a concept of sociogenesis, it seems far more promising to view the mastering of cultural tools as only a tiny part of the transmission of culture from one generation to the next. Accepting the Janetian-Baldwinian framework we may conceive of a process of sociogenesis as a process in which social relations and attitudes (and modern researchers would add "scripts") are being internalized by the developing child. The mastering of cultural instruments may be, but need not be, particularly appropriate for the development of cognitive skills, but development involves much more than cognition. Even accepting the metaphorical model of the cultural instrument, we should be reluctant to accept the Vygotskian idea of a necessary period of reliance on physical tool use.

An adequate sociogenetic view should show and explain the essential bi-directionality of the process in which children master their culture (Valsiner, 1989). The internalization of human culture by the child involves at the same time a transformation of the tools, instruments, and scripts thus mastered. Likewise, the reciprocal process of externalization connotes activities by which what has become part of the subject's conceptual system is injected back into the environment. In such an account the internalizing process is not seen as an automatic copying operation but rather as an operation involving the coordination of the new with the old and the restructuring of both (Lawrence & Valsiner, 1993. It does away with unidirectional views of child development in which the child's own selective contribution is underemphasized. Or, to put it in Wallon's words:

> The manner in which the child assimilates [culture] can have no resemblance at all with the manner in which the adult himself uses it. If the adult surpasses the child, the child in his way surpasses the adult. (Wallon, 1941/1968, p. 15)

Vygotsky would undoubtedly have agreed with this statement, and he made many valuable contributions to an adequate sociogenetic understanding of the human mind (cf. Ratner, 1991; Van der Veer & Valsiner, 1991). Neither is there any doubt that he understood that culture is broader than cognition and technology. In this chapter, however, we have pointed out that at times he made use of a concept of culture and a view of internalization that were too narrowly defined and led to less adequate views on human sociogenesis as well as to internal inconsistencies in his thinking. A fully adequate and comprehensive view of sociogenesis should correct this one-sidedness and probably requires the integration of the contributions made by Baldwin, Janet, Vygotsky, and various other thinkers.

References

Adams, A.K., Sciortino-Brudzynski, A.P., Bjorn, K.M., & Tharp, R.G. (1987), "Forbidden colors". Vygotsky's experiment revisited. Paper presented at the SRCD meeting in Baltimore.

Danziger, K. & Shermer, P. (in press), The varieties of replication. A historical introduction. In R. van der Veer, M.H. van IJzendoorn, & J. Valsiner (eds.), *Reconstructing the mind. Replicability in research on human development*. Norwood, NJ: Ablex Publishing Corporation.

Gould, S.J. (1981), *The mismeasure of man*. Harmondsworth: Penguin.

Graham, L.R. (1987), *Science, philosophy, and human behavior in the Soviet Union*. New York: Columbia University Press.

Hinde, R.A. (1982), *Ethology*. Glasgow: Fontana Paperbacks.

Janet, P. (1928), *Le développement de la personalité*. Paris: Alcan.

Kevles, D.J. (1985), *In the name of eugenics*. Berkeley: University of California Press.

Köhler, W. (1921), *Intelligenzprüfungen an Menschenaffen*. Berlin: Julius Springer.

Lawrence, J.A., & Valsiner, J. (1993), Conceptual roots of internalization. *Human Development*, 36,150-167.

Leont'ev, A.N. (1931), *Razvitie pamjati. Eksperimental'noe issledovanie vysshikh psikhologicheskikh funkcij*. Moscow-Leningrad: Uchpedgiz.

Leont'ev, A.N. (1932), The development of voluntary attention in the child. *Journal of Genetic Psychology, 40*, 52-81.

Lewontin, R.C., Rose, S., & Kamin, L.J. (1984), *Not in our genes*. New York: Pantheon Books.

Luria, A.R. (1936), K voprosu o geneticheskom analize psikhologicheskikh funkcij v svjazi s ikh razvitiem. In *Problemy nervnoj fiziologiii i povedenija* (pp. 361-367). Tbilisi: Izdatel'stvo Gruzinskogo Filiala Akademii Nauk SSSR.

Luria, A.R. (1937), The development of mental functions in twins. *Character and Personality, 5*, 35-47.

Luria, A.R., & Mirenova, A.N. (1936), Eksperimental'noe razvitie konstruktivnoj dejatel'nosti. Differencial'noe obuchenie odnojajcevykh bliznecov. In S.G. Levit (Ed.), *Trudy mediko-geneticheskogo instituta. Tom 4* (pp. 487-505). Moscow: Mediko-Geneticheskij Institut.

Mirenova, A.N. (1932), Obuchenie i rost u odnojajcevykh bliznecov (OB). Eksperimental'noe issledovanie po metodu vzaimokontrolja A. Gezella i G. Tompsona. *Psikhologija*, 4, 119-122.

Ratner, C. (1991), *Vygotsky's sociohistorical psychology and its contemporary applications*. New York: Plenum Press.

Valsiner, J. (1989), *Human development and culture*. Lexington, MA: D.C. Heath.

Van der Veer, R., & Valsiner, J. (1988), Lev Vygotsky and Pierre Janet. On the origin of the concept of sociogenesis. *Developmental Review, 8*, 52-65.

Van der Veer, R. (1990), The reform of Soviet psychology: A historical perspective. *Studies in Soviet Thought, 40*, 205-221.

Van der Veer, R. (1991), Decreasing use of external means in a memory task. An argument in favor of internalization? In R. van der Veer, M.H. van IJzendoorn, & J. Valsiner (eds.), *Reconstructing the mind. Replicability in the study of human development*. Norwood, NJ: Ablex Publishing Corporation.

Van der Veer, R. & Valsiner, J. (1991), *Understanding Lev Vygotsky*. The quest for synthesis. Oxford: Basil Blackwell.

Van der Veer, R., & Valsiner, J. (1991), Sociogenetic perspectives in the work of Pierre Janet. *Storia della Psicologia, 3*, 6-23.

Vygotsky, L.S. (1925/1987), *Psikhologija iskusstva*. Moscow: Iskusstvo.

Vygotsky, L.S. (1931), *Pedologija podrostka*. Vol. 3. Moscow-Leningrad: Gosudar stvennoe Uchebno-Pedagogicheskoe Izdatel'stvo.

Vygotsky, L.S. (1935), *Osnovy pedologii*. Leningrad: Gosudarstvennyj Pedagogicheskij Institut Imeni A.I. Gercena.

Vygotsky, L.S. (1984), *Sobranie sochinenij. Tom 4. Detskaja psikhologija*. Moscow: Pedagogika.

Wallon, H. (1941/1968), *L'évolution psychologique de l'enfant*. Paris: Armand Colin.

Wertsch, J.V. (1980), The significance of dialogue in Vygotsky's account of social, egocentric, and inner speech. *Contemporary Educational Psychology, 5*, 150-162.

7. Questioning the Mechanism of Sociogenesis

Robert Maier

Pretending to conceive and to know the mechanisms of sociogenesis is to posit oneself in the position of the master of the universe. Indeed, if sociogenesis covers the social and historical forms of individual development, and if the mechanisms point to the ways of producing and transforming these forms, a good theory of these mechanisms can only be established from a central and very powerful position, which would even enable an anticipation of future forms of development.

I acknowledge the temptation to establish oneself in such a position. However, within the very modest aims of this paper, one conclusion will be that no such general theory is available. The aims are to discuss several conceptions of the mechanisms of sociogenesis and to indicate significant insufficiencies of these conceptions. At the same time a series of criteria of evaluation will be established.

Measures and Comparisons

How can we compare the theory of Piaget and the one of Elias, which both use, for example, a concept of assimilation? Or with other theories? For the purpose of this paper I will adopt two procedures that are usually presented as excluding each other.

The first one is a procedure introducing a common language into which all the various theories can be translated. Such a language will necessarily be rather general. Moreover, this language will posit, in a straightforward way, entities in the world. In other words, it will have a distinct realist flavor. The other procedure is a relativistic one. It will approach the different theories purely as stories or as discursive productions, having some inner "logic." This second procedure does not need any presentation; it consists of stepping into the "discursive world" of the story told, looking for bizarre parts, and identifying holes and inconsistencies in the story.

The first approach supposes a new language. This will be the language of actions, conceiving *social and historical contexts* as complex systems of (inter)actions, and *individuals* as a particular system of actions. I will use the language of action as a general frame of reference without any pretention of disposing of a well-elaborated theory of action.

Development can now be formulated as the set of transformation of the system of actions standing for the individual. But, supposing the language of actions as general, these transformations will also be actions of some kind. Social and historical contexts can be defined in a similar way, as systems of actions, which may be transformed by other actions, if the first ones are not supposed to be stable.

A first, extremely simplified formulation of what a mechanism of sociogenesis might be is as follows: a mechanism of sociogenesis is a subset of the complex system of actions having effects in a specific way on individual development. An example would be selection and elimination of an individual according to some specified criterium, such as the color of his hair or left-handedness.

In other words, mechanisms of sociogenesis are sets of actions or production programs that are applied to systems of actions standing for the individual. These systems of actions characteristic for an individual may be comprehended as momentary stable properties of an individual, as for example when saying, "He is a really stupid bastard" or, "She looks very happy." Knowledge, beliefs, and emotions can be translated into this language. For example, a belief can be conceived as a disposition of action in a certain direction, or an emotion can be defined as an action potential, which specifies the context, the aim or the instruments of action. Anger is such a potential; it refers to space which has to be defended, and to actions with a distinctly aggressive character.

If we adopt for a moment an Aristotelian conception of action, we can say that, in sociogenesis, both the instruments used as well as the materials worked on, are actions. This simply means that the scenario is as follows: the transformations of actions occurs through actions of another kind. Therefore, the materials used are actions or conditions of actions. For example, if there is no space left for an individual or no food, this individual, as a system of action, will disappear. But to give no food or to leave no space are specific actions, which act on the conditions of actions. Also the instruments used will have an action component, because the instruments have at least a social relevance; they are not provided by nature. Examples are learning motivations, opportunities to earn money or to have pleasure; these examples are related to social actions, even if they use "things" such as books.

I will stop here with such abstract considerations; an abstract and/or formal theory of action could be elaborated upon in many ways; however, I do not consider that there is at the moment a satisfying definition of elementary actions nor a good theory of the fundamental properties of actions that could be used as a satisfying, general theory.

Simple Cases

With the help of the language of action and the provisional definition of the mechanisms of sociogenesis it is now easy to point out the extreme cases. A first case would be a conception of individual development reduced to growth on which the social system of actions has no effect at all, with the exception of providing some living "space" or eventually supplying specific situations that may activate and release some sleeping feature of the organism. In other words, individual development is reduced to biological growth. Sociogenesis has no proper place in such a conception, there are no specific mechanisms of sociogenesis, with the exception of action providing a *Lebenswelt*.

Such a radical nativist and individualist conception was never absent from the scene of philosophy and from theories of social sciences; it even seems to have regained more influence in some recent "cognitivist" accounts. Nonetheless, I will not use much ink here in rejecting such a conception, because it is, to some extent, quite useless to argue against such a biological foundation which is not based on any detailed theory of ontogeny. Furthermore, I do not see how forms of intellectual cooperation like discussions and communications, can be explained without reference to social interactions. This remark does not exclude the possibility that some forms of interactions are, in some way and at some level, "memorized" and may appear afterwards as properties of the organism. The various theories of evolutionary epistemology have suggested several models of this kind (see for example Callebaut & Pinxten, 1987).

Another extreme case negates the reality of individual development. Development is assimilated to a process of socialization; the social system of action determines completely the form and the identity of individuals. The totality of meaning of the individual is shaped by the social system and attached to the biological support of the individual. Such "over-socialized" (this expression is taken from Wrong, 1961) conceptions of individuals can be found, for example, in some readings of the work of Durkheim or Parsons.

But we should clearly distinguish two interpretations: it is possible to affirm that any aspect of the individual organism might be caught in a social network of meaning, which guarantees expressivity and perceptibility of the given aspect. In this way Parsons (1962), for example, defends himself against Wrong. If, moreover, all aspects of individual development are also seen as (co-)produced by this social network, then we have a clear instance of this extreme case. This, according to Wrong (1961), is what Parsons really meant. Once more, I do not wish to discuss here in any detail such conceptions. I shall limit myself to indicate a line of argument against such a view which I consider to be quite powerful. If we consider such a theory as a story, and if we read it with careful attention, we will always find that the story postulates beginning with some properties of individuals which make it possible that these individuals fit well, at the end, into the social system. In other words, such a conception supposes a potential fit of individuals to society, which is then realized by social means. For example, Moscovici (1988) has, for three sociologists: Durkheim, Simmel, and Weber, shown in detail that each of them presupposes a quite specific psychological makeup of individuals that turns out to be very functional for the social system they elaborate upon.

It would be quite easy to conceive of other simple cases, for example, by postulating one specific action as mechanism bearing on individual development, such as selection according to a specified criterium. I will not pursue such attempts here, because I prefer to introduce a discussion of some more relevant classes of theories.

Directions of Specification

The language of action used up to now has been quite elementary. Attempts to specify and to work out this language will provide a richer collection of instruments, and consequently more possibilities for formulating conceptions of the mechanisms of sociogenesis. My intention is not at all to establish some abstract matrix of the possible theories of sociogenesis. On the contrary, I will limit myself to the consideration of some interesting directions which have already been explored. These are (a) dynamic versus static systems of actions; (b) the points of impact of the mechanisms of sociogenesis; (c) forms of causality; and (d) forms of identity of individuals and groups.

Dynamic Versus Static Systems of Actions

Society, or at least some significant part of it, such as science, conceived as a complex system of (inter)actions can be understood as *static* relative to the time scale of individual development. Depending on the degree of differentiation of this system of interactions, we should expect that a more or less well-defined sub-system guarantees "adapted" forms of individual development.

Indeed, we can find quite a number of theories and popular conceptions which work with such presuppositions. Parsons (1962), for example, conceives the social system and the cultural system as equilibrated and differentiated, and personality systems are formed according to this theory in order to fit into the social system through socialization. The process of socialization has its agencies and its mechanisms, which are controlled forms of internalization.

Also, to some extent, Vygotsky (see R. van der Veer, this volume) uses such a perspective. He supposes that some socially established forms of knowledge, such as mathematics, are established as truths once and for all. To pass on such knowledge to growing individuals can, therefore, be delegated to a specific activity of social transmission, called "instruction."

My purpose is not to deny the heuristic fertility of such presuppositions. I only want to point to one difficulty of such a conception: if one supposes that individuals are individual biological organisms, this presupposition will either steer the theory in a direction of "socializing" biology (that is, for example, what

Parsons does with the Id), or it will posit a duality, namely the biological and the social, and we are left with the problem of how to build a satisfactory bridge. A typical question in this context is for example: is there a satisfactory answer to the question of the relation between the "elementary functions" and the "higher functions" in the theory of Vygotsky? I would say not (see Elbers et al., 1992).

Moreover, it could be argued that it is just plainly wrong to suppose the social system as being static. With the exception perhaps of some so-called "cold" societies, there is no global stability at all, which does not exclude the possibility of social entities with a relative permanence. However, we should be rather modest, because at the moment there is no good "dynamic" social theory, which might help to generate specific models of sociogenesis. Candidates might be the theory of civilization by Elias, the social system theory, or Marxist theories. And indeed, we can find several mechanisms of sociogenesis and also agencies of sociogenesis in these theories.

Elias (1988) explicitly introduces several such mechanisms, such as coloniza- tion, assimilation, differentiation, and emancipation in his theory. For example, members of lower classes are, on the one hand colonized, but on the other hand they try, by assimilation, to "get closer" to the higher classes and their presumed privileges. But if the lower classes are to some extent getting "closer," the higher classes will differentiate themselves even more. This rudimentary summary should not be read as an attempt to banalize Elias' theory; on the contrary, I consider that some of these mechanisms have been worked out in detail in some areas (See, for example, De Swaan, 1989).

A remarkable feature of sociogenetic mechanisms of dynamic social theories is their pervasiveness. If there are no stable social sub-systems, these mechanisms will filter through the totality of the social body. The identities, namely the "we's" and the "I's" (Elias, 1988), of social groups and of individuals are, according to Elias, interdependent. Therefore, the sociogenetic mechanisms have to be exam- ined globally as well as specifically for each individual. In other words, the sociogenetic mechanisms work on a global scale, but their effects are differential for different social groups and for particular individuals.

Individual and group identities are shaped and constructed at the same time; the working of the sociogenetic mechanisms postulated by Elias is therefore self- and other directed, which could not be the case when stability is presupposed. That is certainly an interesting feature, but once we want to know how such a mechanism works, we will quickly be disappointed. There are only few detailed studies and "exemplars," such as in Elias' theory of nationalism, (Elias, 1989). Furthermore, Elias seems to avoid this difficult question of "shaping" and "con- structing" by introducing a general notion of internalization, which is only a universal tool that bypasses the problem.

However, we know that many versions of the dynamic theories, such as Marxism and system theory, affirm the existence of temporarily stable sub- systems. In this case we fall back into regionalized agencies and mechanisms, such as the educational system. The question then is how these specific mechanisms and agencies interact with the dynamic tendencies, which are also considered to be at work in the social system at large. Unfortunately, these theories do not address this question in any detail, which is, in my opinion, a very central one. This is the problem of social integration. In terms of the language of actions, the problem can be formulated as follows: in face to face contacts, the actions of different individuals are connected. These interactions may then influence each of the actions of those present. But actions of individuals who are not in the presence of each other can also be connected by an interaction on another scale, and that is social integration. The theories mentioned recognize this problem, but do not offer any satisfactory solution. (For a discussion of this problem see, for example, Giddens, 1984.)

Indeed, any dynamic system, at least in a mathematical sense, supposes states of relative stability, otherwise it will be chaotic, and life will become impossible.

The Points of Impact of the Mechanism of Sociogenesis

On what kind of entity is a sociogenetic mechanism supposed to act? In a very unsophisticated way, I have introduced the simple idea that such a mechanism works on individual development. But this is evidently a rather problematic formulation. Only when development is reduced to growth is there any sense in using such a formulation, which is then pointless, as I have shown. However, if we suppose that development is co-produced by sociogenesis, we cannot ask how the mechanisms of sociogenesis work on development, as if development would in some way already be given, outside of the workings of the sociogenetic mechanisms.

In other words, the concepts of "individual development" and of "sociogenesis" themselves, the one at the origin and the center of a well-established discipline, developmental psychology, the other more floating, prevent easy access to the problem formulated here. Therefore, it is necessary to start once more at the beginning. Sociogenetic mechanisms cannot "work" on individual development but only on some "developmental potentials." I am well aware of the dangers of using such an Aristotelian concept of potentiality, but I will be careful not to introduce the well-known diseases of this concept in the present discussion.

An apparently simple solution is to affirm that sociogenetic mechanisms work on "growth potentials" manifest in actions or activities of the organism provided by biological evolution. An example would be the "elementary functions" of Vygotsky. In some way the "social" (inter)actions capture the "biological" by connecting the one to the other. Moreover, by some magic, the "biological potential" will then be transformed into a "social reality." I would like to say that I like this story very much, because it has such a magical flavor and it attributes such an enormous power to social action.

However, when I am tired of magic and power, I do not understand anything at all. How could something "social" be connected to something "biological"? Avoiding a difficult discussion about biological organisms and evolution, I jump to the only solution that is, in my opinion, satisfactory: such a connection is only possible if the biological is already "social" in some sense, and, I would also say, the social is also "biological" in some sense. In the language of action we can formulate such an insight as follows: neither the agent nor the action are elementary, but the interactions between social and psychological organisms. There is always some biological correlate. These organisms do not only interact with each other; they also act on other "things," as, for example, objects in the world. These organisms, however, do not have to be conceived as unified centers of actions; they can be rather fragmented (probably babies are quite fragmented psychologically) and nonetheless be involved in interactions.

The problem of the mechanisms of sociogenesis can now be reformulated as follows: the interactions between social and psychological organisms are an integral part of the complex system of interactions which is a characteristic of the social system. But all these interactions are not interconnected, and if they are interconnected, the connection can be realized in various ways. Sometimes there is a connection, sometimes not. Some examples serve to illustrate this point: learning and instruction at home and at school are connected with each other, but not in the same way for different social groups. And there does not seem to be any connection between the "learning" interactions characteristic of these different social groups.

Moreover, there may be hierarchies of connections, and so on. To summarize, we can say that some interactions interact, others do not. The questions are how the interactions between organisms are interconnected, how these connections exclude or strengthen certain interactions, and what kind of effect on the identity of individuals and groups can be found. These questions will be further developed, in a less abstract way, in the following section.

It is now possible to formulate the point of impact of sociogenetic mechanisms more specifically; one point being already established in a previous point, namely that these mechanisms cannot work on everything. That would mean that we are in a situation of total socialization or within a completely dynamic system without any relative stabilities. Consequently, some divisions have to be introduced.

The most elementary solution is to divide actions and interactions into two distinct classes: Piaget (1979), for example, has distinguished the so-called general actions, such as ordering or counting, and the particular actions, such as riding a bicycle. The general actions have all kinds of properties; they are, for example, largely independent of the objects they are applied to, they can be combined in many ways, and so on, whereas the particular actions remain linked to the objects and only few and specific combinations are possible. The problem of sociogenesis can now easily be solved: the general actions are to be found in the handling of "things" in the world by an individual organism, as well as in the interactions between organisms and also in all the connections (or interactions at another level) between these interactions. There is, according to Piaget, a full identity between all these different forms of actions and interactions as far as the general actions are concerned; there is also a strong resemblance with organic connections. Therefore, the "growth potential" of the general action-aspect will be favored in the long run. Sociogenesis, development, history: it is essentially the same story; they reinforce each other because the same mechanism is at work, see Maier (1992). Quite different is the fate of the particular actions. This will depend on contextual factors and on chance.

But there are two serious problems with this solution: first of all, one may question the possibility of classifying actions so neatly either on the general heap or on the particular one. Does such a classification not depend on criteria which are of a social and historical nature? The second problem is more intimately related to this discussion. Even if we accept such a classification, there is some serious doubt that these general actions are present equally in all the connections of interactions. Piaget (1979) defined these general actions as properties of interactions between the organism and objects in the world. And he has extended these properties to interactions between organisms conceived as centers of action without any detailed analysis. Do these interactions not also have other properties? I would say they do, but even if we neglect this question, there remains another possibility: all these interactions are not always connected with each other; some connections may be dominant in a given historical period. Think, for example, of the organization of work in early industry, where each worker did the same work in different places; later this work has been decomposed and recomposed in new ways according to other norms of efficiency. In this example we find two forms of coordination of actions, one prevailing at one time and another form of coordination at a later period. Both belong to the general forms of actions and their coordinations, and both are similar to forms of coordinations found in studies of cognitive development in young children. This would mean that an important category of general actions and interactions can prevail during some time in history. If we reason with Piaget, we should conclude that in this case, these very dominant social forms of interactions will reinforce the equivalent interactions between individual organisms and their actions on or with objects in the world, and at another historical period, other interaction will be reinforced. But if such a differential reinforcement takes place, then cognitive development will vary in different historical periods, because the sociogenetic mechanism will be at work, sometimes reinforcing and sometimes disfavoring the same general forms of actions and their coordinations. Indeed, we can find in Marx (1992), in his history of industry, and in Piaget (1979), almost the same terminology concerning the coordination of actions. That is not astonishing; they both use an action theory going back to Aristotle. This similarity can be used, in a Piagetian way of reasoning, against the generality of cognitive development defended by Piaget. This idea was originally suggested to me by Apostel, and will be developed in another publication.

Piaget's solution of dividing the sphere of actions into two classes is simple and powerful. It also offers a very general solution for sociogenesis. But unfortunately, there are some serious problems with this solution. If we accept this solution and work it out, then the simplicity and the universality of the suggested solution just vanishes, as we have seen.

Therefore it has become fashionable to introduce more classes of actions. All these attempts can be grouped under the heading of modularity. A more or less important number of modules, or classes of actions, have been distinguished. The individual appears more and more as a society of actions. In general, the sociogenetic implications have not been worked out, mainly because the dominant formulations of this view base the modules in biology. However, similar problems, as in the case of Piaget, could be formulated for these conceptions, which are only critical when these conceptions defend, as Piaget, theories of development which are totally independent of the social and historical context.

Still another solution puts forward the role of peer groups as a level of interaction, which exists alongside the other forms of interactions. For the mechanisms of sociogenesis, this would mean that we should take into account these particular forms of interactions as a shock-breaker, which mediates between the particular action systems which stand for individuals and the social coordinations of interactions. But at the moment, none of these accounts have been worked out in detail.

Forms of Causality

How do sociogenetic mechanisms work? The causality has to be found in the relation between actions, which is certainly different from the causality in physical nature. One cannot, literally speaking, paint or break an action. However, one can kill the organism which is, in some way, the siege of action, or one can influence an action causally by changing the context of the action, for example, by removing the objects or instruments which are necessary for the execution of the action.

A first distinction can be made between actions bearing on actions, and actions bearing on the conditions and on the context of actions. The second alternative has been used extensively in the explanation of cultural differences of cognitive development. Because in some contexts there are almost no materials or no practical opportunities for some classes of actions, these actions will not (or to a lower degree) develop, whereas these same actions will develop "well" in "rich" conditions. Intuitively, such a form of causality seems clear enough, but it has to be said that without a detailed account of the actions involved, such explanations remain to some extent ad hoc.

Quite different is the situation when actions "work" on actions. In this case, we can once more distinguish two specific cases: the two actions, where the one acts on the other (which does not exclude the case of reciprocal action), remain either external to each other or not. An action is said to be external to another action if there is no common ground in terms of goals or instruments. Usually, this external relation is called instrumental or strategic. This means that the first action influences the second one without any coordination of the goals of the two types of action. Examples are: salary and profit in capitalism, the search for truth in scientific research, and social legitimation through science.

In this case, the action bearing on another action remains completely external to the area of this action. The most simple way is sanctioning, which means that an action will be either rejected or accepted; this rejection or acceptance constitutes clearly another action. There are positive and negative sanctions; moreover, the sanctions can be realized by many different means, for example physical, economic, emotional, or political means. This form of causality among actions has been widely used in biology: selection is just an instance of sanctioning, and in psychology, where behaviorism used this form of causality almost exclusively.

But there are more complex, and I would say more interesting, ways as to how an action can work on another action, while remaining external to it. An action can accelerate or delay another action, or change the direction of it. Moreover, an action can combine or dissociate other actions. Simple sanctions only accept or reject other actions, whereas this procedure, which can also be based on sanctions, is able to transform, in subtle and powerful ways, given actions. This form of causality has been used for example by Foucault in his analysis of the technology of power (see Foucault, 1975), called "discipline." He shows how actions in many areas (school, production, army) became objects of systematic interventions in the 17th and 18th centuries. These given actions are classified, ordered in time and space, integrated in hierarchical connections, and so on. Evidently, to classify and order actions means executing actions on actions. This procedure is therefore a quite remarkable instance of a causal sociogenetic mechanism, which should merit elaboration in much more detail in sociology and psychology.

In this last category, actions "work" on other actions, but the two actions are from different levels; in other words, they remain external to each other. There is another possibility. Actions on actions can be of the same family and combine, or if they are not of the same family, these actions can be intimately coordinated with each other. In this case there will always be some coordination of the goals of the two actions. This means an action assimilates another action, or is assimilated *to* another action. If we use, for an instance, the terminology of Piaget (1979), we can also conceive forms of accommodations between actions. (As I have already pointed out, this is really an area neglected by Piaget.)

Such a mechanism situates the actions, in principle, on the same level, and the procedure is directed towards reciprocity between the different actions. We could therefore say that this mechanism instantiates cooperation.

I think that Vygotsky and his followers make use of this type of causality. The action of instruction is nothing other than an attempt to assimilate "elementary actions," with the perspective that the elementary action will accommodate to the action of instruction. Moreover, successful instruction means that the elementary actions are transformed, because they will progressively assimilate the aims and the instruments of the action of instruction, which has assimilated them to begin with.

I would suggest that the last two causal procedures, namely complex actions on actions should be explored in much more detail in attempts to formulate satisfactory accounts of the mechanisms of sociogenesis. This is the direction which should be explored in future research.

Forms of Identity of Individuals and Groups

How are individuals and groups conceived? It is rather evident that individual organisms are not mechanical entities. If this were the case, a mechanism of sociogenesis could affect one isolated aspect of the mechanical entity, without any influence on other aspects. Such a conception can be found in some rather crude versions of behaviorism, but experience has shown that the possible range of action on some specific action is bounded by the system of which this specific action is part of. In other words, some more or less explicit model of (relative) equilibrium seems necessary. A simple version of such a model posits that changes in the environment cause, at least in the long-run, transformations of the organism, which reacts as a structured totality in interaction.

The role of sociogenetic mechanisms, conceived as working exclusively on isolated actions will, therefore, be severely limited, because there are boundaries to the variation of one action within the system of actions constituting an individual. These boundaries are a result of inter-relations among the various actions, or in other words, there are regulations between these actions. This idea is at present quite generally accepted, and mostly conceived in analogy to some organic system of regulation. However, there are many possibilities as to how these regulations might work: are there totalizing forms of regulation, as Piaget would have it, for the cognitive system of actions? Or are there various types of regulations, each specific for some module of actions? Is there a centralizing module or not?

In any case, it seems necessary to take into account these regulations; but to some extent we fall back on the same question as in the case of development. Are these regulations co-produced by sociogenesis or not? The situation becomes still more complicated if we attribute to the systems of actions (i.e., individuals, and eventually, but in a different way, social groups), the possibility of self-regulation.

I would not hesitate to do so, without however pretending that this self-regulation has the form of a totalizing self-reflection and self-realization. Moreover, I would suggest attributing this self-regulation to interactions between the social and psychic organisms. (That is, for example, the choice of Habermas (1992) in his attempt to rewrite Hegel, but according to me he has a tendency to "totalize" too much.)

In this case, we have to conceive specific instruments which are needed for this self-reflection, as for example forms of self-consciousness and language. Such instruments are symbolic; they furnish powerful possibilities but introduce necessarily also ambiguities and illusions.

The central question is then to know whether these forms of self-regulation are products or mechanisms of sociogenesis? I would say both, and join, as far as this point is concerned, the conceptions of Elias (1988) and Habermas (1992).

Final Remark

I would like to close this very provisional overview by expressing my own hesitations: Very often, I thought that this was a rather foolish attempt. It is pretentious and dangerous to start such an abstract discussion. However, I do not have the pretention to present a complete overview of all the varieties of conceptions of the mechanisms of sociogenesis nor any worked-out theory. I also think that such an effort is not completely in vain. It can at least give some indications of important directions to be explored, or of specific difficulties once a choice has been made, as in the case of Piaget (1979), or indicate problems one will have to confront.

References

Callebaut, W., R. Pinxten (eds.) (1987), *Evolutionary Epistemology. A Multiparadigm Program.* Dordrecht: Reidel.

De Swaan, A. (1989), *Zorg en de staat.* Amsterdam: Bert Bakker.

De Swaan, A. (1990), *In Care of the State.* Cambridge: Polity Press.

Elbers, E., R. Maier, T. Hoekstra and M. Hoogsteder (1992), Internalization and adult-child interaction. *Learning and Instruction*, 2, 101-118.

Elias, N. (1988), *Die Gesellschaft der Individuen.* Frankfurt/M.: Suhrkamp Verlag.

Elias, N. (1989), *Studien über die Deutschen.* Machtkämpfe und Habitusentwicklung im 19. und 20. Jahrhundert. Frankfurt/M.: Suhrkamp Verlag.

Elias, N. (1991), *The Society of Individuals.* Oxford: Blackwell.

Foucault, M. (1975), *Surveiller et punir.* Paris: Editions Gallimard.

Foucault, M. (1977), Discipline and Punishment. New York: Pantheon Books.

Giddens, A. (1984), *The constitution of society.* Cambridge: Polity Press.

Habermas, J. (1992), *Moral Consciousness and Communication.* Cambridge: Polity Press.

Maier, R. (1992), Internalization in cognitive development. An examination of Piaget's theory. In R. Maier, (Ed.), *Internalization: conceptual issues and methodological problems*. Utrecht: ISOR.

Marx, K. (1992), *Capital*. Harmondsworth: Penguin Classics.

Moscovici, S. (1988), *La machine à faire des dieux*. Paris: Fayard.

Parsons, T. (1962), Individual Autonomy and social pressure: An answer to Dennis H. Wrong, *Psychoanalysis and the psychoanalytic review*, 49, 70-79.

Piaget, J. (1979), *Behaviour and Evolution*. London: Routledge.

Wrong, D. (1961), The oversocialized conception of man in modern sociology. *American Sociological Review, 26,* 183-193.

Part 3

Analysis of Existing Theoretical Frameworks

8. The Constructive Function of Language in the Baby's Development from Sensorimotor Adaptation to Humanity

Christiane Gillièron

The French writer Vercors devotes his whole novel *Les Animaux dénaturés* to the question of defining criteria for humanity. Facing the creatures they named the "Tropis" (an easy way to avoid choosing between *anthrôpos* and *pithêkos*), discoverers meet with a moral, as well as an epistemological problem. If the Tropis are animals, nothing prevents the discoverers from having an instrumental, though decent relation to them. If they are humans, the matter is of course quite different: they are potential interlocutors.

Today, while psychologists try hard to train Washoe, Sarah, Luci, Nim Chimsky, and other apes to attain some communicative know-how, while believers and sceptics argue with each other, incapable of agreeing on the limits of the competences to be credited to these lower brethren, I think it useful to analyze the concept of common sense, or shared sense. This means going beyond the usual discussions on "communication," a dangerous word often used as a mere equivalent for any social dealings. That the baby actively relates to her parents; that she exchanges, transmits; that her fundamental needs grow into affective relationships through some cognitive organization, we cannot but agree. However, let us remain cautious in our attributions. Truly, we know that the baby will grow into a peer, an alter ego; but how different she is, and the genetic method compels to focus on the difference. This chapter is an invitation to look at the epistemic baby, i.e., the "epistemic subject" at her lowest stage, and the baby as knower. Genetic epistemology will provide me with the background for this discussion, since in psychology and sociology the subject-of-an-object is rather ill-defined. I accept, as a starting point, the three following propositions by Borel (1987, p. 87):

[1] There are things; things are what they are....We meet with them while experiencing....

[2] There is a causal (interactive) link between the things and the subject-of-an-object; there is a semiotic link between the object and the thing....

[3] The only way to understand something about the semiotic link between object and thing is to know the causal link: the correspondence between words and things (problem of empirical truth) is not simple, it occurs between strata (levels and moments) of our experience. [Author's translation]

At the core of Piaget's genetic epistemology is the fundamental image of the "circle of sciences," which proposes a general solution to the problem of "strata." Indeed, only a number of arguments transcending individual scientific disciplines allow for a such a solution:

> Man knows the universe only through logic and mathematics, a product of his own mind, but he can understand how mathematics and logic were constructed only by studying himself psychologically and biologically, that is, in function of the whole universe. (Piaget, 1947, p. 148)

Subject, metasubject, meta-metasubject, all lie inside the same organism, or within the same social body. Is it possible to avoid circularity? How can one validate such a differentiation of the objects of knowledge, while taking the viewpoint of a subject to whom it is self-evident? Three relations are to be considered: (1) the relation between the agent who mathematizes reality in order to master it and this reality; (2) since he masters it to the point of reaching the moon, one has to consider the "miraculous" link between mathematics and reality; and (3) the subject's relation to mathematics is no less important, for to him, mathematical beings exist. He can, his neighbor can, his grandchildren will someday be able to compute *pi*, for example, and in different ways. *Pi* is thus a "real" object.

Piaget's solution is well known: the fundamental agreement between mathematics and reality is due to the reality of the "subject," his biological incarnation. In this sense, Piaget is a realist, and, as I have tried to show elsewhere, not a Darwinian evolutionary epistemologist (cf. Gillièron, 1987b). Theories are not "selected" afterward for their adaptive value, which emerge from inside the subject. Empirical confrontations and actual experience (the so-called subject-object, better named organism-thing interaction) are not sufficient to explain the harmony between mathematics and reality. This harmony results from the psycho-bio-physical nature of genesis.

Now, although some objects refer to things, other objects are purely cultural entities which are constructed by means of symbolic systems whose articulation allows for this kind of creation. Properties, concepts, and signs, intimately bound to each other, acquire a type of quasi external existence; the semiotic reference leads to a "thingability" of the referent. It must be evident that such a process is a long-term story, and numerous constructions will take place following the first 2 years of life; "strata" will continually deposit, products of ontogenesis as well as of history. I want to focus on the first stages of the construction of meaning, but let me first insist on how relative, albeit impressive, the achievements of the baby are. Not everything is present at 2 years of age, and internalized speech is not sufficient to explain the "metacognitions" to appear later. While accepting Vygostky's thesis, concerning the reciprocal modifications of speech and practical intelligence due to the internalization of the former, I am reluctant to attribute to the actual social trade the incredible transformations that take place between 2 and 12 years, not speaking of the scientific evolution. For the same reason that actual interactions of the organism with things are not sufficient to explain physics, the child's interaction with others lacks explanatory power. I rather assume a causal function of the interaction with linguistic "things." The evolution from instrumental use to objectification seems indeed a very general process, which ends with new cognitive tools (see Karmiloff-Smith, 1986). Symbols first are tools, they later become objects, and such a reflection is constructive. More-over, from 2 to 12, "reflection" and "construction" are self-modifying. The succession of these meta-levels is very complex and difficult to disentangle for us adults, and psychologists as well: one easily confounds metalanguage and meta-discourse, meta-discourse and operatory activity. In the most general way we can speak of the progress of de-centration. In this sense, Piaget was able to present operatory grouping as the antithesis of egocentrism (see for example Piaget & Inhelder, 1941/1974, p. 201). My own thesis, as it will show, gives much importance to language and semiotic activity. On the one hand, the precocity of vocal production makes it possible for the child to actively map events and names at a very young age (which is not the case for, say, graphic activity). On the other hand, the arbitrariness of the linguistic sign makes it easier to be looked at as an object (but this refers to much later stages). Even adults are prone to confound image and thing, video recording and event....

Psychology: Vernacular and Constructed

An animal (a being endowed with a soul, or *anima*), is a being with inten-tions, an autonomous agent. Acknowledging animality is acknowledging subjectivity, and differentiating behaviors from mere physical movements or transformations. Only living creatures behave. Recognizing beings as animate is expecting behaviors on their behalf. Such expectations are not restricted to humans. Mammals show that they read behaviors according to their own system of meanings. A cat is capable of learning by just looking at another cat solving a problem (Herbert & Harsh, 1944); a Vervet monkey mother expects a fellow mother to react to the (recorded) sounds of her crying baby, the same way she herself reacts to her own child (Cheney & Seyfarth,1980); and young chimps "lie" (Woodruff & Premack, 1979).

The human infant certainly has expectations in front of adults, that is, she has psychological norms. However, at least five to six different stages must be distinguished in the "psychology" of the 2- to 12-year old child (Gillièron, 1988; Thommen, 1991). This points to fundamental differences between mere social animals and Humans. Attribution, projection, and successful interchange are not restricted to the latter. Nor are they sufficient to account for the construction of the self.

The thesis apparent in the title of this chapter gives a prominent role to language. For the human child, as for scientists, knowledge is constructed in and by means of some discourse; and discourse includes the subject in an essential way, for it is predicative. One consequence is that conceptual objects become consistent.[1] They are "real" for they are endowed with the necessities given by the subject, and the kind of externality given by intersubjective agreement. (Mutual understanding, and, better yet, translation (Putnam, 1978), are to be considered as central.) A second consequence could be that discourse, presenting and re-presenting the subject *qua* subject, allows for her self-discovery.

Another thesis, developed elsewhere (Gillièron, 1986), deals with the question of validity. Psychology is the science of subjectivity; it reconstructs meanings from the point of view of the subject. Now, the reconstruction of animal subjectivity only involves first-order attributions, as is shown in von Frisch's (1950) marvellous studies with bees, but dealing with symbolic animals—*les Animaux dénaturés*—makes it mandatory to study not only meanings, but their representations from the subject's point of view. This means the psychologist must work as semiotician.

In consequence, this chapter will provide a semiotic analysis of the "signs" of different levels, from perceptual cue to sentence. I do not aim at a theoretical debate, and will not address the question of causality, which must be very complex. Referring, as Piaget does, to four general factors of development (maturation, activity, social transmission, and equilibration; cf. e.g., Piaget & Inhelder, 1966/1969, ch. 6) seems sound, but quick. Emphasizing one of these factors is no more satisfactory, as long as one does not provide a description of how it works. If the old methodological concept of comparison is still valid, which I believe, only intercultural, interspecies, and "pathological" studies will provide answers. Actually, "answers" are not straight, as was already evident in the Piaget-Chomsky debate (Piatelli-Palmarini, 1979). The astonishing capacities of thalidomide children may be used as an argument against "activity," those of deaf children against language; modularity may be used against constructivism (however, see Karmiloff-Smith, 1985), social interaction against maturation. I cannot offer an explanation of how the child proceeds, but heartily agree with Boesch's (1991) approach. For him, human psychology is inevitably "cultural." However, "cultural psychology" must be incorporated in general theory that acknowledges the biological, functional features of development. Only individuals develop, act, and are motivated. The appropriation of culture by real organisms, with biological needs as well as personal histories, asks for a psychological theory, a subject's theory. In Boesch's case, it is action theory.

Zoom In: The Genesis of Human Subjectivity

Ce qui est donné, ce n'est pas la chose seule, mais l'expérience de la chose, une transcendance dans un sillage de subjectivité, une nature qui transparaît à travers une histoire. Si l'on voulait avec le réalisme faire de la perception une coïncidence avec la chose, on ne comprendrait même plus ce que c'est que l'événement perceptif, comment le sujet peut s'assimiler la chose, comment après avoir coïncidé avec elle il peut la porter dans son histoire, puisque par hypothèse il ne posséderait rien d'elle. (Merleau-Ponty, 1945, p. 376)

As I said, I want to take a look at the baby in order to understand the different types of reference better: the reference of object to thing, of cue to object, of surrogate to what is (re)presented. Thus I will stress the epistemic function of linguistic practices that come before verbal communication. Only when predication occurs, that is, the possibility to associate one's own subjectivity to the event that is described, can language become a means of common representation. Predication "unloads the words from their egocentricity" (Russell, 1940). However, language can commonly present something at an earlier stage, and today's genetic psychology will help update the still marvelous analysis by Cassirer (1929, especially Ch. 2).

Table I is adapted from Gillièron (1987a, 1988). The grand periods correspond to Piaget's six sensorimotor stages, which still hold. The voluminous literature published after Piaget's celebrated trilogy (*The Origins of Intelligence in Children,* 1936/1952; *The Construction of Reality in the Child,* 1937/1954; *Play, Dreams and Imitation in Childhood,* 1946/1951) must be sampled. Four phyla seem important: (1) the development of linguistic capacities, (2) the development of communication, (3) the instrumentalization of the other, and (4) self-recognition. In matters of perception, I adopt Brunswik's (1952) probabilistic functionalism (cf. Hammond, 1966), and I rely upon Saussure (1916/1969), Barthes (1964), and Prieto (1966, 1975) for semiotics.

Meaning and Pre-symbolic Signs

Sensorimotor functioning, proper to every animal, entails access to the external world, with a specific way of dividing it up (assimilation). The first meaning is that which dwells in perception. Hence my first question: what is the meaning of "perceptual meaning"?

	General	Object	Mirror	Practices	Social behaviour	Language
Stage I 1 month	Reflexes exercising				Syntonisation Harmonisation	
Stage II 3-4 months	Learning / Primary circular reactions				First smile Circular play	
Stage III 8-9 months	Secondary circular reactions	Vision-grasping coordination			Specific attachment	Babbling
Stage IV 12 months	Means-end coordination	Object scheme	Looks back towards object	Identification	Triangle Proto-imperatives	Phonological differentiation No more babbling in deaf children
Stage V 18 months	Discovery of new means Experimentation	No more localisation error	Gallup's blob OK	Designation Denomination	Proto-declaratives	One-word phrases
Stage VI 24 months	Invention of new means	Object permanency	Names herself	Communication		Two-word phrases
Sources	Piaget (1936/1952; 1937/1954)		Gallup (1977) Mounoud & Vinter (1981)	Bonnet (1980)	Spitz (1957) Rivière (1990) Rivière & Coll (1987)	de Villiers & de Villiers (1979)

TABLE 1. The six sensorimotor stages.[*]

[*] As is usual in genetic psychology, ages are only indicative. While vertical hierarchies are fairly substantiated, horizontal links are better to be thought of as correlations. Only specific (and difficult) studies may point to interdomain invariants.

Brunswik's (1952) lens model was inspired by Heider's (1926) seminal paper. It represents the organism as a box, with a sensory-perceptual surface (to the left) and a response surface (to the right). The radial lines indicate the multifarious aspects of external as well as internal events. On the stimulus side, the "same" event does not afford the same configuration twice. One presentation of a thing is different from another presentation. Sometimes visual aspects prevail; sometimes olfactory, or auditory ones prevail. Perceptual cues, on the other hand, function precisely as cues in that they (vicariously) indicate more than their own presence. Moreover, for the organism, only proximal cues exist (modifications of the sensory organs). Meanwhile, the functional link between action and perception allows the subject to externalize her experience, since reality "is a *causal texture* (*Kausalgefüge*) in which different events are regularly dependent upon each other. And because of the

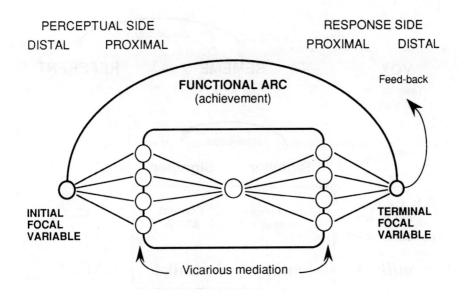

PERCEPTUAL SIDE

DISTAL   PROXIMAL

RESPONSE SIDE

PROXIMAL   DISTAL

FUNCTIONAL ARC
(achievement)

Feed-back

INITIAL
FOCAL
VARIABLE

TERMINAL
FOCAL
VARIABLE

Vicarious mediation

FIGURE 1. The lens model (Brunswik, 1952; Hammond, 1966). This model emphasizes the functional unity of afferent and efferent systems, the *Gestaltkreis* (von Weizsäcker, 1939; see also Heider, 1926).

presence of such *causal couplings* (*Kausalkoppelungen*), actually existing in their environments, organisms come to accept one event as a *local representative* (*Stellvertreter*) for another event" (Tolman & Brunswik, 1935, p. 43). This is true from Stage II onwards. On the action side, the same vicariant functioning is at work: the focus is on the act, and not on the ways it is materialized.

It is worth pointing to the fact that such a description is given from an external point of view.[2] Only an external observer is in a position to link the "stimuli" and the "initial focal variable." For the subject, stimuli are not known independently of the event. Attributes and properties are submerged in a global, undifferentiated experience. This experience is perceptive and motory. As Church (1961, p. 28) puts it: "Both perception and action entail, initially, a total organismic mobilization."

The Saussurian model of the sememe (Figure 2) also involves a double categorization. Recognizing some phonic substance (i.e., assimilating a sound to a signifier class) is correlative to evoking the signified class (opposed to the class which includes everything-other-than-signified). The presentation of

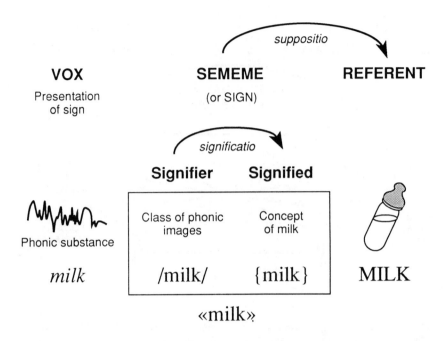

FIGURE 2. The sememe according to Saussure (1916/1969). The typographic forms will be used throughout this chapter: Italics for *vox*, capitals for REFERENT, French quotes for the name of «sememe», bars for /signifier/, braces for {signified}.

a sign (*vox*) is a "real" event, and generally refers to some real thing as well, namely the referent. These two material, external events must be distinguished from the sign itself, and from each of its two components. For the sake of clarity, I use French quotation marks when referring to a sign (=sememe, i.e., the signifier-signified biface); italics when refering to an instance (presentation of some signifying substance): and capitals for the referent. The signifier class is written between bars, and the signified class, between braces. Hence: on hearing milk, the English speaker calls upon «milk» whereby he assimilates milk to /milk/, and thinks of {milk}, perhaps associating the MILK he sees in the mug with what he hears.

The linguistic sign is "the combination of a concept and an acoustic image" (Saussure, 1916/1969, p. 99), and the relationship between the two is usually named "signification." The relation between a sign and a referent, or the "suppositio," is usually named "denotation." What is signification and what is denotation, for the non-linguistic animal? At the very first level of semiotisation, that is, at the level of sensorimotor functioning, the "sign"—the Piagetian

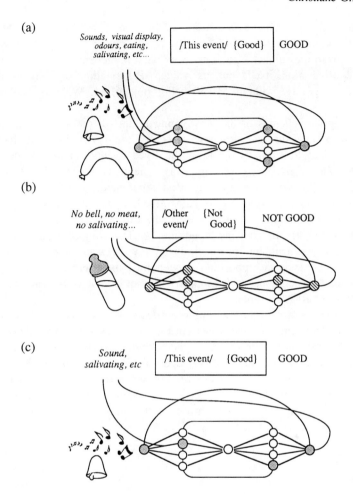

(a)

Sounds, visual display, odours, eating, salivating, etc...

/This event/ {Good} GOOD

(b)

No bell, no meat, no salivating...

/Other event/ {Not Good} NOT GOOD

(c)

Sound, salivating, etc

/This event/ {Good} GOOD

FIGURE 3. The "signal" in Pavlovian conditioning (4) is only differentiated from the point of view of the observer. It is part of a whole event (a) and this event is "known" by the subject in opposition to other events with different values (b). After the learning period the subject is able to recognize the event even when its presentation is partial (c).

scheme—assimilates perceptive configurations and associates the class they form with values such as "good," "bad," "nice," and "to be avoided." In other words, recognition entails opposing the actual experience to different past events, as well as confounding it with similar ones. The actual event (the presentation of the thing, for example) is contrasted with other events, but for this opposition to occur, a necessary correlative opposition is involved, namely, distinguishing the "signified" part of the perceptive sign from other signifieds. From the subject's point of view, what is recognized in the event is not the configuration itself, but its value.[3] Presentation of milk is read through «milk-good», without MILK being objectified. What is known is GOOD.

The perceptual schemes of the very young infant (or the animal) can only differentiate a new substance (a new aspect of reality) if the latter has an immediate value. It is the VALUE of the lived events that determines the class of the /signifier/ of a new «sign». This happens at Stage II, when the subject can be the seat of conditioning. Past experiences, good or bad, dictate how future events are going to be categorized, and which dimensions are going to be differentiated. In other words, the dimensions of reality are not known independently of previous conditioning. The subject must of course have the sensory instruments to discriminate, say, between blue and red, but blueness or redness is an opposition created by experimental conditions, by some historical associations, such as experiences of red-GOOD-events, as well as blue-INDIFFERENT-events.

At this early stage, what the observer describes as "sound of a bell," together with "offering of meat" (two cues of the interesting event), must be described, from the dog's viewpoint, as the following totality: this (perceptual) event «/meat or bell/—{good}»—this (response) event (salivation). This chain exists because of the sensory-motor arc. For the dog, every presentation is partial, and every aspect of the event has the same "symbolic" value. The response is just as much part of the event as the presence of the meat or the sound of the bell. It is part of the *vox*.[4]

Month 8

Without even stopping at Stage III (just mentioning the co-ordination of vision and grasping, which implies a differentiation of the sensory and the motory realms), I jump to the crucial transition from Stage III to Stage IV, around 8 months. In the physical domain, the baby looks for the disappearing thing, and is able to subordinate means to ends. Socially, the "second organizer" (Spitz, 1957) makes her a true partner, able to discriminate between people, and to deliberately use the (more) competent adult. In the linguistic domain, her vocal productions evolve and become closer to the music of her mother's mother tongue (babbling becomes culture-bound: an Italian baby can be recognized from a Russian or a Baoulé babbler).

In terms of subjectivity/objectivity, one speaks of the objectal scheme: that is, for the subject perceptions come to indicate the THING. Things and events

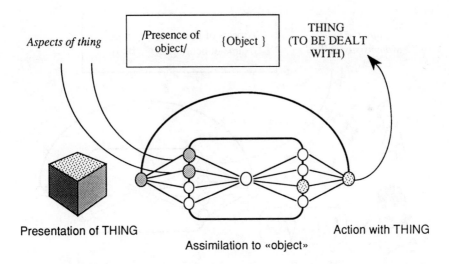

FIGURE 4. The semiotic link between object and THING. THING is known through object, but this knowledge is activated only in the presence of some cue, in "presence of thing." For the observer, the knowledge of THING is indicated by some action, for example, the baby turning the feeding-bottle when the rubber teat is not visible at all. However, the response is now a true response, that is, it is not merely a vicariant aspect of the event.

are externalized (Dallet, 1974). The semiotic link between object and thing comes into existence, even if the baby does not know herself as a subject. The functional bias toward the world (the focus) obliterates the subject, as is shown in studies using mirrors. For the 8-month-old, the subjectivity of the other is very important, but her own subjectivity she doesn't know.

The object of the 8-months-old subject is not our object. It has as yet no permanency. However, the thing is reflected in the baby's experience: the «object» is at the same time the sign of the {thing} and the {signified} of its /properties/, which act as cues. The event presentation-of-thing activates the sign «/aspect-of-object/-{object}». Not only are the experiences valued, but they are recognized. However, this knowledge of the event, or this "image" of the thing in the baby's head, is restricted. It shows up only in certain *hic et nunc* functioning. The THING is more than its appearance, but can only be "complemented" by its qualities in presence of some cue. According to Bonnet (1980), this qualifies the first stage of symbolic representation.

Now, a thing may be physically presented, affording visual, olfactory cues, and so on. But the thing may also be obliquely presented by means of its name. In this case, the physical stimulus, the phonic substance, is no longer

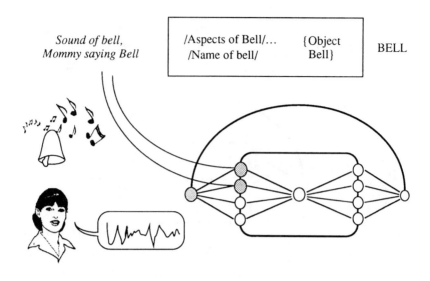

FIGURE 5. The name of THING is known like its shape or odor. The actual experience of vox (Mommy-naming) activates the knowledge of some event (SOMETHING WITH THING). The thing may be absent, and no direct manipulation possible.

spatially attached to the thing. The sound of the bell and the sound of its name are very different: they do not come from the same source. Both are attached to the BELL, and both characterize the {bell}. The /name of bell/, however, is linked to humans as well.

For an animal, even for a mammal, capable of looking for a thing that has disappeared, "an object is anything which moves in unison" in the words of von Uexküll (quoted by Lorenz, 1970, p. 302). For the baby, the object is more than that. Besides having physical qualities spatially attached to its source, it has social qualities conferred by its naming, as by triangulation. The adult names the thing and answers the requests of the baby by using the thing, thus the thing exists for the adult as well as for the baby. The objectively social human Umwelt makes the object a common, intersubjective object for the child.

The changes that take place in her phonic production must be analyzed with this in mind. The music of the child's babbling begins to sound like the music of plain English—or French, Italian, Baoulé—which means that for the child, English is not the same as music. Music comes from things: from bells, doors, cuckoo-clocks. Bell, door, cuckoo-clock come from Mommy, manipulating BELL, DOOR, CUCKOO-CLOCK. The baby does not yet name the thing, but, while babbling, she positions herself as a sound producer just as the adult. Although the child does not yet produce meaning in the way that the adult does, she does show her anglicity.

Month 12

Stage V is characterized mainly by the overcoming of "localization error," and the first words. During stage IV things acquire the status of intersubjective objects; during stage V, events become objectified.

Several authors speak of communication (e.g., Bates, Benigni, Bretherton, Camaioni & Volterra, 1979). However, a closer look at the child's discourse shows that she uses her words in two different situations. Either she "labels" while observing some event (label-words), or she uses words to manipulate the adult (dada-words). In doing so, however, she does not represent, that is, she does not monstrate symbolically to act upon the adult.

The dada-words are imperatives, but what are the label-words? What are they used for? First of all, they are recognized as words by the adult. Secondly, their grammatical status is not simple. Usually they are said to be "holophrases" (see Greenfield & Smith, 1976, for a historical and theoretical discussion of the concept). Thirdly, the so-called "over-extension" phenomenon points to two different characteristics, one of which seems very important to me: Not only does the signified of the label-word, as inferred by the adult, over-extend that of the adult, but it over-extends a single class of referents. What is labeled is an event: mainly, dynamic phenomena, presentations of new things, "representations" of things (quotations as in songs, pictures), presentations of "cues" for known things, "common" things. By naming the event, the icon or the new thing, the child seems to designate it as member of some collection, known as such. The stage IV {object} is an individual; it is the invariant under different presentations of one THING. The label-words of stage V, however, are used only when the referent is absent, or in the presence of some "image" (icon, cue, name); they also refer to events or to vicariant things. This means that labeling has a true "leveling" function. It obliterates differences and shows off the assimilating scheme. Not only does the name classify PRESENTATIONS-OF-A-THING, what was already the case for {object}; it also classifies PROPERTIES. Giving a "common" name is a way of matching events. «Dodo», «pati», «vou-vou» and similar statements use true signs, in spite of Piaget's ambivalent judgment (1946/1951, Ch. 8); were they not, they would not be understood by the adult, and a description such as the following OBS. 101 would be impossible:

> Also at about 1;6, the word *"papeu"* was used to mean "gone away" and was applied to people going out of the room, vehicles going away, matches that were blown out.

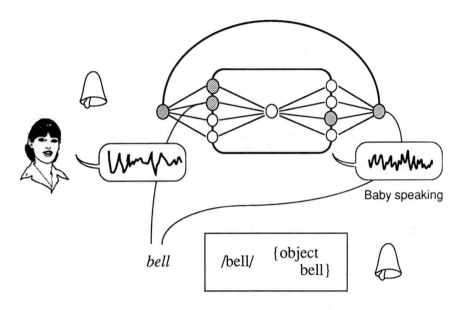

FIGURE 6. If the *vox* produced by the baby may be assimilated by the same /signifier/ as the *vox* produced by the adult, and if they are produced in similar circumstances, it means that the {signified} is common, known and recognized as common by both. This also means that the sign is common.

At 1;6(11) she even used it of her own tongue which she had put out and then put in again." (Piaget, 1946/1951, p. 217).

In particular, the translation, «*papeu*» = «*parti*», would be meaningless. Now, if the adult recognizes what is similar in the events Mommy-leaving-room, match-dying-out, streetcar-disappearing, surely, the child does too, for she is speaking....Naming these events with «*papeu*» is a way of knowing them, and of acknowledging their common physiognomy. Moreover, /papeu/ is taken from /parti/, which means that the sign itself is intersubjective.

Epistemic label-words, expressive dada-words still function independently. Speaking is acting: acting socially when soliciting, acting intellectually when naming. At this stage, however, action is still direct. While exploiting the situation, the child achieves her goal without mediation.

In being focused on the objective world, and in exploring and constructing the properties of things, the child of stage V is self-forgetting. In the mirror situations, for instance, she is able to turn around to reach for a thing reflected in the mirror. However she still explores her own image. Similarly, in pretend play, she acts her own part: theater is a way for understanding the setting, the scenario, the accessories, but not the actor. The child is not an object to herself.

Month 18, Enlightenment

Aha Erlebnis, invention of new means, is one of the 18-month-old's impressive acquisitions. "Means," that is, mediation, is what truly characterizes the "enlightened" baby. She becomes able to subordinate one goal to another goal, she takes roundabout ways. Bonnet (1980) speaks of compounded practices and gives a unified frame for analyzing practical actions as well as "symbolic" ones. Only at this stage does the child truly communicate, that is, her utterances are means to make others act. However, communication is but one aspect of a more general capacity.

On the linguistic side, the appearance of two-word sentences announces a revolutionary shift: the subject is partially introduced into the sign. The name of the thing is still a part of the thing, and saying the name is a way of knowing the thing. But two-word utterances are truly "sentences," they both link and represent.

They link: the two words are not any two words. They do not have the same function. Psycholinguists speak of "pivot" and "open class." One of the most important pivots is negation, for it acts as an illocutionary mark. Deictics have a no less epistemic function, emphasized by Schaerlaekens (1973, p. 169). "From the highly frequent deictic sentences in the early developmental period, a function emerges which simply designates, identifies, or draws attention to objects and events, and in which the child gives no indication that it desires anything from this object that would satisfy some need. Apparently, the child is concerned about disinterested language usage...not meant to control the environment....It would be basically ill-advised to insist that this abstract or disinterested function of language be considered a secondary development of language use as a satisfier of needs" (ibid, p. 170).

They represent: pivots such as «here», «that», explicitly associating the name with the thing, separate the thing from the act of identification. At stage V, naming is a way to know the referent: dog. Saying "That dog" (stage VI) is showing or testing one's knowledge that THAT is a {dog}, and that {dogs} are named /dogs/. It is a way of making dogs (including their property of having a name) autonomous from the speaker. This autonomization is even more visible when we look at the conditions under which utterances are produced: for the first time, the child is capable of mentioning the object in absentia. This truly implies re-presentation, since it means having "in one's head" more than a scheme which is triggered when some "cue" is present. The object is inscribed within the child and for the child. It may be evoked out of the blue, without any presentation.

Re-presenting by means of language might be a way for the child to present herself. She now knows more about herself: she is objectified. She looks at herself in the mirror, and at least as a physical "object" she is like others.

Coda

An animal "calculates," for its *Umwelt* is a *Welt* of "meanings." The duckling who freezes at the vulture's apparition recognizes the presentation of that silhouette. The shadow is identified by the «/vulture/-{bad}» system, which opposes it to other indifferent configurations. However, the computation done by the duck's organism has no experiential residue except the response itself. An object conserver of the animal type has something more "in the head": what is {signified} by the *vox* is the object, it denotes the THING, and not a VALUE. The object is an "image" of the thing, inscribed in the experience of the subject. Some psychologists call this image "representation." I prefer to use the term "representation" in a restrictive sense, the same as Piaget (1946/1951), for whom evocation is of central importance.

As important perhaps as evocation seems to me the fact that what is known by the subject is "common," shared by other people, from the subject's viewpoint. In this sense, the animal's object is not the same as the 8-month-old human baby's object. For the baby, the thing is known to be known by the adult. She may not know that it is the same thing. This will be the case once properties are isolated, designated, and constructed as objects by a similar process.

Washoe's or Sarah's "signs" certainly have a lot to teach us about ourselves. One of the questions I would like answered is: "Are they 'concerned about disinterested language usage...not meant to control the environment'?" (Schaerlaekens, 1973, p. 169) The child, as soon as she talks, is interested in language. She looks at it as she looks at the physical world, she tries to understand the relations between words and things. She uses other symbolic tools: pretend play, and later, drawing (apes do not draw). But language is unique with its predicative structure. By creating an image of the relation between subject and object, language allows for an objectification of this relation, that is de-centration.

Speaking of language sends us twice to sociogenesis. When looking at the social "factors" involved in ontogenesis, we saw that social trade as well as cultural "transmission" are at stake. For the child as for the adult, most objects are cultural constructs, not related to things; meanwhile, the third world of concepts is as real as the phenomenal objects created by our perceptual activity. Obviously language, which allows for the creation and permanency of cultural objects, has a crucial role in the shaping of our *Umwelt*. But this refers to the other face of sociogenesis, that is, the genesis of society as a self-organizing system, and the apparition of language. To this, I will not risk any answer, and only mention the difference. Language does not come to the baby the way it came to the species (cf. Trân Duc Thao, 1973). Should we then speak of phylogenesis?

Meanwhile, coming back to the Tropis, it is nice to look at the answer encapsulated in one of Vercors's (1952) interrogations: "Do the Tropis have taboos? Do they have amulets? Do they have rituals?" It happens that at least one social psychologist was concerned with the same matter, as shown in this quotation:

> All the societies of which we have knowledge possess some form of medicine and some rules of hygiene. In all societies we find personal names, modes of greeting, hospitality, feasting, games, and athletic sports....Facts of this order offer a threat to the belief that the invariant properties of men are to be found *solely* at the earliest stages of development." (Asch, 1952, p. 78) [Italics mine]

They also offer a challenge to developmental psychologists, who could "politely" (Brown, 1990) acknowledge their debt. I suggest "a Japanese word often used to close indebtness routines that says it: *sumimasen*, which means, literally, 'this is not the end,' or 'it is not over.'" (Brown, 1990, p. 36)

References

Asch, S.E. (1952), *Social psychology*. Englewood Cliffs, NJ: Prentice Hall.

Barthes, R. (1964), Eléments de sémiologie. *Communications, 4,* 91-135.

Bates, E., Benigni, L., Bretherton, I., Camaioni, L. Volterra, V. (1979), *The emergence of symbols: cognition and communication in infancy.* New York: Academic Press.

Boesch, E.E. (1991), *Symbolic action theory and cultural psychology.* Berlin/New York: Springer.

Bonnet, C. (1980), *L'enfant et le symbolique: l'accès aux premières structures sémiotiques.* Paris: Vrin.

Borel, M.J. (1987), Discours descriptif et référence. *Cahiers du centre de recherches sémiologiques* (Neuchâtel), 53, 77-89.

Brown, R. (1990), Politeness theory: exemplar and exemplary. In I. Rock (ed.), *The legacy of Solomon Asch: essays in cognition and social psychology.* Hillsdale NJ: Lawrence Erlabum Associates.

Brunswik, E. (1952), The conceptual framework of psychology. In O. Neurath, R. Carnap, C. Morris (eds.), *Foundations of the unity of science*, Vol.I. Chicago: University of Chicago Press. pp. 1-102.

Cassirer, E. (1929), *Philosophie der symbolischen Formen*, Band III. Berlin: Bruno Cassirer.

Cheney, D.L., Seyfarth, R.M. (1980), Vocal recognition in free-range Vervet monkeys. *Animal behaviour, 28,* 362-367.

Church, J. (1961), *Language and the discovery of reality: a developmental psychology of cognition.* New York: Random House.

Dallet, K. (1974), Transactional and probabilistic functionalism. In: E.C. Carterette, M.P. Friedman (eds.), *Handbook of perception, Vol.I.* London: Academic Press.

Von Frisch, K. (1950), *Bees: their vision, chemical senses, and language.* Ithaca: Cornell University Press.

Gallup, G.G. (1977), Self recognition in primates. *American journal of psychology, 32,* 329-338.

Gillièron, C. (1986), La validité en psychologie: première, deuxième ou troisième personne? *Archives de psychologie,* 54, 201-225.

Gillièron, C. (1987a), Du tiers inclus au tiers exclu: le rôle du langage dans la construction du sujet bien pensant. *Revue européenne des sciences sociales,* 25, 115-129.

Gillièron, C. (1987b), Is Piaget's "genetic epistemology" evolutionary? In W.R. Pinxten (ed.), *Evolutionary epistemology.* Dordrecht: Reidel.

Gillièron, C. (1988), Les avatars du non. *Cahiers du centre de recherches sémiologiques* (Neuchâtel), 56, 55-86.

Greenfield, P.M. Smith, J.H. (1976), *The structure of communication in early language development.* London: Academic Press.

Hammond, K.R. (ed.)(1966), *The psychology of Egon Brunswik.* New York: Holt, Rinehart, Winston.

Heider, F. (1926), Ding und Medium. *Symposion, 1,* 109-157.

Herbert, M.J. Harsh, C.M. (1944), Observational learning by cats. *Journal of comparative psychology,* 37, 81-95.

Karmiloff-Smith, A. (1985), A constructivist approach to modelling linguistic and cognitive development. *Archives de psychologie,* 53, 113-126.

Karmiloff-Smith, A. (1986), From meta-processes to conscious access: evidence from children's metalinguistic and repair data. *Cognition,* 23, 95-147.

Lorenz, K. (1970), Gestalt perception as a source of scientific knowledge. In *Studies in animal and human behaviour,* Vol. II. London: Methuen. (Original 1959).

Merleau-Ponty, M. (1945), *Phénoménologie de la perception.* Paris: Gallimard.

Mounoud, P., Vinter, A. (eds.) (1981), *La reconnaissance de son image chez l'enfant et l'animal.* Neuchâtel: Delachaux Niestlé.

Piaget, J. (1936/1952), *The origins of intelligence in children.* New York: International University Press.

Piaget, J. (1937/1954), *The construction of reality in the child.* New York: Basic Books.

Piaget, J. (1946/1951), *Play, dreams and imitation in childhood.* New York: Norton.

Piaget, J. (1947), Du rapport des sciences avec la philosophie. *Synthese,* 6, 130-150.

Piaget, J. Inhelder, B.(1941/1974), *The child's construction of quantities: conservation and atomism.* London: Routledge Kegan Paul.

Piaget, J. Inhelder, B.(1966/1969), *The psychology of the child.* London: Routledge Kegan Paul.

Piatelli-Palmarini, M. (ed.) (1979), *Théories du langage, théories de l'apprentissage: Le débat entre Jean Piaget et Noam Chomsky*. Paris: Seuil.

Prieto, L.J. (1966), *Messages et signaux*. Paris: Presses Universitaires de France.

Prieto, L.J. (1975), *Pertinence et pratique: essai de sémiologie*. Paris: Editions de Minuit.

Putnam, H. (1978), *Meaning and the moral sciences*. London: Routledge Kegan Paul.

Quadranti, P. (1989), *Approche constructiviste de l'intersubjectivité comme préalable à la langue*. Conférence présentée au "Internationales Kolloquium 'Sprache und Denken: Variation und Invarianz in Linguistik und Nachbardisziplinen'," Lenzburg (Schweiz), 17-19 Mai.

Rivière, A. (1990), Origen y desarrollo de la función simbólica en el niño. In J. Palacios, A. Marchesi & C.Coll (eds.), *Desarollo psicológico y educación*, Vol.I. Madrid: Alianza.

Rivière, A. & Coll, C. (1987), Individuation et interaction avec [sic] le sensorimoteur: notes sur la construction génétique du sujet et de l'objet social. In M. Siguan (ed.), *Comportement, cognition, conscience: la psychologie à la recherche de son objet*. Paris: Presses Universitaires de France.

Russell, B. (1940), *An inquiry into meaning and truth*. London: Allen Unwin.

Saussure, F. de (1916/1969), *Cours de linguistique générale*. Paris: Payot.

Schaerlaekens, A.M. (1973), *The two-words sentence in child language development: a study based on evidence provided by Dutch-speaking triplets*. The Hague: Mouton.

Sherrington, C. (1906), *The integrative action of the nervous system*. London: Scribner.

Spitz, R.A. (1957), *No and Yes: on the genesis of human communication*. New York: International Universities Press.

Straus, E. (1935), *Vom Sinn der Sinne*. Berlin: Springer.

Thinès, G. (1977), *Phenomenology and the science of behaviour*. London: Allen Unwin.

Thommen, E. (1991), La genèse de la perception de l'intentionnalité dans le mouvement apparent. *Archives de psychologie*, 59, 195-223.

Tolman, E.C. Brunswik, E. (1935), The organism and the causal texture of the environment. *Psychological review*, 42, 43-77.

Trân Duc Thao. (1973), *Recherches sur l'origine du langage et de la conscience*. Paris: Editions sociales.

Vercors [J. Bruller] (1952), *Les animaux dénaturés*. Paris: Albin Michel.

de Villiers, P.A., de Villiers, J.G. (1979), *Early language*. London: Fontana.

Von Weizsäcker, V. (1939), *Der Gestaltkreis: Theorie der Einheit von Wahrnehmen und Bewegen*. Stuttgart: Georg Thieme.

Woodruff, G. Premack, D. (1979), Intentional communication in the chimpanzee: the development of deception. *Cognition*, 7, 33-362.

Notes

1. This might point to the existence, beyond language, of a functional tertium comparations which stands to the concept as the thing stands to the object (Quandranti, 1989).

2. Such an "external" point of view is analytical and artificial. As early as 1906, Sherrington was insisting upon the Gestalt qualities of natural simulations. He also emphasized the biological importance of precurrent receptors in the evolution of the brain. Sherrrington's physiological work is in deep harmony with modern ethology as with the psychological theories of Brunswik, Straus or von Weizsäcker, and, of course, Buytendijk (see Thinès, 1977).

3. Note the convergence with Prieto's (1966) analysis.

4. Of course, this is not the Pavlovian description of "Pavlovian conditioning", which was discussed for example by Straus (1935).

9. On Learning and Tradition: A Comparative View

Rik Pinxten and Claire R. Farrer

Introduction

We are both anthropologists, working with different American Indian peoples. We have a deep interest in the phenomenon of learning as it is continued through tradition in these peoples. In a very real sense we think that these Indian processes of learning cannot be found in the school type of learning which is prevalent in the West. At the same time, we are convinced that culture specific learning processes and strategies are probably the core of sociogenesis as it is understood in the contributions to the present book. We hold that such an anthropological perspective on learning in a sociocultural context is not in contrast with a Vygotskian view (embraced by many of the contributors), but offers rather a multicultural and comparative expansion of it. In that sense, our conclusions stress two very specific points, both of which are important critical addenda to the sociogenesis approach (in Vygotskian terms or otherwise) of today: (1) the role of history in the sociogenetic approach is typically Western and is not to be found in oral cultures; (2) the analysis of other learning processes (Apache and Navajo) may help to broaden the models presented so far.

The Problem

We focus exclusively on the culturally embedded learning process from the perspective of the learner, whether Apache, Navajo, or Western—the latter being a term we use to signify an individual from one of the Western Europe-an–derived cultures. Teaching techniques and principles are only marginally relevant in our present effort.

A dichotomy, Them and Us, immediately arises by our juxtaposition of Apache and Navajo with Western learners. It is good to keep in mind that we are aware that few dichotomies can be sustained upon closer examination. Nevertheless, dichotomizing can be fruitful to bring out differences and formulate questions.

We are first led to questions of similarity and difference, or comparison and contrast, between Them and Us in respect of aspects of learning process-es, for example, consistency, logical operators (inclusion, exclusion, etc.), paradox, and so on, whether we refer to learning or thinking in their, or our, tradition. It is our belief that the use and format of these aspects of the learning processes differ on several points between Them and Us. Our concern is with the why and how of the differences. We begin our discussion with paradox and its differential meanings.

We use the concept of paradox in the most common sense:

> A statement or proposition which on the face of it seems self-contradictory, absurd, or at variance with common sense, though, on investigation or when explained, it may prove to be well-founded (or, according to some, though it is essentially true). (Oxford Dictionary, 1984, p. 2072)

The notion of a paradox flows throughout Western academic discourse. Nonetheless, our understanding of Western schooled traditions is that paradoxes are problematic and are to be avoided; the occurrence of a paradox is not permitted, if one is to think and operate logically. It is not altogether clear whether this norm (i.e., to avoid or dissolve paradoxes) did or does hold for practical knowledge in the West. Indeed, we often tend to live with "two conflicting standards," or we can be taught to follow conflicting interpretations in our daily lives (e.g., both homeopathy and allopathy in medical treatment). Nevertheless, proper reasoning (as it has been learned in and out of school for generations) does not permit paradoxes: we do not "really" know or we did not learn something "adequately" if we end up with two conflicting opinions about it. Paradox forces the Westerner to choose between two possibilities, for, if paradox exists, we assume that one of the premises is incorrect. We choose one premise and discard the other. Logically, this process is captured in the principle of the "excluded third" (or excluded middle): a statement is either true or false, but it cannot be both at the same time. The standard view on logical reasoning in the West is "the assumption that no contradiction is true, and hence that the reasoning that results in the contradiction is fallacious" (Priest, 1987, p. 30). In his book devoted to the analysis of contradictions and paradoxes, Priest attacks classical logic on this point and aims at preparing the ground for the acceptance of some contradictions as true or valid. He is, however, very conscious of the uncommonness of such a program; in his own words: "[It] is outrageous, at least at the spirit of contemporary philosophy" (1987, p. 7), precisely because the law of non-contradiction has in the West at large "traditionally been endorsed as a priori unassailable" (p. 259). The concurring consistency is considered to be "normal." To these extralogical criteria for proper reasoning Priest adds a last, in our minds clearly sociocultural, explanation: "the sheer weight of orthodoxy" (p. 259 footnote). Of course, the general stance toward contradiction or paradox is a norm in Western thinking rather than a given fact. We maintain that, in learning as an expression of a schoolish or school-directed phenomenon in the

West, it is a guiding norm and serves powerfully to organize not only how we think but also what is appropriate for thought.

A correlate in Western learning processes is that absolute, context, and person-independent truth (in the exclusive sense) is a major principle guiding the development of thinking and learning (see the developmental studies of Piaget, especially in 1937; the later Piagetians stress the importance of the social context in the process of learning itself. However, the role of the guiding principles of logic remains: Elbers, in press). The explanation or justification for this status of paradox is that ultimate truth is, by definition, universal and unchangeable. (Historic changes are not considered here; "progress" is measured with the same rod, be it after the fact.)

In order not to oversimplify the picture we must mention an important addendum here: although it can be said that absolute or ultimate truth is the guiding principle, it is also the case that such truth cannot be reached at all times. The learner often has to settle for less. The long-standing tradition of rhetoric distinguishes between two types of argumentation in the history of the West, corresponding to two concurrent views on truth. Some truths are absolute or universal, and hence do not allow for change or modification: the theological convictions as well as scientific truths (both a priori and factual) have this status. Other beliefs are held or are attained on the basis of persuasion, of shared values and interpretations, and the like. The difference, however, is not fundamental when looked at from the point of view of the learner or knower; indeed, the learner is persuaded to share a certain view on matters through appeal to soundness, evidence, or necessary truth of these beliefs (see Perelman & Olbrechts-Tyteca, 1958, and later rhetoricians on these matters). So, from the perspective of the learner, the guiding role of absolute truth is the vehicle by means of which s/he can be won over to a certain view. Differences in opinion, in the Western mode, are viewed as handicaps of perspective, which are either false in nature or the result of a lack of soundness, intelligence, or information; differences are not seen as a positive value. One either has/knows truth or one does not (see e.g., Pinxten & Balagangadhara, 1989).

The emphasis on norm and on the context of absolute truth leads us to a further clarification on the use of paradoxes. Paradoxes seem to be important for the Westerner first and foremost in what is often called theoretical knowledge. It is this theoretical type of knowledge, which is clearly separate from the often denigrated practical knowledge, that is taught in schools, and which is held by scientists and philosophers to be the real or higher sort of thinking. The learner is believed to get a better grasp on the world by developing a cognitive map or world view, that is, by building a theoretical knowledge frame about the world. In this knowledge frame, true statements have to be absolutely true, irrespective of time, space, person, or situation. An important instrumental feature for the learner of this knowledge is the discursiveness of this knowledge: everything that can be known in such an absolutely true way can be expressed in explicit statements that describe and explain the state of the world. In the tradition of the West, this implies that there is one unique way that reality is and one unique way in which it should be rendered in the language of the learner.

Our observations of the Navajo and Apache lead us to conclude that this situation with regard to paradox does not hold. With both groups, different and apparently conflicting "truths" or opinions can be maintained in harmony with each other. For example, one can follow the Medicine Man's/Woman's view, the white man's view, and the Peyote Way all simultaneously, even though portions of one may contradict portions of another. The conflict is one of non-fit only to Western perceptions, not to those of the Apache or Navajo; indeed, for most Navajo and Apache there is no conflict. Rather, one can choose opinion A at moment *t1* and opinion B at moment *t2*; or one can select the perspective of person X in a certain situation and that of person Y in another, perhaps analogous, situation. For the Apache and Navajo, the value of an opinion is always attached to, or related to, a person and a situation rather than being person and context independent. This does not preclude "logical reasoning," to be sure; rather, it substitutes an emphasis on absoluteness for one on contextuality, or a stress on temporal and spatial universality for one on change. The premises differ, not the structure of reasoning.

The explanation, or justification, for this stance is that one must always be prepared for constant change and have the ability to adapt to it. If differences or conflicts are recognized (as is, for example, the case in witchcraft accusations), they are explained in terms of the difference of persons or circumstances, or as differences in the way in which one was taught/learned or views the situation. Thus, their perception of what Westerners call paradox is that the differences are not in conflict but have a positive value and are intrinsic to reality.[1] In fact, reality will be held by Navajos and Apaches to be changes, processes and differences, rather than objects or image-like phenomena. The Apache and Navajo correlate for absolute truth can be conceived of as being those tenets or beliefs that are differentially distributed throughout the universe. Human beings acquire only aspects or parts of this truth through the medium each of them uses. Thus a seer can have insights from his or her angle and translate them in a poetic vision for a larger audience; a medicine wo/man can manipulate forces in the world in a primarily nonverbal ritual act and evoke or express aspects of truth that way. In general, it is held that higher knowledge is inaccessible to the layman other than through ritual, visionary, and other nondiscursive means in the hand of the so-called holy men (i.e., thinkers, ritual specialists, speakers, seers, etc.). The transfer of knowledge of this kind is through a different medium than is the case for the Westerner. The characteristics of the medium differ: no discursiveness obtains, and thus no necessity arises for a normative use of paradox.

It is clear that, although marked differences between Navajo–Apache and Western attitudes and opinions have been highlighted, a dichotomy between them can only be defended on some points (e.g., absolute versus contextual truth) and not on others (e.g., logical versus alogical reasoning). Thus, we reiterate that our posing of the dichotomy is for heuristic purposes only.

Turning to a consideration of a linked phenomenon, consistency, we again observe significant differences between Westerners, on the one hand, and Navajos and Apaches on the other. In the West there is a high value placed on consistency; it is a structural characteristic of knowledge and hence of the process of learning. It is a norm for the learner. Consistency leads to a dominant preference for an unique, and presumably correct, view: just one.[2]

The authoritative character of an uniquely true rendering, including facts within a consistent theory, is sustained by a specific use of data, written sources (texts), and the like. They have authority over individual and person-bound opinions by virtue of their consistency and within a perspective that sees them accepted as valid, valuable, true, or right, on the basis of the received belief. We Westerners accept that this truth may well be modified, or discarded, at some future time, but for the moment it is canon until there is a revolutionary shift based on new data, new truths, new facts, or increased understanding where previously there had been only partial understanding. In learning, the focus on the unique interpretation of others (in texts and data) is implemented by giving them the imprimatur of authority. Again, our view coincides here with that of the present-day Piagetians, where they stress the role of the social context (those who grant authority) in the development of children (Elbers, in press).

By contrast, Apache and Navajo authorities are always multiple and are dependent upon the interacting persons, the time, the place, the effect, the event, and the topic in any one instance. Hence, authority cannot be used automatically as a coercive force in learning beyond that instance. And consistency cannot be justified by recourse to authority. For Apaches and Navajos, there are a series of truths, none based on literary texts but many based upon the spoken and remembered word. That word, in its multiplicity of possible realizations, is intrinsically flexible and ready to respond to changes in persons, events, effects, and topics. Its consistency, to stretch the term, is its variability. Before exploring these topics in any more depth, we need to explain our own analytic apparatus for approaching them.

The Analytic Tools

It is our conviction that a culture (or a particular aspect of it) can be approached both respectfully and adequately by describing it in terms of its base metaphor and/or cultural intuition. The term "base metaphor" (Farrer 1976, 1980, 1981, 1991) refers, in our understanding, to the result of a sense-making process whereby disparate items are likened to each other through recourse to a rationale, or organizing principle, which is stated, and believed, to underlie the entirety of the culture; the metaphoric move is made with the purpose of defining or otherwise indicating similarities between the items and their consonance with the most basic structural organization in that culture.

Metaphors are usually thought of in terms of literary moves and linguistic forms (as in poetry or with prose symbolism), but they exist beyond the limits of the linguistic medium as well. They can be found in nonverbal artifacts; they can be visional or actional, or they can be mental. (See Hatcher, 1974, for the Navajo; Farrer, 1991, for the Apache; or Fernandez, 1974, for a general statement of metaphoric moves in expressive culture.)

For example, a well-known metaphor in the West is to think and speak about sound or light phenomena in terms of waves. In these cases, the phenomenal form of the surface of water in a river or a lake or sea, which proceeds in waves, is used to describe a physical feature of sound and light, with the purpose of allowing their displacement through space and time to be readily understood. The wave metaphor can be used because we take as a given that the phenomenon of (water) waves is a basic one that everyone in our experience both knows about and believes in as having reality.

A base metaphor serves to organize aspects of culture in general into a harmonious and readily understood whole, in the same way that a linguistic metaphor serves to illuminate a poorly understood or new aspect of an item or thought by reference to another, generally well-known, one. The word "base" is key here in that in order for an understanding to be a base metaphor, it must organize the entirety of a culture for the society or societies forming it. For Mescalero Apaches, the base metaphor may be rendered by o, in its plastic manifestation, or by recourse to stating that the base metaphor consists of the number 4, sound/silence, balance/harmony, and circularity. When Apaches indicate the fundamental principle of orderliness in their culture, they refer to this base metaphor. When they express the way of tradition, the way the world is in the eyes of the people, they use the base metaphor. They use it as well in their everyday lives as when they predicate formal speeches on the principles or when they salt food in accordance with its mandates. A culture has only one base metaphor, although it may have many corrolaries and manifestations of it. While basic to thought, structuring, action, and belief, base metaphors are not necessarily readily apparent.

A very deep distinction in the Western view on the world is that between the subject (knower) and the object. Anything in the world, including the self of the knower can be objectified: that is it can be looked upon as if from the standpoint of the outsider. The general structure of the relationship between a human being and his/her world is a candidate for the position of "base metaphor" in the West, we think. Although we do not deal with it in any great detail here, we are cognizant that this stance also produces a dualistic perception so characteristic of Western thinking and organization.

Within the general structure of objectification we find the so-called "God's Eye View," a common trope, or cultural intuition, in Western cosmological thinking. From ancient times on, the Westerner has built cosmology by conceiving of the cosmos as a whole that can be grasped, seen, or thought of, as if it were one unified object. This view draws on a conception of a God/ Creator who is situated outside the universe, eventually holding it together or contemplating it from His perspective as Creator. When the Western layman or scientist conceives of the universe as a closed or bounded unit, s/he mentally adopts the position of the God/Creator, who is the only one to be able to look upon the universe in this way. The scientist or layman thus comes in his approach to the one that is, in our Western conception, typically the view of God. The likening of God and human being in the observation and knowledge development process is consonant with the Western base metaphor that holds that there is an essential dualistic organization of reality. Thus, we maintain, the Western base metaphor is one of dualism.

What, then, is a cultural intuition? The Oxford Dictionary gives a list of meanings of "intuition." The one that conveys best the meaning of the term as we use it here is from a philosophical tradition and is rendered as, "The immediate apprehension of an object by the mind without the intervention of any reasoning process; a particular act of such apprehension" (1984, p. 1474). When we use the term "cultural intuition," we refer to this act of immediate apprehension which is typical for, or especially powerful within, a particular culture. For example, the field data of one of us (Rik Pinxten) indicate that Navajos conceive of the universe as a home they live, think and act in. They see themselves as actors (i.e., through perceiving, thinking, acting, speaking) within the universe, sharing the cosmos with all sorts of creatures, all of whom, Navajos included, are constantly having an impact on the universe. The view from the outside that we find in the European tradition is simply inconceivable for the Navajo. The Navajo cosmic view and the relationships between the universe and human impact is captured by the formula "the Navajo universe is an action habitat"; the "action habitat" constitutes a cultural intuition for the Navajo cosmology (Pinxten, in press).

Base metaphors and cultural intuitions are linked to each other in our minds. The relationship between them can best be expressed by means of a comparison: a metaphor relates to a cultural intuition in a particular culture in the way a gestalt relates to the particular process that yields the gestalt. Finally, we suggest that both base metaphor and cultural intuitions may, consciously or unconsciously, be used by members of a culture as vehicles for learning. In order to clarify these terms even more, we here resort to a few examples in the cultures under discussion.

Examples of Learning

When John enters the school in Ghent, Belgium, his life is altered in a variety of ways: he will remain inside from morning to twilight; he will sit most of the time at a desk and face the blackboard at the front of the room; he will set his brain to work and read, write, and calculate from books for several hours; he will subordinate himself to the authority of the adult who stands in front of the classroom and teaches what is to be known, quickly and to all students in the room at once. John can ask questions if he does not understand; the teacher will provide more information, correct mistakes, and have him practice things. Sometimes John can go out and look at real things outside school, bring their images back into the classroom, and learn more about them there. Most of the time, the textbooks will hold all the knowledge that is to be known, and trips outside the room are not undertaken. When the bell rings, the lessons are over and John can return home. When you ask him why he goes to school, he says he learns things there in order to be able to live in the real world when he is an adult.[3]

Any child who enters a primary school in the West is roughly given the same curriculum as the next one. All knowledge is collected in teaching guides and children's schoolbooks, which are meant to be used on a national or even an international scale. By the same token, all this uniform knowledge can be taught by any teacher chosen at random. He or she has to qualify in terms of certificates, but the role of teacher is not linked in any way to kinship ties, cultural background, or other more personal characteristics. Learning could hence be summarized in terms of three partners as follows: there are individual minds (learners), mediators (teachers), and the objective knowledge about the universe (the curriculum, most of all in the form of texts). Learning consists of transferring elements from the third partner into the minds of the first partner.

When one of us studied the Navajo school situation, with the goal of developing a curriculum for geometry teaching (see Pinxten et al., 1987), several white teachers complained to us that Navajo children are silent and apparently inactive in the classroom. One striking remark of teachers was that children "never asked questions" in the classroom, the absence of which was often interpreted as a lack of interest or of zeal. Hence, deciding to work on a geometry curriculum, we laid heavy focus on perception and visual exploration of aspects of the environment, which were visited and experienced in situ, outside the school. In the classroom the perceptions were recapitulated and small-scale models of the phenomena were built (e.g., a hooghan, a rodeo ground, etc.). The enthusiasm was great, but most striking to us was the high level of precision and the beauty of what the children built. In this case, learning could be characterized as follows: each individual is confronted with reality and has to build his/her own representation or interpretation of it. Reality exists around the individual and in him/her. Learning is manipulating the real phenomenon with all the risks (of disturbance, disruption, etc.) attached to it.

In the above examples and in other instances, we witnessed that children and adults were learners in a variety of ways, and that teachers had different statuses with respect to both learner and the subject matter. For instance, it proved to be the case that adults had to have maturity or knowledgeability in order to learn more. In practice, learning about the higher knowledge implied that you were at least in your sixties and were ripe and eager to learn the old stories, the sacred knowledge of the Navajo tradition. Transferring knowledge to those who cannot cope with it in an adequate way is dangerous and will lead to abuse of knowledge and threat to the whole community. This rule applies to all ages, including children. The aim is not to transfer as much information as possible, but gather appropriate and beneficial knowledge.

The other author of this paper (Farrer) has had similar experiences in her work with the Mescalero Apache (Farrer 1990, 1991). The research that led to a year's stay at Mescalero concerned the educational process of Apache children and specifically trying to devise ways to make Anglo-dominated schools more relevant to Apache children in order to motivate them to stay in school. The very problem itself was one that was peculiar to Native Americans in that mainstream culture parents believe themselves to be in a superior position vis-à-vis their children and therefore able to command them to remain in school, at least through the early teenage years. Apache parents do not see themselves as having such control over the lives of other individuals, even their own children. While Apache parents may grieve that their children are not staying in school long enough to allow them to be competitive in mainstream American markets or job venues, they do not perceive themselves to have the power to demand that children remain in a place the latter find to be irrelevant. The cultural intuition is that each person, beyond babyhood and prior to senility, is not only capable of making valid decisions but also does so; further, those decisions are not subject to ratification by outsiders.

In a school situation, then, children must be engaged. All too often, the engagement is stifled, albeit unwittingly, by Anglo teachers or those Indian teachers trained by, and committed to, the Anglo model. This model means that the teacher, as authority figure, demands attention and respect, both of which are demonstrated by sitting quietly with eyes-front attention.[4] For Apache children, already well socialized into their culture's proper way of attention paying, there is an immediate problem. The proper way to pay attention is first to be circumspect and quiet; this is demonstrated by lowering one's eyes, for to establish direct eye-to-eye contact is to make a statement that the learner is on par with the teacher. Secondly, Apache children indicate their willingness to be instructed by coming close to the one who has the knowledge or skill to be acquired; thus, especially in kindergarten and first grade, Apache children try to get next to the teacher. When the teacher then sends the children back to their seats, the children feel both rebuffed and conflicted: how is one to learn if not permitted to be close to the teacher in order to observe as closely as possible? Teachers expect to instruct verbally; Apache children expect to be taught by demonstration and their own close observation. Anglo teachers expect questions; Apache children would not presume to question an adult and will speak of their knowledge only when they feel they have fully acquired all the necessary components of a skill or a body of information. Here there is clash of several cultural intuitions.

Similarly, when she was herself being instructed in things Apachean, Farrer found that questions were not allowed. Each questioning attempt was answered by the demand that she "pay attention," with the presumption that by being quiet, observing, and thinking, the desired knowledge would be made abundantly manifest, as indeed it was. After having absorbed information through paying attention, she could be corrected when she made an incorrect assumption or reached an illogical conclusion; also, having paid proper attention, she was included in discussions of esoterica based on the body of knowledge she had been trying to learn. In this way, her knowledge base could be increased without direct instruction. In sum, she was treated as though she were an Apache learner, rather than an Anglo one.

The Dimensions of Learning

When we look at the examples given in the previous section, we begin to see that very different ways of learning are emphasized in the Navajo-Apache and in the Western traditions. Different procedures for learning, therefore, are inculcated and developed in the learner. Again, no dichotomy will do the job, but rather we propose that different values on a set of bipolar[5] dimensions can be identified in both traditions:

1. The Apache-Navajo place more emphasis on qualitative ordering and aesthetic aspects and less on quantification and universal statements or conclusions from ancient times; they do not emphasize universal truth at the cost of particular experiences. One only learns what one understands, at one's own pace. In Western schools the emphasis on quantification and universal truth yields techniques of rote learning rather than learning by insight. One often "takes in" information that is said to be important without understanding it. We cannot say that the particular and different types of knowledge in these cultures causes or induces the different learning strategies, but we claim that there is a correlation between knowledge characterization and learning strategies.

2. The Apache-Navajo learners stress detail and orthopraxy, with less

concern for sharing exactly the same contents (or orthodoxy). An implication of this difference is that for them the constant awareness of the contextuality of knowledge guides the learner in choices between relevant and irrelevant meaning or information. The Western learners are led by orthodoxy and attend less to differences in practice; they emphasize general features at the cost of details. Hence, relevance for them can be largely decontextualized or even formal at the extreme limit (see Sperber & Wilson, 1987). Thus, the Western learner learns to reason in a purely abstract, psychologically "unreal" world (perhaps culminating in the recent new math pedagogy). This kind of decontextualization can only be done because there is a belief, for learners and teachers alike, that decontextualized thinking trains the mind and that "coming down to concrete instances" is always possible. Apache and Navajo learners are wary of decontextualized learning and stress the idea that contextual details matter at least as much as general features. A different balance between abstract and concrete seems to obtain, although both, of course, practice abstract and concrete reasoning.

3. Apache and Navajo learners depend heavily on personal experience and on person-ladenness of knowledge. The interpersonal learning situation is both discrete and unique, while the personality of the teacher is an integral part of every particular learning process. In the Western case the emphasis for the learner is more on authority and less on experience; hence, texts are used extensively as substitutes for personal experience. In correlation with these features, knowledge is considered to be preferably, or optimally, of a decontextualized kind. The personality of the teacher in the interpersonal learning situation is secondary: any qualified teacher will do, eventually even a machine (cf. programmed instruction).

4. For the Apache and Navajo learner, all knowledge gathering is a process of negotiation and interpretation, within the appropriate context for knowledge transmission. In the interpersonal learning situation, the knowledge given by the teacher is not mere data or information, but also the process of transfer is one of negotiation, interaction, and so on, with other interpersonal aspects. The model is that of storytelling rather than that of transfer of information. This turns the knowledge into the personal reconstruction by the learner of the "traditional" rendering by the teacher. Hence, we have here the basis for differing interpretations of the same event or differing understandings of the same process. In the Western case, any knowledge transfer focuses more on the data, or elements as such; the act of interpretation consists mainly of the integration of these bits and pieces into the uniform frame or theory or into the hierarchical organization of knowledge that is deemed to be closest to the truth, irrespective of the personal features of the teacher. There are a correspondingly divergent set of procedures for learning among Western learners. Very generally, we see more emphasis on perception and exploration for the Apache and Navajo learner; for the Western learner, we perceive more

emphasis on the verbal transfer of knowledge, with the consequent reliance on written reports of verbal behavior, that is, texts.

Base Metaphor and Cultural Intuition

How do the base metaphor and cultural intuitions function in these different kinds of learning processes? Again we will start from our data about Apache and Navajo cultures and build the Western case by conceiving it as being in contrast.

An important cultural intuition for Navajos is the "action habitat" view of the universe: the cosmos is a home or habitat for everything living in it (including human beings). At the same time all living beings in the cosmos have a constant impact on it through their thoughts and actions, which threaten to unbalance it (Pinxten, in press). This intuition is not learned or taught in any abstract way, but is worked towards by every individual Navajo from an early age, by means of observation, exploration, and story listening. The first and most important auxiliary in this learning process is the hooghan, or homestead, which manifests, in its structure and in its way of construction, the elementary features of the universe. No straightforward or formal teaching takes place, but rather innumerable occasions occur when aspects, instances, and details of the hooghan, or any other perceivable global structures (such as a landscape, a rainbow, a sandpainting) are explored by the learner or referred to in a story. Gradually, the intuition becomes more manifest in the mind of the learner, although it need not become fully conscious; the Navajo does not and cannot properly label such an intuition. Nevertheless, it seems to be working as a guiding principle in the stories and in the sacred acts of the Navajos, that is, in those contexts where references to the more encompassing aspects of the world are dealt with most explicitly. The learner is always and directly involved in a dialogue between his/her own view of reality and reality itself. This is possible because of the fact that learning, and thinking in general, *has* an impact on reality; more properly, learning and thinking *are* reality (see Witherspoon 1977). Hence, learning is not making a re-presentation, but building links and units *in* reality. In this particular way, all learning is subjective, in a non-Western sense.

Similarly, Apache children learn to expect things that are deemed to be most proper to be in circles. That is not to say, that squares, rectangles, and other shapes do not exist: they do indeed. Rather, it is to aver that there is a cultural intuition encouraged that sees primary beauty, and certainly important efficacy, in that which is circular. Thus, Apache children, from Head Start programs onwards, fill up the circular tables first and only secondarily, and reluctantly, seat themselves at square and rectangular ones. Apache men will build round corrals, even though square ones are easier to construct and hold horses every bit as well. Adults inculcate this cultural intuition through stories, through example, through implicit instruction (as when teaching children how to salt food properly, in a circular motion), and by themselves being seen to prefer the circular, whether in body contour or in speech construction.

The Western learner is confronted with an objectified representation of reality in actual texts and in the presupposed or virtual encompassing "text" comprising all there is to know about reality. The teacher is directive. When the learner reaches a right or "true" view, that is, one that is congruent with the objectified representation, the end of the learning process is reached. The learner is engaged in a dialogue between his/her own (partial) representation and the objectified representational system. Only so-called creative thinkers challenge the correctness or truth of the objectified version and hence create new concepts and models going beyond the received view.

If our analysis is a valid description of learning processes, then it is clear that both the status of knowledge and of knowledge acquisition differ markedly in the Apache-Navajo and in the Western traditions. In the Western case, knowledge stands on its own and has a "history": changes are integrated in the global, historical, and objectified body over the generations. In the Navajo and Apache case, the learner is always manipulating reality itself in the learning process: no cumulative structure prevails, and what is learned is relevant and insightful with respect to person, situation and time. Hence, ritual, mythical, or ancestral representations of reality are as present as the result of any individual involved in a learning process. Ancestral knowledge serves as just one more element of present reality, not an objectified, distant, inert position of wisdom or truth. Two important consequences follow from the status of learning. Firstly, any individual learner's insights exert power on—or better still, in—reality. Any particular item of anyone's knowledge is therefore a part of that person's power. Any transfer of knowledge is, by consequence, a giving away and hence loss of power. Secondly, history is not an attribute or vehicle of an objectified representation of knowledge about reality. Hence, an Apache-Navajo correlate to the Western notion of history would be something like "the process of what is constantly in the making."

The consequences of our present interpretation of these differences are considerable. History can only be used as a justifying and power-laden reference (or indeed as a source for learning in the Vygotskian sense) in the West, because history is attached to the objectified version of reality, irrespective of any "true" reality. There is a presupposition of privileged correspondence between objectified rendering and reality itself. This again leads to discussions of the power impact of knowledge in terms of the indirect relationship between objectified knowledge and reality, not of the individual learner in his/her relationship to reality, as for Apaches and Navajos. In the Apache-Navajo case, the learner's power's impact on reality is direct and history does not enter the picture. Reality existed now as it did in the past and does in the future; actions and thoughts impinge on reality, whatever its temporal setting. Since objectification in the West makes primary use of texts as solid, dependable, and unchanging renderings of the objectified version of reality, the power struggle in the Western culture often takes the form of rhetorics with textual arguments or of whose history qualifies for the term "history" and which "history" is correct. The Navajo and Apache argument refers to reality itself with the learner as an intimate correspondent of it in its existence at the moment of the interlocution.

What is the relevance of all this for the sociogenesis perspective? In our understanding the sociogenesis approach explains the growth of knowledge, and hence the forms and procedures of learning, in terms of the social and historical particularities of these phenomena; it emphasizes a (re)contextualization of knowledge and learning by tracking down their social character and historical roots. The point we want to raise here is one of anthropological sophistication. First of all, history, or for that matter temporality, is an altogether different dimension for the written culture of the Westerner and for the written culture of the Muslim, let alone for the oral cultures of Navajo and Apache Indians. Hence, sociogeneticists have to work on the notion of "genesis" to broaden it or to specify its meaning for the culture they are dealing with. At present, we know little of the temporality of other cultures and a supposedly new "general" approach should take this lack of knowledge into account, lest it fall into the trap of "colonial" or "Eurocentric" hegemony. In the second place, the "social" aspect of sociogenesis offers some problems. It is clear from the present contribution that, for example, learning may be quite different from one culture to the next, because the premises, the habits, the interpersonal relations, and so on are different. In our opinion, we can identify a Navajo-Apache type of learning that diverges in general and in some particular features from Western (school) learning. Hence, we propose that, at least until one would reach a general, universally founded theory of learning, it is scientifically warranted to differentiate and take into account the diverse sociocultural settings and build culture-specific theories of sociogenesis. Our suggestion, then, is to consider the anthropological contribution to sociogenesis as holding a message of diversification and caution.

In elucidating this structural characterization of Western and Apache and Navajo considerations, we make no statements concerning the rightness or wrongness of either perspective. We merely sketch the differences in approach and thus hope to illuminate some of the fundamental misunderstandings that are apparent in the confrontation of them in metaphysical and in political struggles. Finally, by focusing on these differences we want to dissuade the adherents of the dominant Western perspective from blindly promoting their own view as the only one, or even as the only salutary one.[6]

References

Cole, M., Cole, S. (1989), *Children in Development*. New York: Freeman Press.

Elbers, E. (in press), *The Development of Competence and Its Social Context*. Educational Psychology Review.

Farella, J. (1984), *The Main Stalk*. Tucson: Arizona University Press.

Farrer, C.R. (1976), Play and Inter-Ethnic Communication. In D.F. Lancy, B.A. Tindall (eds.), *The Anthropological Study of Play*. Cornwall, NY: Leisure Press.

Farrer, C.R. (1980), Singing for Life: The Mescalero Girls' Puberty Ceremony. In C.J. Frisbie (ed.), *Southwestern Indian Ritual Drama*. Albuquerque: University of New Mexico Press.

Farrer, C.R. (1981), Living the Sky: Aspects of Mescalero Apache Ethnoastronomy. In R.A. Williamson (ed.), *Archaeoastronomy in the Americas*. Los Altos, CA: Ballena Press.

Farrer, C.R. (1990), *Play and Inter-Ethnic Communication. A Practical Ethnography of the Mescalero Apache*. New York: Garland Publishing Inc.

Farrer, C.R. (1991), *Living Life's Circle: Mescalero Apache Cosmovision*. Albuquerque: University of New Mexico Press.

Fernandez, J.W. (1974), The Mission of Metaphor in Expressive Culture. *Current Anthropology,* 15, 119-174.

Hatcher, E.P. (1974), *Visual Metaphors*. Philadelphia: Pennsylvania University Press.

Latour, B., Woolgar, S. (1979), *Laboratory Life*. Los Angeles: Sage Publications.

Perelman, C., Olbrechts-Tyteca, S., (1958), *Traité d'Argumentation*. La Nouvelle Rhétorique. Paris: PUF.

Philips, S. (1972), Participant Structures and Communicative Competence: Warm Springs Children in Community and Classroom. In Cazden et al. (eds.), *Functions of Language in the Classroom*. New York: Wiley.

Piaget, J. (1937), *The Child's Construction of Reality*. London: Routledge.

Pinxten, R. (in preparation), *Comparative Study of Knowledge*.

Pinxten, R., Balagangadhara Rao. (1989), Rhetorics and Comparative Anthropology. In R. Maier (ed.), *Norms in Argumentation*. Leiden: Foris.

Pinxten, R., Dooren, I. van, Soberon, E. (1987), *Towards a Navajo Indian Geometry*. Ghent: KKI Books.

Priest, G. (1987), *In Contradiction*. Dordrecht: Nijhoff Publishers.

Sperber, D., Wilson, R. (1987), *On Relevance*. Oxford: Oxford University Press.

Witherspoon, G. (1977), *Language and Art in the Navajo Universe*. Ann Arbor: Michigan University Press.

Notes

1. A good description of the meaning and relevance of difference in Navajo knowledge is given in Farella (1984, Ch. 4), while an analogous one for Apache is in Farrer (1991, Ch. 6).

2. We are not concerned, for the present, whether this is an effect or a cause of consistency.

3. This description is inspired by the "laboratory studies" of authors such as Latour & Woolgar (1979), but it equally matches the prescribed pattern of a learning-in-school situation which may be found in any textbook on pedagogy (e.g., Cole & Cole, 1989).

4. See Susan U. Philips (1972) for an excellent discussion of cultural ways of paying attention in Anglo-dominated schoolrooms.

5. We admit, with chagrin, that we here follow the Western base metaphor in structuring the following statements in a dualistic manner.

6. A previous and somewhat longer version of this text appeared in the journal *Cultural Dynamics,* (1990).

10. Sociogenesis: Subject-Forms Between Inertia and Innovation

Willibrord de Graaf

As far as I am aware, no clear and unequivocal description of the concept of sociogenesis exists. Sometimes one refers to the historical-societal development of human action and knowledge, and at other times to the interactional processes in human development, and still on other occasions to the social construction of individual and collective representations. I will not discuss the problem of disentangling such definitions or the difficulties of finding a language with which to formulate satisfactory perspectives in this field. I will simply mention what is the point for me: if we may assume that subject-forms always represent particular historical figures, how can we understand the processes which constitute subjects according to the "dominant fashions," and in what ways do such processes co-produce the forms and contents of onto-genesis?

In my view, the study of sociogenesis involves two questions: the first concerns the socio-historical construction of subject-forms, and the second concerns the corresponding variations in psychic development. Both problems immediately raise the question of the mechanisms which are at play in sociogenetic processes. In the first case, the question is how transformations of cultural and psychological lifestyles or "scripts" do occur, and, in the second case, the question implies the possible changes in the structural or epigenetic individual development.

In this paper I will confine myself to the first question, and I will approach the matter by examining the solutions and difficulties which are offered by the works of Bourdieu and Moscovici. Although they do not have explicitly formulated theories on sociogenesis, their work on the genesis of practices and of representations offers many elements which may be fruitful in a discussion of sociogenetic mechanisms.

Transfer and Change

The theme of long-term shifts in both societal and psychological forms and contents has already been posed by Elias, when he researched the changes of the human affect and control structures towards what is called "civilization" (Elias, 1981). One may object to his explanation, especially based on psycho-analytical insights (from *Fremdzwang*, coercion by others, to *Selbstzwang*, coercion by the self) in correspondence with changing power structures in state and society, but the problem of the relationship between social changes and subject-forms remains intriguing.[1] On the one hand, the process of growing into a given socio-historical context, into already established moral orders, implies a process of transfer and of learning how the world is (has been), a process, which in the first instance, brings to the forefront the element of the known, of the familiar, or of inertia. On the other hand, there are social and individual conflicts and changes, small and large innovations which create new familiarities. A crucial question is who or what produces such innovations: are they the product of acting subjects who carry out more or less planned projects, or do they happen "behind the backs" of the people and are these subjects nothing more than particles in historical whirlwinds?

These questions are the more pressing because social theories tend to offer both an overdose of structural or functional mechanisms and a surplus of unexplained individual exceptions to the rules. The reverse is true for psycho-logical theories, which present too many endogenous and individualistic universals or too many unexplained determining "environmental conditions" while limiting themselves to very special micro-situations.

Furthermore, a simple "interactionist" solution fails because the social cannot be reduced to interpersonal relations, which, in principle, are based on the primacy of individuals as the cornerstone of interaction. Equally unsatisfy-ing is the idea of mentalist constructivism in which individual actions obtain a social dimension by "internalizing" external forms and contents. The interac-tionalist or interpersonal realm cannot be equated with the socio-historical, and internalization of external givens remains a term which maintains the split between the individual and the social without satisfactorily explaining it (cf. the criticisms of Valsiner on sociogenetic theories in psychology elsewhere in this book). There is also the problem as to the extent to which internalization is a useful concept, or is rather a container-concept for an uncomprehended process.

In this theoretical field of forces, which continually risks breaking into the binary options of 0 or 1, efforts have been made to surmount this polarity by rejecting, in advance, the opposition between individual and society. I shall confine myself to a selective discussion of two efforts. One is of sociological/ anthropological origin, that is, the constructivist structuralism or the structural-ist constructivism of P. Bourdieu (1990b, p. 123), and which is also referred to as reflexive sociology. The other is of psychological origin, that is, the theory of social representations of S. Moscovici (1984). In my selection I looked for themes which are discussed in both theories, and I have selected a discussion of the place of science and of the problems of action and structure.

In the course of my discussion I hope to present and comment on some central concepts in their theories.

The Role of Science and the Scientist

The cultural embedding of science is attracting more and more attention in the social sciences, as, for instance, in developmental psychology (Kessen, 1983; Valsiner, 1987). What is particularly at stake is the role of basic assumptions about objects of knowledge and directions of explanation and about methodological principles which guide theoretical approaches.

In the works of Bourdieu and Moscovici, the role of science and scientists is also considered on two levels: epistemological problems and theoretical contents. On the epistemological level, the question concerns the construction of the object of knowledge connected to the problem of the relation between scientific activity and common sense thinking and acting. This regards matters which are also discussed in the so-called constructionist movement (Gergen, 1985) or are analyzed in social studies of science (Latour, 1987; Woolgar, 1988). On the level of content, the problem of the influence of science on common sense is central. Such questions can also be found in studies on "psychologization," such as the one by Donzelot (1979) on the development of the family as the object of interventions or the study of the spreading of the therapeutic institution and the rise of proto-professionalization (Brinkgreve, Onland, & de Swaan, 1979).

On the epistemelogical level, one can find in Bourdieu what has become namegiving for his sociology: the necessity for reflection on the role of (social) theory and its conditions of production in order to avoid intellectualism, and to prevent an opposition between objectivist and subjectivist approaches. Bourdieu sees subjectivism in approaches like ethno-methodology, (symbolic) interactionism, and social phenomenology, which try to relate to daily experiences and presentations of the actors by means of methods such as participant observation, ethnography, discourse analysis, etc. Bourdieu's objection to subjectivism is that, in this way, social science reduces social reality to a construction of constructions, an account of accounts. Surely, the daily experiences are taken seriously, but their power as phenomenological evidence and immediacy remains unexplained because the conditions for their possibility are not being reflected. The same problem obtains to the social relation which is established in the effort of understanding primary experiences: how can one escape in the theoretical analysis from common sense once its primacy has been accepted?

In the search for objective regularities which determine the behavior of individuals apart from their will or consciousness, objectivism breaks positively with common sense and establishes a split between theoretical knowledge and practical knowledge. It refers individual representations to the field of rationalizations, ideology, and the like. But then the objection against objectivism is the failure to objectify this objectifying relation and with it the possibility of a caesura with common sense. In this way one pretends the possibility of objective knowledge (epistemocracy) in which scientists can have a complete picture of reality but the actors cannot.

Intellectualism in theoretical analyses follows thus from the lack of an analysis of the subjective relation of the scientist to social reality and the objective social relation based upon it (Bourdieu, 1990a). On the one hand, Bourdieu locates the way out of this in a dialectical combination of a subjectivist and an objectivist moment in the theoretical analysis, and, on the other hand, in the use of sociological means against sociology itself: a historical and social-critical analysis of science as institution and institutional practice. Thereby theories must give a place to the role of science and its symbolic power. This is necessary because the lack of such a reflection not only leads towards a substantialization of the object of knowledge, but also towards "substituting the observer's relation to practice for the practical relation to practice" (Bourdieu, 1990a, p. 34). In other words, the scientist projects his own distance—as product of a social division of labor—into the object of knowledge. The scientist assumes the same type of attitude, characterized by the idea that an action can only be fully understood when it is completely planned or thought out, and so the actors are attributed with forms of rationality and systemacy which "in practice" do not exist. An example of this is the definition of kinship as a system of closed and logical relations, where, in practice, the use of these rules is more flexible and differentiated, whereby some figurations are more recurrent than would logically be expected. The abstract model to explain practices gets, in this way, a determinist force: there is a silent transition from observed regularities to consciously designed and applied rules or to unconscious regulating mechanisms, or from a model of reality to a reality of the model (Bourdieu, 1990a, p. 39). With that the epistemological problematic pertains directly to the contents of theory: the practical activities of actors are thus removed from the analysis.

Where Bourdieu stresses the constructive significance of scientific theorizing (without otherwise disclaiming the pretension of universal laws, etc.!) in the field of forces between common sense and objectivation, Moscovici situates the role of science particularly in the content of common sense. That is not to say that he does not discuss epistemological aspects. But he confines himself to a plea for social representations as the appropriate object of social psychology, and thereby for these representations as the raw materials for common sense and as ways of creating reality. His focus is less the scientist, but more the envisaged object of a discipline. Moscovici is opposed to a conception of information-processing individuals who react to an autonomous reality. He replaces it with a conception of the relation between individual and environment as determined by the social representations of this environment and the corresponding reactions. In short, he transforms the classical psychological scheme of S causing R (with or without an O) into a scheme within which S does not cause R by means of internal representations, but within which social representations define both S and R.

In fact, Moscovici does not seem interested in the social place of science other than in its role as origin of social representations (Moscovici, 1988). This impression is strengthened by his characterizing of two universa. He distinguishes a reified and a consensual world. The first is constituted by the unchangeable laws of (natural) sciences and by bureaucratic orders; it is a world in which individuality and identity have no meaning and things are the measure for men. The second world consists of the daily conversations in which social "truths" are constantly made in equal relationships; in this world man is the measure of things (Moscovici, 1984). The division in these two universa is the historical substitution of the division between the sphere of the sacred and the sphere of the profane. As authorities, priest and prophet are replaced by the scientist and the professional expert. In the consensual world people can act as "amateur-scientists," as interested participants, and can create their own meanings. But they do so depending on the modern "myth-makers": scientists, artists, doctors, social workers, media and market specialists. Common sense as "first-hand knowledge" and as a source for scientific reflection has become "second-hand knowledge," derived from scientific insights and concepts (Moscovici & Hewstone, 1983). Such common sense transforms scientific knowledge by personifying it (for instance Freud and psychoanalysis), by representing it through (analogous) terms and images (for instance, curing diseases as a kind of warfare), and finally by ontologizing or objectifying it (for instance, "he has an inferiority complex"). In this process the informative meaning of scientific thought is transposed into a representative meaning, composed of images, ideas, perceptions, etc., and used to explain the why of the world. Social representations are thus common-sense theories about central aspects of society, and are, on the one hand, cognitive vehicles for interpretation and, on the other hand, schemes for action.

Moscovici's characterization of science as a source of common sense looks fruitful because it takes into account the social and symbolic power of scientific knowledge and the ways for "laymen" to assimilate those often strange and abstract ideas. Moscovici's own study of the reception and spreading of psychoanalysis in France shows, for example, that in the process of assimilation other ways of looking at problems and dealing with them may arise. The studies on psychologization mentioned above, also occupy themselves with the effect of scientific and professional practices in health care on the experiences and lifestyles of (future) clients. But I am not convinced of the rather unilateral relationship between science and common sense in the

190 10. Sociogenesis: Subject-Forms Between Inertia and Innovation

way Moscovici presents it.

Firstly, the split in a reified and a consensual world looks very simple: it is unclear why material and economic worlds do not have a part in it. Neither is much attention paid to the institutional processes, which may intersect both worlds (for instance, technological innovations, audiovisual communications, political reforms). Secondly, there is no elaboration of the reasons of the one-way direction of science to common sense. This lack causes problems, because Moscovici's claim that individuals and groups themselves think ("the thinking society") and are not followers of dominant ideas and ideologies, is inconsistent with his thesis of a one-way direction of influence (common sense as second-hand knowledge). I will return to this question later, but I would like to stress here that it also raises difficulties for the pretended status of science. For it may be evident that scientists themselves are co-constructors and participants in social representations, and that, as a group, they are subject to the same mechanisms in the formation of social representations: social representations are cognitions which, amongst others, create a distinction toward groups and establish the identity of the group. So it looks quite "natural" that scientists who operate in the reified universum (with professional hierarchy, strict rules, production of truth, etc.) are involved in the same processes of making representations in the construction of their object of knowledge. But then Moscovici bites his own tail: the impetus for Moscovici's theory was his criticism of a social psychology which projected an information-processing rationality, characteristic for science, into its object of knowledge!

In short, the unilaterality which Moscovici assumes in the relation between science and common sense illustrates the processes of assimilation of scientific knowledge, but leaves how science and scientists could avoid being influenced by social representations in the dark.

In this respect, Bourdieu's reflexive sociology is more satisfying. He analyzes the practical relation of the social scientist to his object of knowledge by proposing a dialectic between a subjectivist and an objectivist moment in theorizing. But there is a problem: his claim of unchangeable, universal laws (of field) does not seem to be compatible with the process of objectifying objectification: where or when would that possibly come to a halt? So his refusal to take a more relativist stand threatens to destroy the dialectic he wishes to introduce.

On the other hand, he has in fact tried, in his studies of the functioning of schools and the academic world (Bourdieu, 1988, 1990b; Bourdieu & Passeron, 1990c), to combine epistemological criticism and social criticism of scientific practices and institutions. These researches even result in an outline of at least two specific subject-forms:

> This privileged [=school] instrument of the bourgeois sociodicy which confers on the privileged the supreme privilege of not seeing themselves as privileged manages the more easily to convince the disinherited that they owe their scholastic and social destiny to their lack of gifts and merits, because in matters of culture absolute dispossession excludes awareness of being dispossessed. (Bourdieu & Passeron, 1990c, p. 210)

This analysis shows some correspondence with the one made by Willis (1977), which demonstrates how boys from the working class who form an intuitive (class-determined) disbelief in the promises of upward mobility through schooling, resist the demands of education and thus contribute to their reproduction as manual laborers.

Summarizing this discussion of the role of science in the theories of Bourdieu and Moscovici, I would propose three possible elements for theorizing about sociogenetic processes. This proposal stresses the fruitful dimensions of their theories while acknowledging that big problems still remain.

1. It is necessary to explicate the assumptions which form the base for the direction of explanations and which may result from social representations about development, socialization, situational, or individual causation etc. Furthermore, a reflection is needed on the practical relation of science to the object of knowledge in the moment of objectifying. Precisely the problems which I have indicated in the theories of Moscovici and Bourdieu, who try to analyze these matters positively, show the importance of coherent reflection of the socio-historic development of social science.

2. Science has an influence on the formation of the contents and activities of common sense. This influence concerns not only the processes of cognitive assimilation of strange and incomprehensible notions, but also the institutional practices with which science, on the symbolic level and by way of its expertise, exerts authority and (d)evaluates behavior. But common sense also has an influence on science: it is both an object of knowledge and a source of explanations. This leads us to the third point.

3. The access to the practice of science supposes a complex process of societal selection based on social divisions and individual dispositions. The results of this institutional process not only determine a factual role competence, but also produce a certain attitude toward the acquired position and its hallmark is the "forgetting" of the process of acquiring. So social scientists tend to substantialize their acquired position and to project themselves as the measure of thinking and action into their object of knowledge. More generally, this process of selection points to the construction of at least two subject-forms, with cultural-academic and cultural-pragmatic orientations as the poles.

Between Action and Structure

Simple endogenous (biological or psychological) and monocausal determinations of human development are disputed more often. Such explanations are, at least more than marginally, substituted by conceptual schemes for interactional dynamics, socio-cultural processes, historical structures, and semiotic and symbolic activities. Within this perspective, individual activity and its socio-cultural embeddings must be studied together as both motor and form of development. So the point is to sail between the Scylla of the autonomous individual and the Charybdis of determining structures.

Bourdieu brings the concept of *habitus* to the fore as dissolution of the antinomy between determinism and freedom, subjectivism and objectivism. On the one hand, there are objective structures (conditions of existence) which form the base of subjective representations and circumscribe the margins for interaction. On the other hand, these subjective representations are important for a good understanding of the daily individual and collective struggles to maintain or to change these structures. The habitus is the system of durable dispositions, which is the product of a specific group of conditions of existence. As a system of structured structures, these dispositions are predisposed to function as structuring structures and generate and organize practices and representations (Bourdieu, 1990a, p. 53). The habitus is a system of cognitions and motivations which produces schemes of perceptions, appreciations, and action. The habitus is closely linked to the body (as locus of and vehicle for accumulated experiences) and so with language and time. Depending on the ways of locating the body in the (social) space, a body-scheme develops in correspondence with the divisions of positions in the social space. In the development of this system, early experiences have a great weight because the habitus strives for constancy, selects new information which fits as much as possible in with already existing knowledge, and tries (unconsciously) to avoid deviant experiences.

Human beings are actors, subjects of construction of the social world, but the social genesis of the principles of construction are to be found in the social world. The fact, however, of genesis tends to be forgotten: "Genesis implies amnesia of genesis" (Bourdieu, 1990a, p. 50). Therefore, the correspondence between social structures and mental structures leads to the *doxa*, the evidence of the common sense, in which the social genesis of the principles of construction is misconceived in the cognitive activity of constructing the object. The practical knowledge, generated by the habitus, is built on classifications, judgments, etc., which are made unconsciously.

Precisely because the habitus is "incorporated history," the practices following from it are attuned to the conditions in which the habitus has been acquired. Structures are thus through the habitus producing the "correct" practices, and this does not imply a mechanical reproduction in which structures determine the actors completely. This is so because actors act according to perceptions and cognitive structures which were constructed with principles external to the constructed object or situation. A crucial characteristic of the habitus is its strategic nature without being a conscious strategy. As embodied past, the habitus provides "the sense of practice" which produces the unconscious correspondence between practices and structures and the belonging degrees of freedom for deviancies and innovations. The habitus thus generates, in advance, an adaptation to the conditions of existence in as far as these have not been changed. When these conditions are changed the persistence of the habitus may result in a failed adaptation or in revolt. However, Bourdieu presupposes in the habitus a kind of ontological complicity with the social world, a compliance with the rules of the game and the involved stakes: the distribution of the different kinds of capital which have been accumulated in a certain field and which form the relations of force and power in the field.

The concept of "field" refers to a social space with specific interests and properties and to the division of positions within it. So there are, for instance, the fields of science, fashion, religion, etc. Each field has its own rules, stakes, and interests, its own forms of capital and power relations. Capital as accumulated labor can be distinguished in three kinds: the *economic* capital, which is directly convertible into money and is linked to the member institutions (property, stock exchange, etc.); the *cultural* capital which refers to the educational qualifications, and the *social* capital, which results from the involvement in a network of social relations (family, party, class, etc.). All three kinds of capital may appear as *symbolic* capital, that is, when they are acknowledged as legitimate and evident by the actors in the field, an acknowledgment that follows from the internalized position of the actors. Symbolic capital consists of the representations of the different kinds of capital within the acknowledged relations of force and power in the specific field. The forms of capital are, in principle, convertible in each other, but the economic capital is the base for the others.

It goes too far to discuss the dynamics of this specification of conditions of existence (field, position, capital) for the different social spaces such as science or culture. This short description is meant to illustrate the thesis of Bourdieu that structures do not just determine their own reproduction, because each structure is always a temporary equilibrium of the force relations in a field. The habitus establishes a comprehensible and necessary relation between a given situation in the field and practices, because the habitus produces an attuned action through perception and appreciation of the situation. Bourdieu even offers a formula: [(habitus) (capital)] + field = practice (1984, p. 101), which underlines that habitus, as embodied past, also implies incorporation of capital, and that the body scheme expresses the relation to the social space. Or in other words, the field is history made into thing, and the habitus is history made into a body: the relationship between these two modes would have to substitute the "naive relation between individual and society" (Bourdieu, 1990b, 190-191).

The dilemma between individual autonomy and determining structures is transformed by Bourdieu into a dialectic within which the habitus fulfills an essential role. The habitus establishes both continuity and opens a certain freedom of activity for the actor. These margins may pertain to a more or less evident future or to a more conscious projected plan, but absolute subjective freedom does not exist. Although Bourdieu recognizes the specificity of the individual habitus (as unique accumulation of experiences and dispositions) he points out the correspondence between the individual habitus and the habitus formed by social class, so that in the end the individual habitus is nothing more than a particular instance of the class-habitus.

All in all, this analysis satisfies, on the macro level, the social and cultural embodiment of actions through the introduction of the habitus. But there is also a problem: the sociogenesis of patterns of thought, action, and perception seems to deliver the actor completely up to the dynamics of the field and one cannot imagine what innovating influence actors (individually or collectively) may have on the field. In a recent publication (Bourdieu, 1992), this question of the negation of innovation is taken up again. Firstly, Bourdieu stresses the point that the refusal of the acceptation of any social determination might be the consequence of the illusion of the intellectuals who see themselves as original originators. Secondly, he repeats that the habitus is durable but not unchangeable, but immediately he adds the statistical determination that people will meet the same circumstances in which their habitus was constituted. The habitus is primarily dominated by former experiences, but the thus built dispositions are only *relatively* closed. Whether the habitus can produce different practices depends on the structure and stimulations of the field. Thirdly, Bourdieu points to the fact that actors are determined insofar as they determine themselves. So there is a possibility of reflection on dispositions, on the ongoing complicity. This government on dispositions requires a continuous and methodical effort to self-examination, to explication. Without such a reflection one makes him/herself an accomplice to the unconscious effects of the dispositions. This kind of reasoning, however, seems to presuppose a subject which resembles Bourdieu himself as a professional intellectual, because he does not specify in what ways "common" people have access to the kinds of capital to reflect on their position.

This flaw in Bourdieu's theorizing is reinforced by his reduction of the different kinds of capital to one: the economic, and by his neglect of the multiple character of the individual habitus. If the habitus is linked to positions in a field, and if individuals may simultaneously occupy positions in different fields, then the habitus of an individual person must be a very complicated system to be attuned to a diversity of possibilities in different situations. It may even be possible that precisely the genesis of this "multi-determination" is the condition for individual creativity and innovation. But unfortunately Bourdieu does not pay much attention to this problem. So despite his claims, Bourdieu seems not to have escaped from a structuralist determinism and leaves the actor rather helpless.

Moscovici appears to tackle the problem of action and structure in comparable ways. But in addition to terminological differences, there is also a distinction in the conception of the subject as actor. Social representations have, as the product of human actions and communications, a relative autonomy, a "material" existence, and as such, influence in their turn human thought and activity. So people are influenced by representations, but in the end they are also the persons who construct these representations (the thinking society). Moscovici uses the metaphor of a decision committee in which each member has a vote in the process of construction, and where the result is the collective product on the condition that individual initiatives fit into the common line (Moscovici, 1988, p. 200). (What happens when someone operates outside this line is not mentioned.) Social representations develop, so it seems, in the exchange of individual representations, and when a collectively shared social representation has been formed, this representation exerts, in its turn, influence as an objectified figure of evident patterns of thought and action. This influence is mostly unconscious and rather limits the possibilities for constructive activities.

Moscovici thus poses the acting subject alongside the structure, and the subject is cut into two parts: one part is the active (co)constructor of social representations; the other part is the social individual determined by these representations. How both parts relate to one another remains unexplained. This lack of clarity is strengthened because Moscovici, as I mentioned before, depicts representations as "second-hand knowledge" developed at the instigation of professionals and scientists. What's more, he discerns three kinds of representations: *Hegemonic* representations can be shared by a group without being produced by it, and are present in all symbolic and affective practices. They are uniform and coercive, and are the expression of homogeneity and stability of the group. *Emancipated* representations are developed in a more or less free exchange between subgroups of society (for instance professionals and laymen), and have a relative autonomy with respect to these groups. *Polemic* representations, which result from social conflicts, are not shared by society as a whole and are mutually exclusive. Each representation presupposes a different role for the actors involved (passive participation, active participation, and conflict), and furthermore actors seem to be groups.

If the role of the actor is unclear, Moscovici is much more explicit about the genesis and functions of social representations as structures. Social representations are structures of knowledge and ideas developed in the communication of people trying to make sense of their world. Their purpose is to familiarize the unfamiliar, to conventionalize it, to assimilate it in existing frames of thinking. This process of familiarization is based on two mechanisms: anchoring and objectifying. Anchoring of the unfamiliar implies classifying and naming it with the aim of fitting it into the present cognitive schemes, and interpreting it. This procedure most often means a reinterpretation of the unfamiliar in known terms with the help of analogy, or a personification of it, or the formulation of certain prototypical characteristics. Such representations then acquire a life of their own in the visible and tangible world, the images replace the imagined, and take on a "material" form. The "figurative nucleus" thus formed is the result of the objectification of the representation. Images are transformed into realities. In this respect, representations are both in the world and in the head of human beings; they are psychological phenomena which themselves can be studied. Social representations create realities because they define situations in language and symbols, prescribe appropriate actions, and deal selectively with information, persons, and objects and thus maintain the communication of the group.

The genesis of social representations through this process of familiarization shows the importance of memories and of the inertia of feelings and concepts. Changes and innovations are the product of familiarization; they are transformed unfamiliarities which transform, in their turn, the existing contents of social representations. The unfamiliar is, as already mentioned, to be found in the reified world of science. According to Moscovici, the theory of social representations has adopted the perspective of the consensual world and presents, from that point of view, the reified world as reality. What might be the status of actors in that reified world, and what kind of relations exists between the subject-forms of both worlds, remains unexplained. These problems may be connected to the reduction of representations to linguistic realities and the neglect of the relation between representations and concrete behaviors.

Finishing this discussion on action and structure, I would conclude that, regarding the problem of actorship and structure, Bourdieu's theory seems to be more consistent than Moscovici's. Bourdieu gives the acting subject a clear-cut and circumscribed position in fields with different kinds of capital, and tries to avoid a mechanical determinism by the introduction of the habitus. But his dialectical solution risks ending in the construction of an over-socialized subject. Moscovici offers a less precise insight in the dialectics of action and structure, and seems to hesitate between the subject as an autonomous actor and a socially determined individual.

But both bring to the fore the importance of the daily evidences (doxa, common sense), which, as products of the social genesis of patterns of action and of class and group structures, must be the object of the social scientist. Studies of sociogenesis should, therefore, be especially concerned with the principles and processes of construction of daily worlds. In other words, it is important to look at the narrative accounts which are formed out of private and public experiences and their constituting activities.

Sociogenesis and Ontogenesis

Moscovici's theory of social representations aims to build a bridge between the individual and the social world and to establish a connection with the changing world. It is striking that he, just like Bourdieu with the concept of habitus, points to the conserving character of the dynamic structure which manages the "mediation" between conditions of existence and subjects. The habitus produces the "sense of practice" (the feeling for the game and an ontological complicity), and social representations provide for the anchoring in the existing collective. Innovation is, for both, something that results from a break with the known and from the dynamics involved in the process of transformation of the new givens and of the adaptation of the existing structures of knowledge and action. The comparison with Piaget's theory of accommodation, assimilation, and equilibration seems natural, and both theorists do refer to Piaget.

But then new problems arise. Piaget's theory concentrates on the development of an active, problem-solving individual in a certain context, and mentions little on the social and historical character of that context and the implied dynamics. On the contrary, Piaget claims that the development of cognitions results from the dynamic interaction between an active subject and a problem-posing context and is not dependent upon the specific social nature of the context. But both Bourdieu and Moscovici postulate that structure and content of cognitions are specific in different social contexts and that sociogenesis of cognitions, perceptions, and actions must be related to the sociogenesis of groups and classes. In other words, there is no neutral, value-free problem-posing context: different tasks or problems do not only have different social values and meanings, but there are more or less limiting or coercive constraints in the search for solutions and in the direction of this search (Goodnow, 1990, Valsiner, 1987). This implies the need to look more precisely at the domain-specific ontogenesis of cognitions and actions. But Bourdieu and Moscovici do not discuss this matter, and nowhere do they describe the process of learning or adopting the habitus or social representation. They refer to concepts like internalization (mostly), conditioning, mimesis, or inculcating. Furthermore, Bourdieu has something interesting (also for developmental psychologists) to say about the importance of the body in psycho- and sociogenesis. He points at the preverbal and verbal forms of interaction and instruction which produce a bodily scheme based on the existing gender stereotypes or on the division of labor. But in spite of this, the problem

remains that both theories, occupying themselves so much with the sociogenesis of psychic and social structures, pay too little attention to an articulated
formulation of ontogenetic processes (see also Haste, 1987). The problem of
the multifaceted determination of what is going on in, for example, the
process of internalization may, perhaps, indicate the direction in which to look
for answers. With internalization the point is not simply the interiorization of
socially constructed and explicit cognitive strategies, but at the same time the
implicit appreciation of what is important for whom. At stake is, therefore,
not only the process of identification and appropriation of the problem and its
possible solutions, but also the significance of the social values of certain
problems and their solution, and of the limits which social interaction poses
for exploration. The question is whether different social values and limitations
could imply different processes of internalization and different subject-forms.

Conclusion

As one of the aspects of sociogenesis I have chosen the problem of the socio-
historical construction of subject-forms, and especially the question of
innovation versus inertia: in what ways are subjects actors of change? I have
attempted to outline and to comment on some answers which have been given
by Bourdieu and Moscovici. Firstly, I discussed the necessity to include the
socio-historical forms of scientific practice and the role of the scientist as a
subject in the objectifying relation to his object. Without such an analysis one
cannot take into account the dialectical relation of common sense and science,
where common sense may be the source of scientific assumptions and the
object of scientific theorizing. Both Bourdieu and Moscovici give convincing
arguments for such a reflective position to science, even when some of their
claims seem exaggerated.

Secondly, I have tackled the problem of action and structure. Both theorists
formulate approaches which strive to overcome the classical opposition of
individual and society, and of subjectivism and objectivism. Furthermore, they
wish to establish the subject as an actor of practices, while at the same time
acknowledging the sociogenesis of content and forms of action. Paradoxically
they underline the rather conserving traits of the dynamic structures which
they propose are at work in the interface of society and individual, of history
and future. Both the habitus and the social representations aim at social
stability, at keeping things familiar, and at doing things smoothly. External
disturbances (new information, change in field forces, for instance) necessitate
these structures to adapt themselves, to develop new schemes of interpretation
and action. These structures enable actions according to the demands of the
situation, where these demands are constantly interpreted within already

established schemes of perception and cognition. Innovations then do not seem to be the result of consciously acting subjects, but of external social developments which instigate processes of assimilation. This image of "puppets on a string" is reinforced by the ontological status of the habitus and the social representations: Moscovici explicitly claims that social representations have a life of their own, adopt a kind of materiality, and are in the world as well as in the head of people. Bourdieu does not say it in so many words, but he also seems to view the habitus as a structure which is bound to positions in fields, and "inhabits" a person (see, for example, the relation of body and habitus). It is not quite clear how these structures (habitus and representations) can then be connected to acting human beings.

These comments are not intended to dismiss these theories: they offer stimulating approaches, and propose new solutions in long-lasting debates. But these solutions themselves seem to be caught in the oppositions they want to overcome. The difficulties of defining a satisfactory concept of the subject as actor show just that. Maybe the problem can be tackled from a different point of view. Thus far I have discussed the problem of innovation in the terms I feared at the beginning: zero or one, too much of this, too little of that. In my comments I have stressed inconsistencies and shortcomings. At the end I would like to propose the following thesis, thereby risking the danger of an abstract and simplified solution.

In sociogenetic theories the attention was focused on the socializing of individuals or on individual contribution to sociality. But what about the individual as acting upon him/herself in order to become a constituent agent of sociality? Although I am not sure about the possibility to generalize, I would like to defend the proposition that at least our Western culture has produced the "deep structure" of the person and its identity as the figure who has to act upon her/his abilities/strivings/emotions, etc., in order to realize a civil and personal status, to be a "character," a "personality." This culture of "individualism" results from a combination of socio-economic and socio-cultural practices. My point of view implies a shift in attention toward the practices with which individuals create themselves as persons and toward the domains which are seen as constituting personhood. Of course, the materials and domains for these practices are given in culture, in socio-moral codes, and in economic constraints. So the problem would be to define the "technologies of the self" which are constructed in the process of sociogenesis. This concept, borrowed from Foucault (1984; see also Martin, Gutman & Hutoon, 1988), expresses the "active" and "passive" positions of the individual: as an individual he/she may practice several "techniques" to constitute a self-identity, but at the same time such practices of individuality are the outcome of historical processes. Reformulating my question at the beginning of this contribution, the problem of innovation and inertia, would be: Under what conditions, what kinds of (combined) individual actions may have any impact (even unintended) on social regulations of subject-forms? Innovation is only possible within the dynamics of historical, conjunctural conditions. The forces of inertia are included in these dynamics. The problem is not the individual as acting or reacting, as spontaneous or conditioned. The question is to analyze in what ways self-practices are both reconstituting and recombining forms of personhood or individuality.

References

Brinkgreve, C., Onland, J.H., & Swaan, A. de (1979), *De opkomst van het psychotherapeutisch bedrijf.* Utrecht: Het Spectrum.

Bourdieu, P. (1989), *Opstellen over smaak, habitus en het veldbegrip.* Amsterdam: Van Gennep.

Bourdieu, P. (1984), *Distinction, a social critique of the judgement of taste.* Cambridge, MA: Harvard University Press (orig. *La distinction.* Paris: Minuit, 1979).

Bourdieu, P. (1988), *Homo academicus.* Cambridge: Polity Press (orig. *Homo academicus.* Paris: Minuit, 1984).

Bourdieu, P. (1990a), *The logic of practice.* Cambridge: Polity Press, (orig. *Le sens pratique.* Paris: Minuit, 1980).

Bourdieu, P. (1990b), *In other words. Essays towards a reflexive sociology.* Cambridge: Polity Press (orig. *Choses dites.* Paris: Minuit, 1987).

Bourdieu, P., Passeron, J.C. (1990c), *Reproduction in education, society and culture.* London: Sage.

Bourdieu, P. (1992), *Réponses (avec L.J.D. Wacquant).* Paris: Editions du Seuil.

Donzelot, J. (1979), *The policing of families.* New York: Pantheon (orig. *La police des familles.* Paris: Minuit, 1977).

Dreyfus, H.L., & P. Rabinow (1983), *Michel Foucault, beyond structuralism and hermeutics.* Chicago: The University of Chicago Press.

Elias, N. (1981), *Uber den Prozess der Zivilisation. Soziogenetische und psychogenetische Untersuchungen.* Frankfurt: Suhrkamp.

Foucault, M. (1984), *Le souci de soi.* Paris: Gallimard.

Gergen, K. (1985), The social constructionist movement in modern psychology. *American Psychologist,* 40, 266-273.

Goodnow, J.J. (1990), Using sociology to extend psychological accounts of cognitive development. *Human Development,* 33, 81-107.

Haste, H. (1987), Growing into rules. In: Bruner, J., Haste, H. (eds), *Making sense, the child's construction of the world.* London: Methuen, 1987.

Jahoda, G. (1988), Critical notes and reflections on "social representations." *European Journal of Social Psychology,* 18, 195-209.

Kessen, W. (1983), The child and other cultural inventions. In: Kessel, F.S., Siegel, A.W. (eds.), *The child and other cultural inventions.* New York: Praeger.

Marková, I. (1987), *Human awareness, its social development.* London: Hutchinson.

Martin, L.H., Gutman, H., & Hutoon, P.H. (eds.) (1988), *Technologies of the self, a seminar with Michel Foucault.* London: Tavistock.

Moscovici, S., & Hewstone, M. (1983), Social representations and social explanations: from the "naive" to the "amateur" scientist. In: Hewstone, M. (ed.), *Attribution theory, social and functional extensions*. Oxford: Basil Blackwell.

Moscovici, S. (1984), The phenomenon of social representations. In: Farr, R.M., Moscovici, S. (eds.), *Social representations*. Cambridge: Cambridge University Press.

Moscovici, S. (1988), Notes towards a description of social representations. *European Journal of Social Psychology*, 18, 211-250.

Moscovici, S. (1990), Social psychology and developmental psychology: extending the conversation. In Duveen, G., Lloyd, B. (eds.), *Social representations and the development of knowledge*. Cambridge: Cambridge University Press, 1990.

Potter, J., & Litton, I. (1985), Some problems underlying the theory of social representations. *British Journal of Social Psychology*, 24, 81-90.

Valsiner, J. (1987), *Culture and the development of children's action. A cultural-historical theory of developmental psychology*. Chicester: John Wiley & Sons.

Willis, P. (1983), *Learning to labor*. Aldershot: Gower.

Woolgar, S. (1988), Science the very idea. Chichester: Ellis Howard/London: Tavistock.

Note

1. A discussion of the relation between Elias and Bourdieu can be found in the introduction of D. Pels in *Opstellen over smaak, habitus en het veldbegrip*, (Bourdieu, 1989).

Part 4

Empirical Case Studies

11. Becoming a Conscientious Objector: The Use of Arms and Institutional Accounting Practices

Viveka Adelswärd and Roger Säljö

Introduction

Social institutions are powerful agents in the creation and maintenance of discursive practices in modern society. In a sociocultural perspective this implies that institutions also play a vital role for the formation of linguistic categories and forms of thought adopted by individuals when acting in such settings. In this chapter, our interest will be focused on studying some aspects of dialogues in an institutional context with an emphasis on analyzing what counts as valid forms of argumentation. The particular setting we have chosen as our subject of inquiry is one in which the decision is taken whether or not to grant a conscript the status of conscientious objector. As part of this bureaucratic procedure there is an interview between a representative of the authorities responsible for the enrollment procedures (usually a psychologist) and the conscript. The purpose of this interview is to establish whether the arguments presented by the conscript are sufficient for him to be exempted from carrying arms.

In the following some aspects of the outcome of the analysis of these interviews will be reported. The issue we want to discuss concerns the fact that the conceptual tools used by the individuals in the dialogues, and the accounting practices (Shotter, 1990) that are considered relevant must be construed as genuinely social in nature. Even though the act of refusing to carry arms is a highly individual decision at one level, the discursive practices used in the dialogues by both parties reflect collective, although conflicting, forms of argumentation. To understand the sociogenesis of mind in complex societies, it may therefore be fruitful to seriously consider the role of social institutions in providing accounting practices which shape individual cognition.

Expressed differently, the purpose of this chapter is to discuss, in a preliminary fashion, aspects of what could be referred to as a non-mentalistic understanding of human communication, cognition, and interaction. The issues that concern us reflect an interest in how human activities are organized in complex societies, and how the relationship between the individual and the surrounding culture can be construed without resorting to the most frequent types of reductionism. Avoiding reductionism, in this case, implies trying to refrain from theoretical positions that portray the individual either as a free-floating entity who processes information and makes choices entirely at his/her own will and with no anchoring in the social and cultural circumstances in which he/she is acting, or, alternatively, as someone who is programmed by his social or biological resources to behave in predetermined ways.

Our interest is thus focused on understanding forms—or genres (Luckmann, 1989)—of communication in society. Communication will be used as a primary, and in some sense primitive, term that is genetically prior to the individual and/or social group in accounts of social phenomena. In line with Vygotsky's (1986) dictum about the role of the "inter-psychological plane" for the formation of the "intra-psychological plane" of mental functioning, we will postulate that the individual's participation in communicative encounters is a fruitful background for understanding not only human interaction but also mental phenomena. Following this perspective, we will deal with two issues at two different levels of inquiry: institutional discourse (Agar, 1985), that is, how people communicate in a specific social setting, and how what is said is construed to mean something in that particular setting, and, secondly, the problem of the relationship between the individual and the social context in which he/she is operating. This latter point is thus an epistemological and ontological issue about how, to put it metaphorically, to delimit the individual and the institution; where does the "mind" (or cognition) begin, and what is the sociogenetic origin of individual mental and linguistic action? This question, in turn, relates to the fundamental issue of what constitutes the unit of analysis for understanding human interaction and cognition.

Institutional Discourse: The Conscientious Objector

In the communicative tools—to use socio-historical language—that people use in modern societies, the traces of social institutions are highly visible. We describe ourselves and others with linguistic categories such as clients, customers, taxpayers, employees, patients, husbands, and all of these terms depict our positions vis-à-vis particular social institutions. The terms carry connotations that imply specific expectations and social obligations. The interactional power and the rights to make claims and argue one's point will differ between, let us say, a client at a social welfare agency and a bank customer, even though the very same individual may be involved in both settings and even though both encounters may involve the transfer of money from the institution to the individual (Cedersund & Säljö, in press).

The institutional setting that we will focus on with some observations is very special and operates on the basis of several tacit, as well as explicit, cultural and social assumptions. In Sweden, all men are called up for national service in the armed forces at about the age of 19 or 20. For those who do not want to carry arms, there is a special procedure which they can go through in order to be accepted as what is called a conscientious objector (CO). This formal procedure has, as its most decisive step, an interview, or a dialogue, with an "investigator," who is usually a psychologist, and who is to hear and scrutinize the arguments presented by the conscript and see if they are sufficient. The interviewer then writes a summary of the interview and this summary is presented to the conscript for his approval. As the next step, the psychologist makes a written recommendation to a board that takes the final decision. The decision generally follows the recommendation given by the psychologist.

This situation has all the necessary features to qualify as an instance of institutional discourse. The representative of the institution is a professional who is familiar with the logic of the procedure and who knows the legal definition of what gives an individual the right to be exempted from the obligation to carry arms. The conscript is a layman with a strong view but with more or less clear insights into how the institution operates and what counts as valid modes of argumentation. This difference in power and expertise is also clearly visible in the dialogues; the psychologist asks questions, controls and shifts topics, etc., and the conscript answers questions and subordinates himself to the initiatives taken (Adelswärd, in press).

The Interview

What the interviewer has to establish is whether the motives against carrying arms qualify as valid in a legal sense. The law prescribes that the individual is entitled to be exempted from using arms if it can be shown that carrying arms is so incompatible with his "firm personal conviction" that he will be unable to complete a military training in the armed forces. The most common basis for argumentation is from the religious stance, where the conscript claims that carrying arms is against his faith.

The interview may be carried out as part of the rather extensive enrollment procedure that individuals go through at the age of 18, that is, a year or two before one is called up for national service. It may, however, also take place when the conscript has already done part of his national service, and several of the interviews that we have access to are of this kind. In these interviews the conscript declares that after being enrolled into the armed forces he has found out that he sees it as conflicting with his beliefs to carry arms and to, for instance, fire at targets that look like human beings.

In all interviews the psychologist asks general questions about the motives for refusing to carry arms, about the denomination that the conscript belongs to, if any, and about his religious activities and attitudes. There are also standardized hypothetical and projective questions which the interviewee has to answer:

Whether or not, for instance, it would be legitimate to use arms in situations where he himself, his relatives, or innocent people would be threatened to be killed by aggressors, or if he could see himself joining a resistance movement if Sweden were to be occupied by a foreign army. An interesting aspect of these hypothetical questions is that the conscript is not asked how he would act in such situations, but rather what actions he would consider ethically justifiable. The interviewers are instructed to ensure that the conscripts realize this crucial distinction. It is crucial since if there are situations (of the kind presented below) in which the applicant would find it likely that he would use arms and in which he would find it ethically justifiable to do so, he may not qualify as a CO.

The Institution and the Individual: Who Tells the Story?

As commonly construed, the act of presenting oneself as a CO is a highly personal and individual one. The individual examines his conscience and arrives at the conclusion that it is impossible for him to carry arms and participate in practices that are preparatory to using arms against other people. What the psychologist has to establish is if it is reasonable to assume that this personal conviction will make it impossible for the conscript to complete the military service. The individual is facing an institutional norm, and he has to argue his case in order to be granted a particular definition, which, in turn, will have certain practical consequences. An interesting issue then is, how does one argue one's case and how are we epistemologically and theoretically to construe what the person is doing? What stories are being told in situations like this, and in what sense are they produced by individuals?

In our view, an analysis of the dynamics of such phenomena must rest on a mediational view of language (Vygotsky, 1986; Wertsch, 1985) and on a socio-historically founded understanding of the background of the particular process that is being studied. What we are observing in the dialogue between the two interlocutors is an artifact and cannot be sensibly understood without making reference to the wider set of circumstances in which they are acting, nor without reference to issues such as how individual responsibilities and duties are construed in language in a particular culture.

Even a very superficial analysis of the interaction in the interviews reveals that the stories that the two parties tell each other are grounded in institutional realities and in the definitions of human activities and motives endorsed by those institutions. By focusing on language, it becomes evident that the object of analysis has to be construed as what Shotter (1990), drawing on C.W. Mills, refers to as "accounting practices" that are used by the interlocutors and through which the particular course of events reported and discussed is filtered and rendered socially meaningful. There is thus an institutional basis for individual action and also—perhaps even more significantly—for individual identity construction (Shotter & Gergen, 1989).

The Use of Arms: Conflicting Accounting Practices

At one level the conflict between the CO and society could be construed as a simple one; through one of its institutions society expects every man to use arms, if necessary, to defend the country against aggressors, and the CO fails to live up to this norm. Value laden statements such as "the nation remaining a free country," "defending the Swedish lifestyle," and "democracy" are rhetorical tools that make up the ideology that results in the particular outcome that all men should carry arms. Similarly, there is an accounting practice which construes military service as a duty and as an act of solidarity; being in the army is nothing anyone desires, but one has to do it, and it is important that no one is let off. In the interviews, the psychologists introduce questions that draw on this social construction of military service as an act of solidarity; for instance, they ask how it would feel "to see all the others go to the front and defend the country, and be left alone at home" or maybe "to risk being seen as a coward or as someone who runs away from his duties."

On another level, however, this mode of construing the ideology advocating military service for all men is caught up in a web of conflicting assumptions and premises that are also recognized by society, and that are endorsed by rhetorically powerful social institutions such as a broad range of religious denominations and peace organizations. The CO's refusal to carry arms can thus be, and generally is, grounded in arguments that it is ethically unacceptable to use violence and to kill other people.

I(B:110):	I see. But that is when you made up your mind. How long have you been thinking about these issues?
Ivar:	Well, I guess I have been brought up with, well maybe not brought up...but at home they have sort of, sort of always said that "you shouldn't fight 'cause this here violence does not solve anything." (P: No, no) And then, I don't know, when I tried to play with toy warriors and soldiers, I guess I have felt like that then (P: Hm) not really in the same way 'cause I was smaller then but in principle yes...
I (111):	Hm (inaudible) at that age or something like that?
Ivar:	Yes, something...
I (112):	And you think that it's partially in one of these norms "do not fight, do not use violence, do not..."
Ivar:	Hm
I (113):	Is there anything that has inspired you to take this stand in this way, any other influences or something you've seen or read, or...personal experiences?

Ivar:	Yes, I've read, now that I have got, now that I've got older I have read a lot of things.
I (114):	What kind of literature?
Ivar:	Books
I (115):	Books about war then, or?
Ivar:	I have sort of read about different things. Yes, Gandhi, for instance, he succeeded quite well with his non-violence (P: Hm) what's it called (inaudible) in India. They got independent and such (P: Hm). And then it's obvious that one does not have to use arms then to achieve certain results.
I (116):	Hm. Anything else that has inspired you, you think?
Ivar:	Yes
I (117):	Events or experiences, or?
Ivar:	But no concrete sort of experience, I can't say that. It's sort of grown step by step (P: Hm) since I've sort of understood more and more (P: Hm) what it amounts to.

The principles of not fighting and not using violence when solving conflicts, and the reference to Gandhi as an alternative model for how to act in critical situations, are all arguments that have wide support not only from religious quarters and from peace organizations but also from many other significant social actors such as political parties, the women's movement, and the school and the preschool where the official rhetoric would be almost identical to the one used by Ivar in this excerpt. The ideological conflict between Ivar and society can thus be more conceived as an issue of internal tensions in "ways of world-making" (Goodman, 1978) within a complex society containing many different institutional accounting practices. What Ivar is arguing is not a position that society does not accept—most people would say that they do not want to kill or solve conflicts through violence—but rather one that is problematic in this particular sociocultural setting.

In a similar vein, it is too simplistic to construe what is happening in the institutional interview as a matter of the candidate CO presenting his faith and his arguments and the psychologist listening and recording what is being said. In many respects the encounter is highly interactional in nature and by asking questions and presenting different scenarios, the psychologist is an active co-teller of the story that the interviewee is presenting. In the following excerpt, the dialogue continues after the interviewer has introduced an ethical dilemma that is used to challenge the respondent's position that he would never be willing to use arms. The situation that is being talked about concerns whether it would be morally defensible to save lives by killing one individual, a soldier, who was about to kill many innocent people.

| I(C:92): | That is what I am thinking of. If you save the lives of many human beings by taking one, you may perhaps get gratitude from the people you've saved? |
| Magnus: | Oh yes (laughs) but I don't think I will feel any gratitude inside myself (P: |

No). Human gratitude that's probably good to have, sort of, but I don't really think...those are the kinds of things that wear off.

I (93):   But maybe then instead you see a number of innocent people, defenseless people lose their lives. How would you feel then?

Magnus: Yes, but I think that according to my faith, it can't be any other way.

I (94):   Can God intervene into this?

Magnus: Yes, 'cause he's done bigger miracles than that.

I (95):   Yes, so this is really not any difficult choice for you since you trust in God?

Magnus: Yes, you have to do that 'cause that's the only way out.

I (96):   Yes. You said that God has done miracles, have you seen that yourself?

Magnus: Yes, I've seen it.

I (97):   Let me hear.

By presenting the scenario and by intervening in the story told with comments and questions on how God can act and if he can do miracles, the interviewer actively contributes to the dialogue, and, in fact, to the moral position articulated by the conscript. In this sense narration is a genuinely social and dialogical affair. What the interviewer does is give the story of the CO the socioculturally appropriate form; the former assists the latter in telling a version of a moral position that will qualify as a basis for making a decision on whether the conviction felt is sufficient to be granted the status of a CO.

Magnus' interviewer pays considerable attention to the issue of how God can do miracles. He listens attentively to the long story that follows and he obviously construes this particular aspect as important and relevant for judging Magnus' moral convictions with respect to using arms. On the other hand, it is obvious that in other cases almost identical stories may be considered as irrelevant. In the following excerpt, another psychologist does not encourage a continuation of a story that would imply a possibility for the conscript to articulate his position with respect to how God can do miracles. Again the conscript, Anders, is facing the question as to how he would act if a soldier were about to take the lives of many innocent people.

Anders: I (laughs) am not...I can't say that I have sacrificed all those people (5 secs) I can't...I don't feel as if I'd do that but in such a situation, they must (4 secs) Either there must be a miracle, if you know what that is (giggles) but

I(A:174):   So you're hoping for miracles sort of?

Anders: Hoping, yes. I believe in miracles (P: I see, have you...) I have seen them myself.

I (175):   I see.

At first the psychologist is amused by Anders' introducing his belief in miracles in this particular setting. Then, when she realizes that he is serious, she cuts him short and does not encourage a continuation of the story. The issue of beliefs in miracles is not on her agenda.

An element of the communicative features of the dialogue is, therefore, that one has to produce a story that is relevant. To achieve this, the parties carry a joint responsibility, and they actively co-construe the version that will form the basis for the further processing of the case. As has been discussed by, for instance, Jönsson, Linell, and Säljö (in press; cf. Linell & Jönsson, 1991) in the case of police interrogations, the expert is often a very active agent in institutional hearings, and the story that is presented as an account of what has happened or, as in our case, of someone's views and opinions, is often heavily determined by the expert's contributions.

To become accepted as a CO, the candidate thus not only has to present his conviction, he also has to tell a story that makes a number of clear points. These points have to be institutionally appropriate and fit the criteria of what it means to have a deep conviction against carrying arms. In subtle ways the interviewer not only helps the interlocutor to construe an appropriate story, he also makes on-line decisions on what aspects of particular elements of the story are relevant and what are not. In the following excerpt, the interviewer wants the interviewee to tell what it was like being in the army and to comment on his experiences of life under those circumstances. The respondent however embarks on a rather lengthy story about his religious attitudes and values that he feels important as a background for understanding his position, but the interviewer intervenes and tries to restore the topic he wants discussed.

I (A:91):   What I was meaning to ask you here—that was really that, well you joined up,...and your reactions, and experiences, collective living and discipline and such.

Carl: Yes, I was meaning to go into that.

I (92):   Yes, I see, I'm sorry.

Carl: Um. No, but, as I said, as you grew older you started to...one started to learn more and most of all to learn more about people. And...I can sort of say that when I was at that age, round 17, 18 years old, then it was often...one had the attitude that religion, one really looked down on that. One saw it almost as a weakness, sort of.

I (93):   In other people?

Carl: Yes, now I can say that now I see it in a different way. I see it as a strength in people. I'm not a believer myself in the conventional sense (P: No), but I value those values about loving your fellow human being and such that religion means. I, I think that if religion is the conscience of mankind and then it in some way shows us something that we all have inside ourselves, a lot of unwritten laws that—maybe got learned too—Yes, they are probably learned—this here that one is to be kind, one should act towards others as one wants to be acted towards, and...yes what else should I say. Yes all these values...which religion stands for. Most importantly then love of your fellow human being then and yes...

I (94):   (pause) If we think about, if we stick to eh...if we, if I should explain a bit how I have thought that we keep a bit to precisely this thing—the enrollment procedure/military service.

Love of humanity and the necessity of acting in ways that you yourself would like others to act towards you, although central topics in Carl's discourse and major reasons why he refuses to carry arms, are not of interest for the institutional process. Only when these values form part of an ideology that prevents the person from using arms will these rhetorical tools gain some significance. To argue at a general level for the value of these principles is thus not the appropriate form of discourse even though this would be relevant in, for instance, a political debate or in a discussion between friends.

The interviews contain many examples of how the appropriate coherence of a story and the socioculturally relevant interpretation of how one makes one's point, have to be embedded in the institutional discursive patterns in specific ways in order to be recognized. It is thus not only the contents of the arguments or their form which are the sole determinants of their relevance to the issue. Rather, it is a subtle combination of what is said, how it is said, and in what context it is said. The arguments that are valid should have certain features, and general complaints or accusations against the army do not count. In the following passage, Carl voices his criticism of the claim made by the army when referring to itself as "Sweden's biggest peace movement." He argues that what it in fact does is systematically create contempt of the people of another nation.

Carl:	Yes, there was an awful lot [of conflicts] (laughs)...I can exemplify with such a thing as there is an awful lot of discussion about Ivan, the Russians, I mean.
I (A:124):	Yes...
Carl:	Yes, just that it was such a stupid thing. First we are a yes, the Swedish army is called the biggest peace organization in Sweden (P: Um). In certain situations they say that. They, they argue that themselves too—certain people and then it doesn't sound right then that one...'cause it's all really about creating contempt towards another people, like the Russians then. That one sort of really did not know anything about more than just this here then that one felt, they argued that they were a threat, sort of. They always all the time assumed that it was from the East that the threat would come, sort of, and they showed a lot of films about how they behave sort of (P: Mm) "this is what they do," sort of (P: Mm). And I just thought it was wrong, first then starting out by insisting (P: Mm) that it is some kind of peace organization, and then go out and run down a people and teach a contempt of a people (P: Hm). That doesn't fit at all, it doesn't.
I (125):	I see. But if we think about that we stick for a while to this here change at the camp or at your regiment—You thought this (a set of conflicts that involved fights and threats between soldiers) was difficult if I understand you correctly.
Carl:	No, that situation was not specific to me 'cause that is something that happens to everyone.

Thus even though the attitudes created by the army—according to Carl—against other people are essential for his argumentation and for his refusal to carry arms, they are not immediately relevant to the psychologist or the institutional actor.

Carl's objections do not form a valid basis for becoming defined as a CO, and therefore the psychologist in his position as a representative of the institution closes the topic.

The fact that the particular point of how Carl experienced life in the army is repeatedly brought back into the discussion can be explained by the psychologist's attempt to check that refusing to carry arms is not a result of the conscript's inability to cope with the not too comfortable conditions of life in the army, or that he might have had problems with his fellow soldiers. Should this be the case, Carl would not qualify as a CO. The very last remark by Carl in the excerpt above is very significant in the particular institutional context that this dialogue takes place. What Carl is doing here is making a conversational move that is grounded in his understanding of the fact that you have problems of that kind with the officers, with living conditions in large dormitories in regimental buildings, or with fellow soldiers, will not help you to achieve the definition of a CO. On the contrary, difficulties of this kind are bound to raise suspicions as to why you want to be a CO. By arguing that those kinds of difficulties are something that everyone has to expect under those circumstance, Carl is in fact "making known" (Rommetveit, 1974) that he is not building his argumentation on those incidents.

Discussion

To understand the sociogenesis of mind, it is, in our view, important to pay attention to the role of institutions in the mediation of reality and their capacity to shape our linguistic tools and discursive practices. When the representative of the institution and the conscript interact, they are not free agents who ask questions and formulate answers on their own. They are operating in an institutional setting with specific assumptions about how arguments should be construed in order to be considered valid and to the point. The particular form of dialogicality—to use Bakhtinian language—that is being established is achieved within an institutional voice (cf. Wertsch, 1990) that is invoked by the interviewer. The latter uses the conceptual framework of the institution to control the dialogue and to elicit statements that are relevant for arriving at a decision. The collective nature of this "social language" (Bakhtin, 1986) is obvious, and the psychologist falls back on discursive forms that are not his own inventions but have a long tradition and do a concrete job in society.

On the other hand, the conscript is also acting within the framework of a collectively construed version of the world. Just as the psychologist "rents meaning" (Holquist, 1981) from an institution, the CO enters into a language and uses arguments that are institutionally grounded and collective in nature. By referring to the Bible and to his religious conviction, and by using this background as a discursive resource in his argumentation, the interaction in fact becomes a dialogue between different institutional realities. In a very real sense, this reduces the asymmetric nature of the dialogue (Linell & Luckmann, 1991). Expressed differently, the CO's rhetorical position is considered reasonable by the fact that it is grounded in a powerful social institution whose line of argumentation has to be recognized. The position of the conscript is defended by the presence of an institution which provides the tools for arguing that one should not have to use arms.

The individual is thus using rhetorical genres and accounting practices as a resource from which to argue a position. At the same time it is obvious that accounting practices are dynamic and change as they are continuously reproduced and negotiated in social encounters. An interesting shift in perspectivization of the ideological meaning of becoming a CO in Sweden is visible if one compares the relevant legal documents from 1966, 1978, and 1991 respectively. In 1966, it was stated that the conscript should be exempted from joining the armed forces if "the use of arms against another person is incompatible with the serious personal conviction of the conscript and would lead to a deep moral conflict for him" (SFS, 1966, p. 413; our translation). What is at stake here is the individual and his moral conviction. In 1978, on the other hand, the law has, as it were, de-moralized the issue, and it is sufficient if the personal conviction of the conscript will make it difficult for him to complete his military service. Thus, the individual will be granted status as a conscientious objector "if it can be assumed that the use of arms against another person is so incompatible with the firm personal conviction of the conscript that he will be unable to do his military service." (SFS, 1978, p. 524; our translation). This change in perspectivization between 1966 and 1978, as mirrored in the legal documents, has moved the issue from being one of moral conflicts within individuals to one of pragmatic problems of functioning within an institution, the army. In 1991, finally, the mobilization of rhetorical resources from peace organizations and activist groups has resulted in a situation where the interview has been abolished as part of the enrollment procedures. The conscript now only has to answer a set of standardized questions, in writing, in which he presents his arguments for refusing to carry arms. And acceptable formulations of the arguments are readily available in a number of books and pamphlets published by peace activist organizations.

The rhetorical conflicts between institutions, and the successive mobilization of arguments and counter-arguments over time, has made the discourse about when someone should be exempted from using arms socially and ideologically visible, and an arena in which the problematic notion of "speaker," discussed by Goffman (1981), is easily recognized. In these rhetorical conflicts two speakers argue, both as "authors" and as "principals." In Goffman's language, the "author" selects the views being expressed and he gives them a linguistic form in a communicative context. The "principal," on the other hand, is the person or the institution that is the ultimate source behind the particular view of reality endorsed. The speaker's individual voice and his way of presenting his arguments are thus discursively intertwined with those of a principal. As a consequence, and using Goffman's language, the individual in his role as "speaker" in this context is no longer necessarily the "author" of his own position. His conviction is formulated in a language provided by a "we," by a principal, with which he at the same time can identify himself.

In our view, our observations illustrate how language and cognition are socioculturally situated. It is by accepting the simultaneous presence of institutions and individuals that communicative encounters in institutional realities can be fruitfully explored and understood. Communication is thus neither an individual act, nor completely determined by features in the situation or social structure. The agency of the individual *and* the constraints of sociocultural institutions somehow have to be conceptually accounted for if we are to understand human communication in complex societies.

References

Adelswärd, V. (in press), Interviewer styles—on interactive strategies in professional interviews. In A. Grindsted, et al. (eds.), *Language for special purposes/ Fachsprachliche Kommunikation.* Tübingen: G. Narr Verlag.

Agar, M. (1985), Institutional discourse. *Text,* 5, 147-168.

Bakhtin, M.M. (1986), *Speech genres and other late essays.* Austin, TX: University of Texas Press.

Cedersund, E., & Säljö, R. Bureaucratic discourse, conversational space and the concept of voice. *Semiotica* (in press).

Goffman, E. (1981), *Forms of talk.* Philadelphia, PA: University of Philadelphia Press.

Goodman, N. (1978), *Ways of worldmaking.* Indianapolis, IN: Hackett.

Holquist, M. (1981), The politics of representation. In S. Greenblatt (ed.), *Allegory in representation.* (pp. 163-183). Baltimore, MD: Johns Hopkins University Press.

Jönsson, L., Linell, P., & Säljö, R. Reformulating the past. Remembering in the police-interrogation. *Activity Theory* (in press).

Linell, P., & Jönsson, L. (1991), Suspect stories: Perspective-setting in an asymmetrical situation. In I. Marková & K. Foppa (eds.), *Asymmetries in dialogue.* (pp. 75-100). Hemel Hempstead: Harvester Wheatsheaf.

Linell, P., & Luckmann, T. (1991), Asymmetries in dialogue: Some conceptual preliminaries. In I. Marková & K. Foppa (eds.), *Asymmetries in dialogue.* (pp. 1-19). Hemel Hempstead: Harvester Wheatsheaf.

Luckmann, T. Prolegomena to a social theory of communicative genres: In memory of Toussaint Hocevar. In A. Lokar (ed.), *Essays in memory of Toussaint Hocevar, Slovene Studies,* in press.

Rommetveit, R. (1974), *On message structure.* London: Wiley.

SFS (1966:413), *Lagen om vapenfri tjänst* [The law about national service for conscripts refusing to carry arms].

SFS (1978:524), *Lag om ändring i lagen (1966:413) om vapenfri tjänst* [Law concerning change in the law (1966:413) about national service for conscripts who refuse to carry arms].

SFS (1991:719), *Lag om ändring i lagen (1966:413) om vapenfritjänst* [Law concerning change in the law about national service for conscripts who refuse to carry arms].

Shotter, J. (1990), The social construction of remembering and forgetting. In Middleton D. & Edwards D. (eds.), *Collective remembering.* (pp. 120-138). London: Sage.

Shotter, J., & Gergen, K. (eds.) (1989), *Texts of identity.* London: Sage.

Vygotsky, L.S. (1986), *Thought and language.* Cambridge, MA: MIT Press.

Wertsch, J. (1985), *Vygotsky and the social formation of mind.* Cambridge: Cambridge University Press.

Wertsch, J. (1990), *Voices of the mind.* Cambridge: Cambridge University Press.

Note

1. The data for this study consists of 20 authentic interviews conducted by four interviewers (referred to as A, B, C, and D). All the interviewers' turns are numbered.

12. Sociogenesis and Children's Pretend Play: A Variation on Vygotskian Themes

Ed Elbers

In a recent study, Lev Vygotsky's intellectual work has been characterized as motivated by a "quest for synthesis" (Van der Veer & Valsiner, 1991). Vygotsky possessed a broad knowledge of the psychological ideas of his time; he was internationally oriented and personally acquainted with many psychologists outside the Soviet Union. His persistent concern was to transcend the contemporary state of knowledge in psychology and to bring to a synthesis the theoretical ideas which he found in the intellectual community of the 1920s and 1930s. He did this by creating novel ideas in an effort to bring others' intellectual achievements together. Van der Veer and Valsiner write that "his best-known contributions...are all reflections on and developments of the original work of his predecessors and contemporaries" (1991, p. 397). Among these "best-known contributions" is Vygotsky's theory of sociogenesis, which he borrowed to a large extent from Pierre Janet (Van der Veer & Valsiner, 1988).

The results of this persevering "quest for synthesis" are nonetheless mostly fragmentary. Vygotsky was a restless thinker whose creativity and passionate interest in psychology led him, in his short life, to many subjects and areas. His intellectual legacy lacks cohesiveness and is unfinished. One reason for this is that Vygotsky was an inspired speaker who, in his lectures, developed many brilliant and innovative thoughts which he never developed further or finished. Some of these thoughts have been preserved because somebody among the audience kept stenographic notes, which were later transcribed and published.

In this chapter, I shall be concerned with some of these unfinished and inconsistent themes. In particular, I shall reflect on a tension in Vygotsky's work between his cultural-historical theory and his idea of intellectual development as involving novelty construction. In the first part of this chapter, I shall argue that, in Vygotsky's work, two themes can be heard, which he never really succeeded in bringing into harmony. Many current interpretations of his theory focus on one theme only: in doing so, they ignore part of Vygotsky's writings. They emphasize the transmission of knowledge from adults to children, but they neglect children's own contribution to their development. I shall argue that Vygotsky's lecture on play, dating from the very end of his life, brings together the two themes in an interesting way (Vygotsky, 1933/1976). The second part of this chapter is a variation based on these Vygotskian themes and has in particular been inspired by Vygotsky's text on play. It presents observations of children's pretend play. I shall show that children's pretend play is not to be considered merely a developmental phenomenon, but that it has an impact beyond this and contributes to the re-creation of the culture. Elaborating on Vygotsky's unfinished work, I shall try to show the interdependency of ontogenetic and sociogenetic processes.

Vygotskian Themes

Vygotsky's Theory of Sociogenesis

In his theory of sociogenesis, Vygotsky connected individual development with cultural historical development. A central part in this theory is the idea that the higher psychological functions are originally social: social relations underlie mental processes such as thinking, reasoning, remembering, and volition. Vygotsky (1930/1978, p. 57) expressed his theory of sociogenesis in a "general genetic law of cultural development": "Every function in the child's cultural development appears twice: first, on the social level, and later, on the individual level; first, *between* people (*interpsychological*), and then *inside* the child (*intrapsychological*)."

As Van der Veer and Valsiner (1988) have shown, Vygotsky, in forging his ideas on the development of the higher psychological functions, leaned heavily on Janet. Both Janet and Vygotsky viewed the intellectual functions as the result of the application of social activities to oneself. Vygotsky went beyond Janet in emphasizing the role of signs and social tools as mediators in the development of these functions. Moreover, unlike Janet, Vygotsky studied the internalization of social activities in children (Van der Veer & Valsiner, 1988).

In his texts on sociogenesis and internalization, Vygotsky did not describe a symmetric relationship between equal collaborators. Rather, he envisaged the interaction and cooperation of children with more experienced members of the culture. In their cooperation with adults, children learn to use symbolic means for the regulation of their behavior. These means are then internalized and become psychological abilities. The external dialogue between a child and an adult is internalized and this process of internalization creates the possibilities for the child to enter into an internal dialogue. Dyadic interaction between children and adults, in many parts of Vygotsky's work, is presented as the mechanism of the psychological transmission of the culture from one generation to the next.

The internalization process makes available to the child activities and skills which already exist in the culture: "The internalization of socially rooted and historically developed activities is the distinguishing feature of human psychology" (Vygotsky, 1930/1978, p. 57). Vygotsky's vision went so far as to believe in a progressive growth of human psychological capacities in history. This growth was, he believed, a result of the development of the culture at large, leading from the primitive mentality in pre-literate societies to scientific and logical thought in industrialized societies (Van der Veer & Valsiner, 1991).

In order to grasp what happens in the interaction between adult and child, Vygotsky coined the concept of the "zone of proximal development." The zone of proximal development is defined as: "the difference between the mental age of a child derived from the child's solitary performance and his or her performance when assisted by an adult" (Kozulin, 1990, p. 202). In formulating this notion, Vygotsky pointed to a level of potential development: a zone of activities which are still beyond the child's capacity for independent performance, but which he or she can carry out with the help of a more experienced member of the culture. The zone of proximal development covers activities that the child is about to master. It shows the direction that the child's development will take.

The concepts of internalization and the zone of proximal development form one theme in Vygotsky's theory: they depict the way the culture is transmitted to children. The idea of a zone of proximal development is easily applicable to the field of education. The recent popularity of Vygotsky has resulted in empirical studies in fields such as adult-child interaction (e.g., Wertsch, 1985) and instruction (e.g., Van Parreren & Carpay, 1980). Vygotsky's theory, in the light of this theme, is often posed against Piaget's: the former, unlike the latter, can provide a theoretical base for including social context variables in the study of human development.

If this was all Vygotsky had to say about the process of children's cultural socialization, there would be a dissatisfying aspect to Vygotsky's theory. Van der Veer and Valsiner (1991, Ch. 13) criticize this part of Vygotsky's psychology quite rightly in their discussion of the concept of the zone of proximal development and Vygotsky's attempts to predict development. If we view development only as the adoption of the existing culture by the child and if we take the adults' role to be the passing on of the cultural experience to the younger generation, then the possibilities of the younger generation are confined by the limitations of the existing culture. In that case, a new generation can never go beyond the possibilities of a former generation. Developing is just copying what is already available (cf. Van der Veer & Valsiner, 1991, p. 343).

However, Vygotsky's theory of sociogenesis should be read in the context of an ambiguity in his writings (for a discussion of this ambiguity, see

Davydov & Radzikhovskii, 1985; Elbers, Maier, Hoekstra, & Hoogsteder, 1992; Wertsch, 1985). Vygotsky's ambiguity is conspicuously present in his work *Foundations of Paedology,* a series of lectures, delivered in 1931 and after, and published in 1935 after Vygotsky's death. (I base my account on Van der Veer and Valsiner, who give an extended summary of this text in chapter 12 of their 1991 book). In this text, also transcribed from stenographic records, Vygotsky begins by explaining the law of sociogenesis and the origin of the higher mental functions in the child's cooperation with others. In talking about cooperation with others, Vygotsky explains that adults represent ideal forms or possible end products of development. These ideals guide the child's interaction with others and with the world.

Then, another theme is introduced in the *Foundations of Paedology* (Van der Veer & Valsiner, 1991, p. 315ff.), which emphasizes, not the reproduction of the existing culture in the child, but the creation of novelty. Vygotsky, in these passages, reflects on the role of the child's personal history. A child's past experiences, he argues, do not determine development, because, in that case, there would be no novelty. They guide the child's actions and the child's construction of what Vygotsky calls the "new present" (Van der Veer & Valsiner, 1991, p. 310). Vygotsky emphasizes that the environment has no direct influence on the child. The working of the environment, both the social and the physical, is mediated through the child's signification, or, as we would say nowadays, his or her definition or perception of the environment. It is "the personally meaningful experience" of the environment which guides the process of development of a child (cf. Van der Veer & Valsiner, 1991, p. 317, who point out that this idea in Vygotsky's writings has been borrowed from William Stern).

This means that two themes appear in Vygotsky's texts. The first theme is the idea of the child's appropriation of the existing culture and the transfer of cultural experience from one generation to the next. A concentration on this theme leads easily to a neglect of the child's own contribution to his or her development. The second theme treats the child's construction of meaning in his or her life; it is the theme of his or her interpretation of the environment and the creation of novelty. These two themes deal with child development in quite different, not to say opposing, ways.

Following Vygotsky's motive for a "quest for synthesis," the burden is on us to connect these loose ends and try to elaborate a theory of sociogenesis in which the child's contribution to socialization is taken into account. Vygotsky's theory of play (Vygotsky, 1933/1976, 1933/1978) combines the two themes in a promising way. Before discussing Vygotsky's text on play, I will show the consequences of ignoring the second theme in Vygotsky.

Vygotsky himself did not present empirical studies of internalization. In recent years, James V. Wertsch took this task upon himself (a review in Wertsch, 1985). In a cross-sectional study, he analyzed how mothers helped their small children to do a puzzle task. The different degrees to which children of various ages were dependent on their mothers' assistance was interpreted by Wertsch as a development from "other regulation" to "self-regulation" (Wertsch, 1979). However, Wertsch did not analyze what means the children themselves bring into the field for making the step from an inadequate level of understanding to a more advanced one. In describing the mother as "luring" the child into her situation definition, Wertsch suggests that children are passively led into making correct performances. In Wertsch's view, understanding is the result of guided performance, instead of the product of a joint effort by mother and child (for a critique of Wertsch's adult-child interaction research, see Elbers, 1991a, 1991b; Elbers et al. 1992; Maier, Elbers, Hoekstra, & Hoogsteder, 1992; Wertsch's latest publications come quite close to the view expressed in the present chapter, cf. Kanner & Wertsch, 1991).

Criticizing Wertsch's study, Elbers, Maier, Hoekstra, and Hoogsteder (1990, 1992) observed parent-child dyads collaborating in a task similar to the task used by Wertsch (1979). We observed children who were very actively involved in these interactions. They took initiatives, they questioned the adults' instructions, and they sometimes refused to follow the lead of the adult; in short, they participated significantly in the shaping of the interpersonal level and the solution of the task. The internalization process does not rest on "other regulation," in which the child passively accepts the mother's situation definition, but on "joint regulation" of the task by two active collaborators. Wertsch (1979, 1985), obviously, has been guided by the cultural transmission theme in Vygotsky, whereas Elbers et al. (1992) have made an attempt to include the children's contribution to their own development in the analysis.

Now, my argument has been developed sufficiently to make two proposals. First, Vygotsky's theory of sociogenesis is not to be read as a theory of cultural transmission, but as a theory of children's construction of their development in the context of social relationships. In putting less emphasis on the cultural transmission theme, space has been made to acknowledge the contribution of the child. The second proposal is that the internalization process does not rest solely on children's interaction with adults, but also on their relationship with peers. This second claim may be deemed problematic, because Vygotsky places his explications of the law of sociogenesis in the context of asymmetric processes of cooperation between adults and children. However, in one major text, Vygotsky discusses the contribution of children's collective play to development. We now turn to a discussion of this text: the study of children's imaginary re-creation of reality in their play will point the way to a less ambivalent approach to the cultural socialization of children.

Vygotsky's Theory of Play

Vygotsky's article, "Play and Its Role in the Mental Development of the Child," is based on a transcription from a stenographic record of a lecture given in 1933 (Vygotsky 1933/1976, 1933/1978). Vygotsky's ideas on play are the outcome of his reading of the works of Karl Groos, Charlotte Bühler, Kurt Lewin, Jean Piaget, and others. Van der Veer and Valsiner (1991, p. 345) mention Vygotsky's text on play only briefly and read it as an expression of his interest in imitation. In my opinion, however, its importance goes beyond this, if it is viewed in the context of Vygotsky's ambivalence and adherence to the two themes.

Vygotsky, who restricts himself globally to a discussion of pretense, posits play as an intermediary stage between the sensorimotor activities of the infant and the thinking and imagination of the adolescent. Infants are still bound to the immediate situation: they cannot distance themselves from the stimuli in the environment. They are, in a sense, left to the mercy of the circumstances. However, as children grow up, they develop means to reflect and mentally represent the world. Play is "the first manifestation of the child's emancipation from situational constraints" (1933/1978, p. 99). The end result of this process is in the ability of abstract thought, inner speech, and imagination, found in the adolescent.

As an intermediary stage, play combines characteristics of the two stages it bridges. The function of play is reflection, but this reflection does not take the form of thinking or mental imagination, but it still needs the support of real objects, of familiar actions, and of well-known situations. For example, children use a piece of wood as a doll, or, in representing horse riding, they stamp with a foot and use a stick to sit on as on a horse. In play, children create a situation of meaning in which objects and actions no longer have their normal meaning, but are subordinate to the meaning given to them in the child's fantasy.

According to Vygotsky's theory, the creative element in play increases as children grow older. Young children playing father and mother may still copy their own father's and mother's behavior, but, as they get older, the playful representation of family life will take a freer and more creative form. They will model their play less on examples than on more general ideas of what parents are. There is a move from the imitative character of the young child's play, characterized by Vygotsky as "memory in action" (1933/1978, p. 103), to the active fantasy of the older child and adolescent.

The function of play is reflection. How is this to be understood? Vygotsky points to a paradox in play. On the one hand, it is free: children can represent and play anything. On the other hand, an essential characteristic of play is the adoption of rules and the compliance with these rules. A child, playing mother, must obey the rules of maternal behavior, at least insofar as the child knows and understands these rules. An important aspect of playing, therefore, is to reflect on social rules.

Vygotsky refers to James Sully (1896), who observed two sisters (5 and 7 years old) playing at being sisters. Vygotsky comments that, in real life, the children behave without thinking, but in the play situation, they try to be what they think sisters should be. They walk hand in hand and they dress and talk in the same manner; in short, they do their best to create a difference between themselves and the rest of the world. Sameness is an essential part of sister-hood, and it is this aspect they reflect on in their play. "As a result of playing the child comes to understand that sisters possess a different relationship to each other than to other people. What passes unnoticed by the child in real life, becomes a rule of behavior in play" (1933/1978. p. 95).

Here, Vygotsky singles out as an essential aspect of play, that children enact roles and by doing so, learn to understand the characteristics and implications of these roles. Moreover, they learn to see and understand what, in real life, goes without speaking. They become aware of their own and other persons' places in the network of social relationships, not because they are taught but by representing these roles in play. This process of learning social roles and rules does not entail a mere copying of these roles. For instance, in playing sisters they make real discoveries about what it means to be sisters. Of course, real everyday life provides them also with a lot of opportunities to learn the meaning of sisterhood: for instance, their parents may tell them not to quarrel "because you are sisters." But play adds to these learning experiences. In play, children can reflect freely on the roles of sisters, they can experiment with these roles, and explore their possibilities and limitations; in short, they can discover the social implications of the roles of sisters. In doing so, they transcend their particular experiences as sisters. It is a reflection, not in abstract thought, but in the form of drama.

If play is considered this way, it is a preparation for real life. What children can do now in play, they can do in real life tomorrow. Or, as Vygotsky states in a classical quotation:

> In play a child is always above his average age, above his daily behaviour; in play it is as though he were a head taller than himself. As in the focus of a magnifying glass, play contains all developmental tendencies in a condensed form; in play it is as though the child were trying to jump above the level of his normal behaviour. (1933/1976, p. 552)

Apart from learning specific social roles, play also promotes rule learning in a more general sense. In developing his argument, Vygotsky quotes Piaget's (1932) studies of children's moral development approvingly. Piaget described a stage of moral realism in children's construction of morality. In this stage, they do not discern between laws of nature and moral rules.

According to Piaget's theory, in mutual cooperation children come to understand that moral rules have a different status from laws of nature. Vygotsky points out that, in situations of playful interaction, with all the conflicts and negotiations involved, children learn that people, including themselves, have a part in the establishment of moral and social rules. In their play, by negotiating about rules and deciding to keep to these rules, children learn that social and moral rules are changeable and that people have to accept them before they are applied.

Thus far, many aspects of Vygotsky's theory of play concur with the views of modern theorists of children's pretend play (see reviews by Fein, 1981; Fein & Kohlberg, 1987; Rubin, Fein & Vandenburg, 1983).

Bruner (1976) and Sutton-Smith (1979), for example, view the creation of novelty and flexibility as an important function of play. When children create an imaginary situation, they can discover and explore new combinations and routes of behavior. These explorations result in a repertoire of behavioral alternatives children can draw from in future situations in real life.

Bateson (1956) emphasized the meta-communicative learning going on in pretend play. He did not so much attribute importance to the actual roles children enact as to the "deutero-learning." In their play, children learn about social roles, not only about particular social roles, but rather about the concept of role itself. In his studies of children's games, Piaget (1932) argues that children, in disputes and negotiations, learn that social rules are not natural, but rest on conventions and traditions, and that the contents of these rules can in part be changed or varied.

Leaning on G.H. Mead (1934), Fein (1984) views play as contributing to the creation of the child's "self." Play involves the imitation of a diversity of social roles. In playing another person, a child appropriates the other's perspective and makes it part of his or her repertoire. In this manner, the child comes to understand the variety of perspectives in the social world and becomes aware of its "self" as a unique part in the interactions with others. Pretend play enacts "imagined encounters" with others. "As these imagined encounters continue, the child's grasp of 'others' becomes organized internally (as well as externally) and as these others become organized, they come differentiated from the 'self' while the 'self' organizes its relation to these others" (Fein, 1984, p. 128).

These modern perspectives on play are compatible with Vygotsky's view. However, Vygotsky goes beyond these positions by comparing play with instruction and using the concept of the zone of proximal development in characterizing both play and instruction: "Play is the source of development and creates the zone of proximal development" (1933/1976, p. 552). Moreover, Vygotsky views instruction at school as a continuation of the pretend play in the preschool period.

It may come as a surprise that Vygotsky characterizes play with the concept of the zone of proximal development. In doing so, Vygotsky clarifies his ideas of both instruction and play. It becomes clear that the idea of a zone of proximal development is not to be interpreted merely as an educational concept. The zone of proximal development is not just the creation of the adult in an attempt to help the child in intellectually mastering a task. In most studies of internalization in adult-child interaction, however, the zone has been considered in this way (Elbers, 1991a, 1991b; Elbers et al., 1992). The child's zone of proximal development should rather be interpreted as the product of the joint activity of the parent and the child.

Moreover, Vygotsky gives play a more privileged place in children's development than instruction. In instruction, children learn intellectual competencies, but play is functional in the formation of the whole personality. In play, children create their motives, their ideals, and their social expectations. They anticipate their future development, not as mere cognitive beings, but as persons (Vygotsky, 1933/1976, p. 552).

In connecting both play and instruction to the zone of proximal development, Vygotsky makes it clear that these activities share a number of characteristics. Now it is easy to see how the two themes of his work are represented in Vygotsky's interpretation of instruction and play. Instruction and play combine both the spontaneous contribution by the child to development and the transmission of the culture to the child. Instruction does not merely involve the transmission of the culture from adults to children; it asks for a creative contribution from the children. And the function of play is not merely in promoting the development of the individual child, but also in contributing to the reproduction of the culture.

I will now present observations of children's play which have been inspired by Vygotsky's article on play. In analyzing these observations, I will try to show, following Vygotsky, that children's pretend play is not just the copying of existing roles, but goes beyond this and contributes to the social change of these roles.

Variation: Pretend Play and the Creation of Culture

I would like to present the transcription of a play sequence in which two children play school. I have chosen this dialogue from a number of audio-recordings I made of my own children and their friends. I started recording their play for sentimental reasons, because I wanted, as a father, to register my children's conversations. Only later did I realize that the recordings could be used for analyzing their playful representation of the world. Among the recordings, I found three recordings that, as a part of the registered play interactions, contain sequences of school play.

These recordings were made without the children being aware of it. Once I had noticed that the children had started playing, I put a small audiorecorder in the room in an inconspicuous place, and left the room. The children knew that I sometimes made sound recordings of them. However, they were usually so absorbed in their play that they did not perceive what I did. I am pretty sure that, in the cases of school play, they did not notice the recording device. There is no conversation on the recordings which indicates that they have realized that their play was being recorded.

An obvious disadvantage adheres to the use of audiorecording when trying to register children's social play. Other studies of play rest on notes made while directly observing play (e.g., Piaget, 1932) or on videotapes (e.g., Fein, 1984). These methods allow a combination of verbal and behavioral observations. My audiorecordings, of course, only register the verbal interaction and the noises produced by the children's movements and their manipulation of toys. However, I have often seen these children playing. I am so familiar with the way they interact that I can reconstruct much of the behavioral context of their utterances. Moreover, as these children at the time of the recordings were between 6 (in fact, close to 7) and 9 years old, the verbal part of these interactions was predominant, although an important part of the play was the handling of toys and other objects. The use of audiorecordings has also an advantage. Because the observations have been made without the children's knowledge, they show spontaneous play uncontaminated by the presence of adults. These recordings give access to a children's world uninfluenced by adults and in which real adults may not be welcome.

Three recordings contain children's representations of school life. In two of the three play sessions the children played with Playmobil figures. The Playmobil figures are toy men and women, boys and girls, which could be provided with various clothes and props (hats, satchels, tools), a lot of animals of many kinds, and the furniture for a hospital, school, house, zoo, etc. The children usually sat on the floor and used the Playmobil figures to impersonate the roles (e.g., teachers, pupils, mothers); they moved and manipulated them and lent their voices to the persons represented by the figures. In these two interactions, the children were girls (respectively 6 years, 10 months and 7 years, 9 months; and 7 years, 3 months and 8 years, 11 months). The third dialogue shows a more direct form of pretend play in which two girls (9 years, 1 month and 9 years, 7 months) played teacher and pupil and used various objects such as pencils, paper, and exercise books.

My children and their friends used to engage in long sequences of pretend play, mostly with the Playmobil material, including the building of houses and castles. Most studies of pretend play involve children younger than 6 years. Some investigators of play locate the end of pretend play around the age of 6

(Fein & Kohlberg, 1987). Although it is true that pretense is gradually replaced by games during child development (Rubin et al., 1983), in my experience children older than 6 years of age engage in social pretend play with much enthusiasm.

The surprising thing is that, in these three play dialogues, no single instructive interaction has been represented. Although the children play teacher and pupils, they do not play teaching. The very heart of school life: learning, teaching, and instructive dialogue, is absent. The theme is rather the social life surrounding learning, and the social patterns and frames of interaction in which teaching and learning occur.

I have chosen one of these play sequences for further analysis. The appendix gives excerpts from this play sequence of Margreet (7 years, 9 months) and Elisabeth (6 years, 10 months) playing with the Playmobil figures. The recording has been transcribed and translated from Dutch into English. All passages of school play from this transcription have been included in the appendix. The children dressed some figures as Indians, and they put a number of wild animals on or in a box. Margreet and Elisabeth manipulated the figures and while doing so lent their voice to the particular figure. During the interaction Margreet and Elisabeth negotiated repeatedly about the figures that each of them will manipulate and about the places of the various figures. Moreover, they discussed how to dress the schoolchildren in order to distinguish them from the other figures (using hats, satchels).

In transcribing this interaction I have indicated the various impersonations of the children. The children's utterances have been indicated with just M (for Margreet) and E (for Elisabeth), if they were only preparing the course of the play and negotiating about themes and roles. During the school scenes Margreet is mostly the teacher (MT) and Elisabeth the schoolchild (EC), although Elisabeth occasionally takes the role of the teacher (ET) and Margreet the role of a child (MC), in one passage identified as Whitey (MW). Of course, the ascription of roles is based on my interpretation, but the interpretation was facilitated because the children use various distortions of their voices in impersonating the roles of teacher and pupils.

The school theme is first mentioned by Margreet who proposes to make a school for the Indian children (Line 1). The Indian chief brings the children to school in a boat (8–18); the dangers of the wild animals are pointed out (8–12; 35–36; 98–101). Several themes from life at school are represented in the play interaction:

- the teacher attempts to start a normal school day, an uncooperative child (61–64; 88–95);
- talking children and the reaction of the teacher (30–35; 84–85; 124–136);
- a child being late (39–40);

- children being privileged as monitors (77–81; 114–116);
- sick children (46–51; 53–59; 68–69; 72–73; 85–87; 113);
- the distribution of desks (30–35; 54; 60; 117);
- the toilet episode, in which the pupil gets locked up in the toilet (88–101).

It is apparent from this list of themes that the children have a fancy for representing interruptions in school life: they invent episodes which keep the pupils from learning. These episodes are violations of the rules and normal practices at school.

Example 1 (Lines 88–101):
MT: Children, sit down.
EC: I have to go to the toilet, Miss.
MT: Now, children, be quiet.
EC: I have to go to the toilet.
MT: I want to tell you something.
EC: (loud) I have to go to the toilet!
M: (chuckles) Wait a second.
EC: (with emphasis) Miss, I have to go to the toilet!!
MT: Okay, you can go.
EC: (cheekily) Where is it? (laughs)
MT: Over there, under that box, the one with the animals on, where the dangerous animals... (chuckles) under there.
EC: Really?
MT: Yes.

The teacher wants to start the lesson, but the pupil interrupts her because she wants to go to the toilet. The teacher, at first, tries to ignore the request, but as the child insists—so there is obviously a real need—the teacher has to give way. It is easy to interpret this passage as a reflection by the children on the rules regulating the activities in the classroom. In normal circumstances a teacher has to be obeyed, but having to go to the toilet is probably acceptable grounds for interrupting the course of the lesson.

The toilet scene has a comical sequel. It is the very first day at school for the pupil, so she has to ask where the toilet is. Margreet seizes the opportunity to take revenge for Elisabeth's lack of cooperation in starting the lesson. The play teacher points out that the toilet is in a dangerous place, near the wild animals. Later, the pupil gets locked in the toilet and has to be freed by somebody coming in a car with a siren.

Another scene about the order in the classroom concerns the disruption of the school activities by talking children.

Example 2 (Lines 120–136):
E: And then school is finished.
M: No.
E: (unintelligible)
M: You, over here.
MC: Hullo, I have a question, I am somebody...
EC: Talk, talk, talk, tralalalalala.
M: No, don't do that.
E: Yes, but the whole class was talking for a bit.
EC: Lalala laaaaaaaa.
MT: I'm fed up with it. Come here.
EC: (imitates) I'm fed up with it. Come along.
E: Give the culprit... (unintelligible). Then I rowed away.
M: Nooooooo! can't do that.
MT: Now, you. Come here.
EC: Lelelelleel.
EC: They are talking, all of them.
MT: But you're the worst of them all.

The talking is Elisabeth's reaction to Margreet's refusal to have the school finished. Margreet clearly wants to continue the school play, but Elisabeth has found another way to disrupt it. The pupils talk and the teacher does not succeed in silencing them. It is remarkable that this scene has been prepared earlier in the play session. In selecting the figures and giving them a place in the classroom, Margreet and Elisabeth have agreed on this theme. In accordance with a familiar teachers' practice, they have provided talkative children with seats at the front of the classroom near the teacher.

Example 3 (Lines 30–35):
M: You should choose four children who always talk the most; those
       children must sit at the front near the teacher. It'll be fun if they talk.
E: You, you sit here and talk, right?
M: The desks are behind each other, then they can only...then I have to
       turn them round all the time, if the children talk.

These episodes in which the normal course of things in the classroom is disturbed can be interpreted as the playful construction of situations of accountability. Much and Shweder (1978) define "situations of accountability" as behavioral episodes in which some breach of social expectation occurs and which therefore are the occasion of accusations, accounts, and discussions on the acceptability of the behavior. The children's fantasy play reveals their fascination with the rules and regulations of school life. In these play interactions, cultural norms are employed, created, tested, and negotiated. Although there is no elaborate argumentative accounting, as there would be in the case of adults, these episodes explore the justifiability of the pupils' conduct. In staging these episodes, the children explore the rules imposed on them by the adult world and their implications. Besides, they explore how they can violate these rules, and how they can find a justification for making a breach of these rules.

In daily life, accounts follow actions which are unusual or in some way unacceptable or wrong (Potter & Wetherell, 1987). In their study of a nursery school and a kindergarten (children between 3 and 6 years of age), Much and Shweder (1978) found 628 situations of accountability during a total of 60 hours of observation. None of the examples cited by Much and Shweder originated in pretend play: their examples come from the discussions and interactions of the children and their teachers as a reaction to the occurrence of unacceptable or unexpected events. The resulting accounts relate to social rules and conventions such as: one has to return a greeting, it is not right to damage others' property, and it is not allowed for children to be unaccompanied in the basement. Much and Shweder observed incidents followed by accounts.

However, in my observations of pretend play, the situation is reversed. The breaches do not simply occur, they are not mere incidents: they are willfully created, because they give an opportunity for reflection on social regulations. Here, Vygotsky's theme of play as a form of reflection is particularly useful. If children want to reflect, one way of doing this is by creating breaches of social expectations in pretend play. These two girls playfully reflect on rules such as: if a child has a real need to go to the toilet, she may disturb the lesson (Lines 88ff), children have to be silent in the classroom when the teacher wants to start the lesson (88ff, 124ff), school is not for fun (61ff), being late on the very first school day is not too serious (39ff). Adolescents and adults would verbally discuss these rules and their justifiability. Children from about the age of Margreet and Elisabeth begin to question the social conventions in a more direct way, but play is also at their disposal as a powerful means to reflect on the social world.

Much and Shweder found that their observed children, among themselves, did not give accounts of school rules: their discussions were mostly about more general cultural conventions and morals. According to their observations, discussions about school rules were initiated only by the teacher, who wished to call the children to account when a rule had been broken. As a contrast, in the enactment of school life by Margreet and Elisabeth, it is precisely the school rules which are represented and reflected on. The play teacher, in these children's representation, is an upholder of the school rules, at the cost of other functions of a schoolteacher. The difference between my observations and the ones by Much and Shweder might be explained by the ages of the children involved. I would, however, suggest that the fascination with rules and regulations, expressed in the play of Margreet and Elisabeth, also meets their need to think about the rules of the adult world among themselves, without the supervision of adults.

These children's playful reflection on social rules are a part of their appropriation of the culture. As I shall attempt to show, in representing and questioning social rules, the children prepare their own lives as persons and as members of a generation, and at the same time contribute to processes of cultural change.

It is useful (cf. Corsaro, 1985) to introduce here a conceptual distinction made by Erving Goffman in his study on mental institutions (Goffman, 1961). Goffman distinguishes between two reactions of the inmates of mental hospitals to the institution: primary and secondary adjustments. Individuals have a primary adjustment to an organization if they cooperate to realize the goals of the organization, if they are prepared to accommodate to the standards of the institution. In contrast, secondary adjustments represent ways in which individuals deviate from the roles prepared and expected for them by the institution. Some secondary adjustments are "disruptive" and disturb the normal functioning of the organization. But mostly, secondary adjustments are "contained" ones and do not generate a radical change of the institution's standards. In total institutions, such as prisons or mental hospitals, secondary adjustments lead to a real "underlife," such as an informal economy or a strict distribution of statuses and privileges, revealed by Goffman, but sometimes completely unknown to the establishment's staff.

In a more general sense, Goffman believes that our sense of selfhood derives to an extent from the secondary adjustments we construct. Being totally committed to the official roles society has in store for us leads to "a kind of selflessness. Our sense of being a person can come from being drawn into a wider social unit; our sense of selfhood can arise through the little ways in which we resist the pull" (1961, p. 280).

William Corsaro (1985) uses Goffman's distinction for interpreting young children's peer culture. In a study based on participant observation and videorecordings, Corsaro reconstructed the "underlife" of young children in a nursery school. Corsaro takes children's creation of a peer culture to be an answer to the restrictiveness of the rules and expectations imposed on them by adults. It is a creative mixture of elements originating from cultural contacts between children and adults. This peer culture strengthens the feeling of a distinction between the children and the adult world and consists of secondary adjustments, which Corsaro, disagreeing here with Goffman, does not see so much as promoting an *individual* identity but as promoting "a way of developing and maintaining *group* identity" (my emphasis, Corsaro, 1985, p. 267).

Corsaro's interpretation of childhood culture is in accordance with my understanding of children's pretend play. By playfully exploring the freedom they have in relationship to the schoolteacher, Elisabeth and Margreet prepare their contribution to the peer culture at their school. These scenes of school life can plausibly be interpreted as an anticipation of the secondary adjustments or even the "underlife" in their classroom.

However, Corsaro views children's participation in peer cultures as a transitory phenomenon. In his view, children have to move through a series of peer cultures, until they have eventually reproduced the adult world (Corsaro, 1985, pp. 270, 281, 307). For Corsaro, the study of peer cultures is important because it helps to understand the way children learn and the way the culture is reproduced. I would claim that children's construction of their identity is not just a temporary and transitory phenomenon. Children will not simply reproduce the adult culture: they will create something new, something of their own. Their peer culture consists of elements which will help to shape their sense, not just as an age group, but as a new generation. The secondary adjustments these children create in their play and in the classroom, as an answer to the official rules and regulations of the adult world, will be part of the experiences of their generation and will color their future life as a generation.

Children's attitude to cultural rules and their knowledge of how to breach these rules is not merely part of their sense as a generation, but contributes to processes of cultural change. The appropriation of school rules by the children among themselves will influence their behavior in the classroom, and this behavior will call forth reactions by the teachers. It is again Goffman who wrote about the adaptations of the representatives of an institution to the unofficial culture of the inmates: "Organizations have a tendency to adapt to secondary adjustments...by selectively legitimizing secondary adjustments into primary ones" (1961, p. 178f). In the light of this, it can be said that children's creation of a peer culture will influence the official culture in the classroom. Teachers will have to look for answers to the children's handling of the school rules and to their life as a peer group. In this way a connection can be made between the children's inventions of accounts and rules in pretend play and the change of rules at school.

In short, children's pretend play contributes to two connected processes. Firstly, it helps children to create themselves as a generation, because they shape their own peer culture as a reaction to the adult culture. Here, they do not only learn the content and impact of the adult rules, but also in what circumstances they might violate those rules. Secondly, the official culture has to adapt to the children's culture, or, in Goffman's terms, to their secondary adjustments. In this way, children's pretend play contributes to the change of the rules at their school and to the change of the culture in a wider sense.

Conclusion

This study of children's social pretend play has been inspired by Vygotsky's theories of internalization and play. Vygotsky did not propose a theory of the transfer of culture from one generation to the next. He rather envisaged children who actively contribute to their development and create novelty. However, Vygotsky did not succeed in integrating in a satisfying manner the two themes of his work: the cultural transmission theme and the theme of children's active contribution to development. Vygotsky's lecture on play points the way to analyzing children's contribution to their own development as members of the culture. Therefore, this text by Vygotsky was at the base of a study of two girls, 6 and 7 years old, who represented school life in their play.

These children did not so much explore the "official" sides of the roles of teacher and pupil as the cultural activities in which teaching and learning are embedded. In playfully reflecting on the rules, children at the same time learn the social rules of the classroom and the means to violate these rules. The children created situations of accountability, in which they could playfully reflect on the justifiability of the rules and prepare their reaction to the teachers' authority. In their play, children invent elements of the school culture, not only as an "official" culture, but also as an unofficial culture, which may come into collision with the official culture. In forming a peer culture, children create themselves as a generation and make a contribution to the reproduction and change of the culture at large.

Culture is not a static phenomenon, which is passed on from one generation to the next in a fixed way. The culture is changed, re-created and reconstructed continuously by all its members. Valsiner's concept of bidirectionality (Valsiner, 1989) is one way of expressing the idea that internalization involves novelty construction and, instead of being a unidirectional process of cultural transmission, contributes to a change of the culture. The two themes of Vygotsky are not opposed as long as we are prepared to see culture as changing, and are willing to study how children, among themselves or jointly with adults, contribute to this process. Play is one situation among many in which children contribute to creating themselves and the culture.

Appendix

Transcription of a Play Session (Translated from the Dutch)
Date of recording: August 28, 1988
Material: Playmobil figures—children and adults that can be dressed in various ways, (wild) animals, pieces of furniture (including school furniture).

M: Margreet (7 years, 9 months)
E: Elisabeth (6 years, 10 months)
MI: Margreet in the role of Indian chief
MT: Margreet in the role of teacher
MC: Margreet in the role of an unnamed child
MW: Margreet in the role of Whitey
MS: Margreet imitating a siren
ET: Elisabeth in the role of teacher
EC: Elisabeth in the role of an unnamed child

M: Let's make a school for the Indian children, because school starts tomorrow.

[They arrange desks and chairs; figures are selected which will be the pupils; E and M negotiate the number of figures each one may dress and manipulate]

5   M: Look what, I take a big one with an Indian. He also isn't...he also will be [at school] today for the first time. You should take that boat. Oh, it is already there.

MI: Oh...the feather from my headdress. I'm ready. Animals. Children, it is very dangerous. There are herds of dangerous animals. So, don't ever

10   go out by yourself, always [go] with me.

E: The crocodiles are swimming nearer.

M: No, they can't go too far.

MI: We have to go to school in the boat. I go first, yes, children?

EC: Me as well.

15   MI: No, you can't go yet.

E: The two of us can go.

M: Yes.

MI: I have to sail there and back.

[M and E negotiate which children may go]

20   M: No, the children with the hats are schoolchildren. Those others are still uhh too small, they can go another time.

     MI?:   Hullo! Hullo!

     M: And the teacher...the child with the satchel must sit next to the big children; the one with the satchel sits next to the big ones, because that

25   is the biggest child.

     MC: Yoo, yoo, yoo.

     E: That one is Diokje, she has a hat too, doesn't she?

     M: Look.

     E: The teacher has a hat as well.

30   M: The small...uuhhm. You should choose four children who always talk the most, those children must sit at the front near the teacher. It'll be fun if they talk.

     E: You, you sit here and talk, right?

     M: The desks are behind each other, then they can only...then I have to

35   turn them round all the time, if the children talk. The herd must be put a bit further away, else the school would be too dangerous.

[M and E discuss how dangerous the wild animals are; then they discuss the places of the children in the classroom]

     MC: Hey hullo, I'm a bit late.

40   ET: It doesn't matter.

     MC: But I've only, I've only..., I haven't got a hat.

     MT: It's not winter, children, you don't need a hat, but it's for the jungle, to prevent the animals catching us.

     E: Here's another hat.

45   EC: No, that's mine.

     M: One child was sick, right?

     E: Which one is sick?...this one.

     MC: There is a sick child, Miss. She wants..., she is looking now, you see, she is looking now.

50   MW: Hullo. I'm Whitey, Miss, I am sick. [waits]

     MT: That's too bad.

[Negotiations about who plays with which figures]

     C: Miss, Liny, Liny is sick.

     MT: Then you have a desk all to yourself.

55   E: It was Whitey, who is sick, isn't she?

     M: What?

     E: Whitey is sick.

     M: Whitey is sick.

MT: Too bad.
60 M: Whose is this...It is your own thing, you have a seat all to yourself.
MT: Now, children, what are we going to do today? What do you want to do?
EC: I don't know. Have a party!
MT: No, no, no.
65 M: You must play this one, so you must say what are we going to...
M: I want to play with the map, then it's ebb.
E: I don't want that.
M: Then I can call you. Now, Liny, then you play with the children at the back, then one of you is sick, right?
70 E: I'll play...the little Indian.
M: You have to get that thing then.
MT: There's one child missing today, why?
EC: Whitey is sick.
MT: Oh, now you know what we're going to. Have you all got a pencil? I
75   don't think so.
EC: No.
MT: Now, uuhhm, I start by saying who is the monitor, for she hands out everything for me. Welcome to Class 4 by the way. You two with the chain, do you want to be the monitor for a whole year? Then we can't
80   forget.
MC: Yeaaaaaaaaa.

[Further negotiations about who plays with which figure]

M: Oooooooh, I've got, I think, four boys. Four, four, four.
E: No, those at the back and those at the front are talking. Right? All of
85   them are talking. No, this one is sick, isn't it? This one was sick, but she had to go to school on the first day.
M: No, this one was not sick.
MT: No, no....Children, sit down.
EC: I have to go to the toilet, Miss.
90 MT: Now, children, be quiet.
EC: I have to go to the toilet.
MT: I want to tell you something.
EC: (loud) I have to go to the toilet!
M: (chuckles) Wait a second.
95 EC: (with emphasis) Miss, I have to go to the toilet!!
MT: Okay, you can go.
EC: (cheekily) Where is it? (laughs)
MT: Over there, under that box, the one with the animals on, where the dangerous animals... (chuckles) under there.

100	EC:	Really?
	MT:	Yes.

[EC goes to the toilet and makes the noises of flushing it]

	EC:	Hey, I can't get out.
	M:	No, she *could*.
105	E:	That thing was suddenly shut, those animals had a little machine in the there...
	M:	Then you must call for help.
	EC:	(in a weak voice) Help, help, help.
	MS:	(imitating a siren) Ttttrrll, ttrrll.
110	EC:	Help, help.
	MT:	No, I've told you, I have also that fastening, so it's open.
	E:	(unintelligible)
	EC:	Miss, I don't feel well.
	MT:	Hey, hey, who wants to be monitor of these two desks?
115	EC:	Uuuuuuhhh, me.
	E:	You must put your hand up.
	MT:	Don't move the desk. Okay. You'll get something. But that thing must go then.
	EC:	Go, what must go?
120	E:	And then school is finished.
	M:	No.
	E:	(unintelligible)
	M:	You, over here.
	MC:	Hullo, I have a question, I am somebody...
125	EC:	Talk, talk, talk, tralalalalala.
	M:	No, don't do that.
	E:	Yes, but the whole class was talking for a bit.
	EC:	Lalala laaaaaaaa.
	MT:	I'm fed up with it. Come here.
130	EC:	(imitates) I'm fed up with it. Come along.
	E:	Give the culprit... (unintelligible). Then I rowed away.
	M:	Nooooooo! can't do that.
	MT:	Now, you. Come here.
	EC:	Lelelelleel.
135	EC:	They are talking, all of them.
	MT:	But you're the worst of them all.

[E and M negotiate again about who can play with which figure. The school is moved and arranged again. No more teacher-pupil interaction.]

References

Bateson, G. (1956), The message "This is play." In B. Schaffner (ed.), *Group processes*. New York: Josiah Macy Foundation.

Bruner, J.S. (1976), Nature and uses of immaturity. In J.S. Bruner, A. Jolly, & K. Sylva (eds.), *Play—Its role in development and evolution* (pp. 28-64). Harmondsworth: Penguin Books.

Corsaro, W.A. (1985), *Friendship and peer culture in the early years*. Norwood, NJ: Ablex.

Davydov, V.V., & L.A. Radzikhovskii (1985), Vygotsky's theory and the activity-oriented approach in psychology. In J.V. Wertsch (ed.), *Culture, communication, and cognition* (pp. 35-65). Cambridge: Cambridge University Press.

Elbers, E. (1991a), The development of competence and its social context. *Educational Psychology Review*, 3, 73-94.

Elbers, E. (1991b), Context, culture and competence. Answers to criticism. *Educational Psychology Review*, 3, 137-149.

Elbers, E., R. Maier, T. Hoekstra, & M. Hoogsteder (1990, July), *How can we analyze adult-child interactions?* Poster presentation at the 9th European Conference on Developmental Psychology, Stirling, UK.

Elbers, E., R. Maier, T. Hoekstra, & M. Hoogsteder, (1992), Internalization and adult-child interaction. *Learning and Instruction*, 2, 101-118.

Fein, G.G. (1981), Pretend play: An integrative review. *Child Development*, 52, 1095-1118.

Fein, G.G. (1984), The self-building potential of pretend play or "I got a fish, all by myself". In T.D. Yawkey & A.D. Pellegrini (eds.), *Child's play: developmental and applied* (pp. 125-141). Hillsdale, NJ: Erlbaum.

Fein, G.G., & L. Kohlberg, (1987), Play and constructive work as contributors to development. In L. Kohlberg (ed.), *Child psychology and childhood education. A cognitive-developmental view* (pp. 392-440). New York: Longman.

Goffman, E. (1961), *Asylums*. Harmondsworth: Penguin.

Kanner, B.G. & J.V. Wertsch (1991), Beyond a transmission model of communication. *Educational Psychology Review*, 3, 103-109.

Kozulin, A. (1990), *Vygotsky's psychology. A biography of ideas*. New York: Harvester.

Maier, R.M., E. Elbers, T. Hoekstra, & M. Hoogsteder, (1992), The puzzle of Wertsch. *Cultural Dynamics*, 5, 25-42.

Mead, G.H. (1934), *Mind, self, and society*. Chicago: University of Chicago Press.

Much, N.C. & R.A. Shweder (1978), Speaking of rules: The analysis of culture in breach. In W. Damon (ed.), *Moral development* (pp. 19-39). San Fransisco: Jossey-Bass.

Parreren, C.F. van, & J. Carpay (1980), *Sovjetpsychologen over onderwijs en cognitieve ontwikkeling* (Soviet psychologists on instruction and cognitive development). Groningen, The Netherlands: Wolters-Noordhoff.

Piaget, J. (1932), *Le jugement moral chez l'enfant*. Paris: Presses Universitaires de France.

Potter, J. & M. Wetherell (1987), *Social psychology and discourse*. London: Sage.

Rubin, K.H.,G.G. Fein & B. Vandenberg (1983), Play. In E.M. Hetherington (ed.), *Handbook of child psychology. Volume IV. Socialization, personality, and social development* (pp. 693-774). New York: Wiley.

Sully, J. (1896), *Studies of childhood*. London: Longmans Green.

Sutton-Smith, B. (1979), Epilogue: Play as performance. In B. Sutton-Smith (ed.), *Play and learning* (pp. 295-322). New York: Gardner Press.

Valsiner, J. (1989), *Human development and culture*. Lexington: Lexington Books.

Van der Veer, R. & J. Valsiner (1988), Lev Vygotsky and Pierre Janet: On the origin of the concept of sociogenesis. *Developmental Review*, 8, 52-65.

Van der Veer, R. & J. Valsiner (1991), *Understanding Vygotsky. A quest for synthesis*. Oxford: Blackwell.

Vygotsky, L.S. (1976), Play and its role in the mental development of the child. In J.S. Bruner, A. Jolly & K. Sylva (eds.), *Play—its role in development and evolution* (pp. 537-554), Harmondsworth: Penguin Books. (Original work published 1930.)

Vygotsky, L.S. (1978a), The role of play in development. In *Mind in society*. M. Cole, V. John-Steiner, S. Scribner & E. Souberman (eds.) (pp. 92-104), Cambridge: Harvard University Press. (Original work published 1933.)

Vygotsky, L.S. (1978b), Internalization of higher mental functions. In *Mind in society*. M. Cole, V. John-Steiner, S. Scribner & E. Souberman (eds.) (pp. 52-57). Cambridge: Harvard University Press. (Original work published 1933.)

Wertsch, J.V. (1979), From social interaction to higher psychological processes. *Human Development*, 22, 1-22.

Wertsch, J.V. (1985), *Vygotsky and the social formation of mind*. Cambridge: Harvard University Press.

13. Psychosocial Perspective on Cognitive Development: Construction of Adult-Child Intersubjectivity in Logic Tasks

Michèle Grossen and Anne-Nelly Perret-Clermont[1]

Obviously the concepts used in psychology at the beginning of this century were directly influenced by the then pervasive ideas of the theories of evolution. Looking back to this period it can be seen how such ideas gave a very important impulse to the study of human behavior. However several decades later, it would be well worth reviewing these concepts and either enlarging on them (as seemingly suggested by the organizers of the present symposium through the consideration of "*socio*genesis") or substituting new metaphors and concepts to the existing ones, in order to draw attention to aspects of psychological reality that the preceding perspective might cause to be neglected. This presentation takes as standpoint the crossroad of these two lines of thought. Indeed, in our opinion, suggesting new concepts (e.g., "intersubjectivity") can be fruitful for the advance of science mostly if it can simultaneously account for both the already known phenomena and for newly described processes.

The gradual introduction into psychology of the idea that mind, personality, mental disorders, etc., are the results of a gradual development starting in early infancy and not just "static" gifts of nature, opened the way for innumerable studies on the micro-evolution of behavior. On a different level of reality but nevertheless with somehow similar epistemological assumptions, these studies echo the ongoing research trends in the study of the macro-biophysical world (with the concepts used from Darwin's theory to the big bang theory) and of the macro socio-historical reality (suppositions on the rise of Homo Sapiens, the growth of civilization from "prehistoric to "post-modern," economic development or "under-development," etc.). In this wide variety of cases, some common elements recur, the most important being: evolution considered as progress; change as being not only quantitative, but also qualitative; and hypothesis as to how one stage prepares for the next (constructivism). In nearly all cases the observers (in a quite understandable ethnocentric shortsightedness) regard reality from their own standpoint taking for granted that their state is the present peak of development: other species are, of course, less developed, but often also other civilizations, social structures, or cognitive stages. In fact the observers do not notice that in interpreting reality they introduce value judgments and perspectives that are closely linked with their own present involvement in larger debates and action plans. And the observers' action plans, of course, often differ from their subjects' action plans.

When Piaget refers to "genesis" to describe the course of child development he does not only point to an evolution but much more precisely to an eclosion, to a growth. He wants to account not only for changes but even more so for qualitative structural transformations. And, in doing so, with this term "genesis" borrowed from the famous myth of creation and in particular of the creation of the first human beings, Piaget tries to identify the very profound mechanisms (i.e., equilibration processes within interactive and constructive dynamics) that, in his eyes, tell something about the nature of psychological life, and perhaps even about life and reality in general. In his famous book *Biology and Knowledge,* Piaget (1971) can even be seen, on some pages, to be stirred by the wonder of the "vection of life" that he feels to be revealed in the fine dynamics of biological evolution and cognitive growth that he studies.

The genesis of what? The classical Piagetian response is: the genesis in the individual beings of ever more powerful and stable regulative processes, the most advanced and adaptative ones being cognitive. The growth of cognition is then accounted for in terms of successive structures characterized by their formal logical power. Once developed they can be applied indifferently to the physical or to the social world.

From there on, various researchers have undertaken studies on the varieties of capacities and understandings that these structural progresses elicit in the child. Often these results have been grouped into areas of interest: logico-mathematical competence; understanding of the physical world; and social cognition. Parallel cognitive stages have been tentatively linked with behavioral development in areas such as: socialization, moral judgement, etc. The risk has then been to consider too readily that all these aptitudes influence each other reciprocally (a possible understanding of the meaning of the concept of "sociogenesis") and in doing so, to forget the standpoint of all this research that sets, at the start, a model of development, value laden by the observer, which a priori considers development as progress, formal logics as adaptative, stages as logical, the search for equilibrium as the dynamic cause, equilibrium as understanding, and all these processes as primarily located in individual beings—within a micro-history that forgets the structuring influences of group and cultural processes. Although all these assumptions are interesting starting points for research (and indeed they have proved their heuristic value), they are not necessary nor are they the only ones possible. For instance, Vygotsky's (1962) partially opposite perspective can be seen as giving more importance to cultural mediations and interpersonal processes and then describing development as an external reality, progressively interiorized by the subjects during their socialization. However Vygotsky's view, no more than Piaget's, questions certain value-laden characteristics of what he considers to be the final stages of development and the role of socialization agents, notably in defining what the cognitive and social tasks are and what their solutions are.

This contribution will present another starting point: stepping back from a normative definition by the adult of what a given task is about and what solving it means, methodological approaches will be described that permit observation of the social and cognitive processes in which subjects are involved in classical tests. It will be seen that the activity displayed by the individual child is the *product* of an interaction between his understanding of the situation and his adult partner's understanding. Furthermore the understanding that might emerge is due to socio-cognitive processes whereby the adult and the child come to more or less negotiate an intersubjectivity.

The Test Situation as a Context for Developing the Logical Abilities of the Child

By what logical and social process does a child acquire new logical abilities? Is the answer a child gives when he is questioned on a logic problem the expression of cognitive abilities which he has already developed, or does it depend on the particular social context in which it was produced? Does this context have a catalytic effect which will or will not allow the child's abilities to become revealed, or is the definition of the context itself the result of an interpretation of the subject? These questions concern firstly the *epistemological status of the cognitive abilities* of the child such as they can be perceived by an observer: are they preconstructed individually, or, on the contrary, do they develop *hic et nunc* in the testing situation? Secondly, the *epistemological status of the social context*: does it consist of a group of *external* factors which influence the subject's cognitive activity, or is it a subjective *internal* construction? Let us note that these questions implicitly assume that cognitive development results from a *bi-polar* interaction between *subject* and *object*.

By confronting two lines of research to which we ourselves contributed (research on the role of social interaction between children, and research on the role of the social context in cognitive development) we propose to show in this chapter how we were gradually led to reconsider this bi-polar perspective, and to view development as the result of a *tri-polar* interaction between the *subject*, the *alter,* and the *task*. Firstly a rapid presentation of the main results of the two lines of research mentioned will be given, then studies whose aim was to understand through which psycho-social processes the child constructs his/her responses will be presented. Finally we will examine how the two socio-cognitive processes mentioned, namely the socio-cognitive conflict and the construction of intersubjectivity, lead to the acquisition of a new logical competence.

The Role of Social Interaction Between Children in Cognitive Development

Research in this field shows that under certain conditions the child can take advantage of an interaction session with a peer to restructure his/her answer, and give an answer which is more complex from a logical point of view. An interaction session can be beneficial individually, even when none of the children in the group has the correct solution to the problem: the fact that children have different perspectives on the solution to a problem is sufficient to generate a conflict known as *socio-cognitive conflict* because it is provoked by the peers' differing points of view and leads to a social confrontation between children. This socio-cognitive conflict may account for the positive influence of social interaction on cognitive development (Doise & Mugny, 1984; Emler & Valiant, 1982; Doise, Mugny, & Perret-Clermont, 1975; Gilly & Roux, 1984; Perret-Clermont, 1980, among others).

Research describing the social context which allows a child to derive benefit from a social interaction session, has also showed that, before the interaction session (pretest), individual performances are often correlated with social origin and/or sex of the children, with children of high socioeconomic status performing better than children of low socioeconomic level. However these differences tend to diminish or disappear after an interaction session. These results show that the cognitive behavior of the subjects is likely to be modified during the *experimental micro-history*; in this respect they concur with results concerning how the social context affects the display of cognitive competence in children (Donaldson, 1978; Grossen, 1988; Perret-Clermont & Schubauer-Leoni, 1981).

The latest research in this field concerns not only the effects of the interaction session between children on their individual performances, but also the *problem-solving strategies* used by the children (Blaye, 1988; Zhou, 1988) and the *specific modalities* of interactions between children. It seems that interactions in which there is a co-construction of the correct solution lead to greater individual progress. It appears that more individual benefit is derived when, during the interaction, the children cooperate equitably by trying to understand each other's point of view (Bearison, Magzamen, & Filardo, 1986; Light, Foot, Colbourn, & McClelland, 1987; Taal & Oppenheimer, 1989).

The Role of the Social Context in Cognitive Activity

Research in this field shows that the child's abilities vary according to the social context in which s/he is questioned. Different contextual dimensions operate, such as the child's *interpretation* of the experimenter's actions (Donaldson, 1978; Light, 1986); the *social rules* governing the testing situation (see on this subject, research on social marking: De Paolis & Girotto, 1987; Doise, Dionnet & Mugny, 1975; Nicolet & Iannaconne, 1988; Roux & Gilly, 1984; Zhou, 1988); the *institutional or formal context* in which the task is submitted to the child (see for example Säljö & Wyndhamn, 1987; Carraher, 1989); the respective *roles* of the actors (adult or peer) with whom the child interacts (Schubauer-Leoni, 1986; Schubauer-Leoni, Bell, Grossen, & Perret-Clermont, 1989).

The results of the numerous studies undertaken show that the child's answers are very sensitive to a change in the presentation of a given task and that even a minute change in a classical Piagetian test, for example, is enough to alter the types of judgment given by the child. It also emerges from these studies that different subjects are likely to approach a given social context in a different way. Our own research has revealed repeatedly that the effect of a given social context is not the same according to the sex and social origin of the children and that these differences themselves vary according to the experimental micro-history (Grossen, 1988; Nicolet & Grossen, 1988; Perret-Clermont & Schubauer-Leoni, 1981).

These results suggest that these different dimensions (grouped under the rather vague term of "social context") should not be simply considered as *external variables*. They do not only *influence* the child's cognitive activity, but contribute to define what the activity is about. In order to assess the child's cognitive abilities the experimenter must indeed construct a "staging" of the task and of the encounter. The child's cognitive activity is therefore always a response to this staging and to what s/he interprets about its meanings and aims. Therefore, it seems difficult to affirm, as some authors have, (for example, Bovet, Parrat-Dayan & Deshusses-Addor, 1981; Donaldson, 1978) that the child's real cognitive abilities are elicited by certain situations and that other situations are artificial and not representative of the child's real abilities. What are these "real abilities"? Can they be assessed in any manner other than via a concrete testing situation? And the latter is of course always "artificial" since it is *constructed* by the experimenter. All dialogues are constructed.

If the experimental situation is considered as indissociable from the child's abilities, then new questions arise. What does the child think of the testing situation with which s/he is faced? How does s/he perceive the experimenter's expectations? What is, from his/her point of view, the aim of their encounter? What is the nature of the problem put to him/her by the experimenter? Is his/her definition of the situation and of the task the same as that of the experimenter (Wertsch, 1984)? Such questions call for a change in the object of study and in the unit of analysis considered. It is thus necessary: (a) to extend the study of the subject-task interaction to subject-task-experimenter interaction, that is, *to make the testing situation itself an object of study*, which necessitates including the role and behavior of the experimenter in the observations; and (b) *to re-place the cognitive activity in the communication context in which the subject acts it out*.

It is then necessary to examine the meanings which the experimenter and the child, from their respective points of view, give to the situation and to observe how they negotiate a supposedly common definition of the situation and of the task.

To attain such objectives it was necessary to resort to different observation methods that would provide an understanding of the meanings which the child gives to the situation.

Three main methods were used: the analysis of experimenter-child interactions during a Piagetian test, post-experimental interviews and role playing (Bell, 1986; Grossen, 1988; Grossen & Bell, 1988). A more detailed account of the research undertaken using this latter method is given below.

The Construction of Intersubjectivity Between the Experimenter and the Child in a Piagetian Test: Presentation of an Empirical Study[2]

Introduction

This research aimed at studying the way in which the child interprets the testing situation and how s/he sees the experimenter's expectations. This objective was not an end in itself, but rather a means of understanding the cognitive and social processes through which a child comes to demonstrate his/her logical abilities.

The method used involved asking children, who had just undertaken the Piagetian[3] conservation of liquids test, to assume the role of experimenter with a naive classmate.

Description of Research

Population and Procedure

The population consisted of 114 children aged between 6 and 7. The children were randomly assigned to two groups: (a) the role-players group (RP), made up of 57 children (27 boys, 30 girls); and (b) the naive classmates group, who were later questioned by the RPs, made up of 57 children, (26 boys, 31 girls). The experiment took place in two stages:

Stage 1: The experimenter submitted each child in the RPsgroup to the conservation of liquids test. Of the 57 RPs questioned, 18 children gave non-conserving judgments during the three test items[4] ("non conserving operatory level"), 23 gave judgements which were alternately non-conserving and conserving ("intermediate operatory level"), and 16 gave conserving judgments ("conserving operatory level").

Stage 2: Immediately after Stage 1, each RP played the role of the experimenter with one of the "naive" classmates.

Analysis of Data

Analysis of the role playing[5] concerned the reproduction by the RPs of certain concrete characteristics of the situation, such as the equalization request, the conservation question, the justification demand, the counter-suggestion, the type of glasses used, and the different types of transformations made (through pouring). On the basis of this first analysis, four patterns of behavior were established through which it was possible to assess the way in which the children define the task and the problem.

The three patterns observed will first be presented, and the links between these patterns and the judgments given by the RPs in Stage 1 will be discussed. Finally we shall give the results concerning the RPs definition of the situation.

Presentation of Results

Definition of the Task

Four patterns were established on the basis of the RPs' behavior during their role playing.

1. The RPs defined the task as a question concerning the comparison of the level of juice in two equal or different glasses. Two types of behavior were observed among the seven RPs grouped in this category:

- At the beginning of the role playing, the RPs took two different glasses and poured some juice into them at unequal levels. These RPs did not reproduce the equalization phase in two equal glasses, and proposed directly the result of the transformation after transferring the liquid.

- The RPs took two different glasses and asked their classmates to pour juice into them at equal levels. The RPs seemed to confuse the equalization phase and the pouring phase, selecting only the equalizing of the levels from the first phase and the different shape of the glasses from the second.

In both cases the conservation question[6] contained a non-conserving assumption of the type "Who has the least juice?" and the RPs themselves gave non-conserving judgments during the role playing.

The seven RPs in this category appeared to see the task as a problem of evaluating the level of the liquid, which was not always seen as being the result of a transformation.

2. The RPs defined the task as a problem of non-conservation of levels after transformation. The 21 RPs in this category proposed one or several sequences consisting of an equalization phase in two equal glasses and a phase where the juice was poured into a different glass. The conservation question presupposed unequal quantities (e.g., "Is there a little more juice in your glass?") and the RPs gave non-conserving judgments during the role playing. For these RPs, the equalization phase could have different meanings: some of them for example considered that it was a problem that had to be resolved in itself and asked their classmates several times to improve the equalization of the levels of the liquid. One RP (a girl) even refused to tell her classmate to pour the same quantity of juice into the two equal glasses as if, by doing so, she would have already been giving her the right answer! The fact that the child did not necessarily consider the equalization phase as a premise to the conservation problem set by the experimenter but as a problem in itself is corroborated by an analysis of experimenter-child interactions in the same testing situation (Grossen, 1988, pp. 173-206).

The 21 RPs in this category seemed, therefore, to think that the problem set by the experimenter was to grasp the fact that, after the liquid had been poured into a different glass, the level of the liquid changed, that is, to understand that there was non-conservation of the levels of the juice. For them it was as if the expression "the same thing" did not concern the quantity, but the level of the liquid.

3. The RPs defined the task as a problem of quantity conservation. The 18 RPs in this category, as was the case for those of the previous category, reproduced equalization sequences in two equal glasses, followed by a transfer to a glass which was different. In this case their conservation question presupposed equal quantity as in the following example: "Have we got the same thing?" and they did not word the question in any other way. Out of these 18 RPs, only 3 asked a conservation question which contained the three terms given by the experimenter ("same thing," "more," "less"). For relational reasons which will be examined later, 4 RPs began by asking a conservation question which presupposed a non-conserving judgment and then asked a conservation question centred on equality. Furthermore, most of the RPs gave conserving judgments to their classmates during the role playing.

The behaviors of these 18 RPs led us to think that, for them, the problem was to understand that regardless of the container, the quantity of liquid remained equal, that is, their definition of the task seemed to be the same as that of the experimenter. In this case it was as if the object of the interrogation was to admit at all costs that the quantities were equal, regardless of what actually happened during the interaction: consequently some RPs seemed to expect a conserving judgment even from their classmates despite the fact that a large quantity of liquid fell outside the glass while it was being transferred!

4. The RPs adopted a neutral attitude so that it was not possible to determine how they defined the task. The 8 RPs in this category did not themselves give a judgment to their classmate during the role playing; neither did they give any arguments to confirm or refute the judgment(s) of their classmates. All these RPs asked a conservation question such as "Have we got the same thing?," that is, a question which seemed to presuppose a conserving judgment, except 1 RP whose question suggested alternatives.

These RPs' behaviors concurred so closely with the experimenter's neutrality that it was difficult to determine how they defined the task, even though their conservation question could lead us to suppose that they belonged to the third category.

Relationship Between the Subjects' Answers During Stage 1
and the Definition of the Task
What relationships exist between the subjects' judgments during Stage 1 (their "operatory level") and their definition of the task such as it can be observed in their behavior during the role playing? The results showed that:

- of the 7 RPs who defined the task as a level evaluation problem, 5 were non-conserving and 2 were intermediate at Stage 1;

- of the 21 RPs who defined the task as a problem of non-conservation of the levels after transformation, 9 were non-conserving and 12 were intermediate at Stage 1;

- of the 18 RPs who viewed the task as a quantity conservation problem, one was non-conserving, 5 were intermediate, and 12 were conserving;

- of the 8 "neutral" RPs only one was non-conserving, 4 were intermediate, and 3 were conserving.

The RPs' definition of the task seemed therefore to be closely linked to the judgments given in Stage 1: All the RPs (except one) who were non-conserving in Stage 1, defined the task as a problem of evaluation or non-conservation of the levels, whereas all the conserving RPs defined the task in the same way as the experimenter. Among the 19 intermediate RPs, 12 defined the task just like the non-conserving RPs had done.

The Definition of the Situation
Concerning the definition of the situation, the analysis of the RPs behavior gives rise to three series of comments:
1. Most of the RPs did not reproduce an important characteristic of the role of the experimenter: her *neutrality*. The experimenter tried, as far as possible, not

to judge the subjects' answers and *a fortiori* not to give them the expected answer. However it was observed that out of the 54 RPs in question, 41 (76%) gave one or several conserving or non-conserving judgments to their classmates during the role playing, accompanied more often than not by reasons in favor. In other words, these children gave their classmates the answer they thought to be correct.

2. Nearly all the RPs ended up by obtaining judgments from their classmates which concurred with their own definition of the task. Thus, all the RPs (except one) who defined the task as a level evaluation problem, or as a non-conservation problem obtained non-conserving judgments, whereas all the RPs (except four) who defined the task as a conservation problem ended up by obtaining conserving judgments from their classmates. Analysis of the interactions between the children showed that the RPs used certain questioning strategies to steer their classmates towards the expected answer, and that the latter used other strategies to obtain more information on the expected answer (Grossen, 1988).

3. Very often the RPs *assessed* their classmates' answers by remarks such as "that's right" or "that's wrong"; *gave* them *recommendations or orders* which emphasized the asymmetry of their relationship; or in some cases observed only with conserving children, *misled his/her classmate concerning his/her expectations* as if to ensure that s/he would afterwards be in a position to have to steer his/her classmate to the expected answer!

These three series of comments suggest that the RPs defined the testing situation as a *didactic* situation whose aim was to transmit knowledge to their classmates. The RPs gradually guided his/her classmate towards what s/he considered to be the right answer, taking on the role of *teacher*. It even seemed that the RPs who defined the problem in the same way as the experimenter accentuated this "little teacher" behavior by giving, more often than the other RPs, judgments or supporting arguments. These RPs seemed to use the knowledge with which they had been provided as an instrument which not only ensured them of their legitimate status of experimenter but also reinforced their power with regard to their classmates.

The Production of a Logical Ability as a Social Co-construction

This study showed that, faced with a situation having the same objective characteristics, the child and the experimenter did not define the task and the situation in the same way. Concerning the definition of the situation, it was noted that, if for the experimenter the aim of the liquid conservation test was to test the logical abilities of the child, for the child, on the contrary, it had a didactic aim. This confirms the results of other studies (Bell, 1986; Elbers, 1986; Grossen, 1988; Schubauer-Leoni, 1986), and can be explained not only by the fact that the didactic situation is more familiar to the child, but also by the fact that the institutional scholastic context in which the study was carried out constitutes a frame which induces the child into giving a certain definition of the situation that in turn modulates the cognitive abilities which the child will display (see research by Monteil, 1988, on the effects of social comparison on the performances of pupils in the scholastic context; Säljö & Wyndhamn, 1987; Schubauer-Leoni et al., 1989).

Concerning the definition of the task, our results showed that some of the implicit characteristics of the task gave rise to interpretations which differed between the child and the experimenter. This was the case for example: (a) of the *equalization request* which, as was shown in the analyses of experimenter-child interactions, can be interpreted by the child not as a premise to the problem (of conservation) but as a problem in itself, which consisted of obtaining the most perfect equalization possible; and (b) of the *conservation question*, which could be interpreted as a question concerning liquid level (see also Bell, 1986), its transformation during pouring, or as other observations showed, could even concern the question of drinking the juice (Grossen, 1988).

Everything seems to take place as if, faced with a new situation, the child has to decipher the assumptions on which the experimenter implicitly bases his interpretation of the situation, that is, make an identical categorization of the various elements which for the experimenter constitute "the task." The fact that in our study there was a link between the judgments given by the children in Stage 1 and their definition of the task in Stage 2 seems to indicate that the construction by the child of a conserving judgment is dependent on the construction of a task definition which is the same as that of the experimenter. The answer produced by the child in the test situation is the result of a cognitive and social activity in which the child tries to decipher the experimenter's expectations and to understand the assumptions on which the latter bases his definition of the situation and of the task.

The test situation is therefore the social location in which two actors having a different status and role (experimenter and child) negotiate meanings concerning the object of their interaction and try to construct an intersubjectivity which will lead them to share a common definition of the situation and the task.

As any communication situation, the test situation is governed by implicit and explicit rules which regulate the experimenter-child interactions. Among these rules, some are specific to the immediate interactive situation; others also apply to different social situations, such as the didactic situation. These non-specific rules, taken as a whole, form what some authors call an *experimental meta-contract* (Elbers 1986; Hundeide, 1988; Rommetveit, 1979, 1985; Schubauer-Leoni, 1986), which will allow the interactants to make sense of a situation and set up the experimental contract which will specifically govern this particular situation. Faced with a test situation, the child's task, cognitive and social, will be to understand the nature of the meta-contract in question and to set up the experimental contract specific to this situation.

The type of cognitive activity which the child works out in a test situation thus results from a *tripolar subject-task-experimenter interaction*. This means, firstly, that the subject-task interaction is mediated by a third party (adult, experimenter, teacher, etc.) who constructs a situation and a task for another actor (the subject) with certain aims (teaching, evaluation, play, etc.). Behind the task there is, thus, always an adult who has constructed it (on the basis of certain cultural, social, and scientific assumptions) and who gives it certain meanings; *secondly, the subject-experimenter interaction is mediated by the task* on which they interact. However the construction of this task encompasses dimensions which go beyond the interindividual experimenter-child interactions because they carry meanings which have been culturally, socially, and historically constructed. Consequently, the intersubjectivity which the experimenter and the subject construct during their interaction is not only an interindividual creation, but also a social and cultural one.

The object of the child-experimenter interaction is thus at the same time, to a certain extent, *preconstructed*, since it exists (as a cultural and social object) independent of the encounter between the interactants; and *intersubjectively created*, since it is partly constructed (or reconstructed) in the *hic et nunc* interaction situation, as a symbolic object carrying numerous meanings and mediating the interaction between the interactants.

In this perspective, the development of new cognitive abilities appears to be specifically linked to the social context in which the abilities were developed. The development of new cognitive abilities is the construction of the cognitive instruments which, in the particular social situation in which the problem is put to the subject (via an alter symbolically or actually present), appear to be necessary for solving the problem and also socially and relationally relevant. Just as the understanding and interpretation of the social situation in which the child is questioned (test situation) require the development of a cognitive activity, so the solving of a logic task requires social knowledge and skills which go far beyond the simple acquisition of logical instruments. Therefore, not only do logical operations (or instruments) develop which make it possible to understand certain problems, but a series of social skills also develop which concern the interpretation of the social situation in which a logical activity is required.

The social context, as studied in the research reported in this paper, is therefore an *intersubjective space*, which does not fall entirely in the sphere either of the experimenter or of the subject. It is in this space that the child will produce an answer which, even if it always depends on abilities and knowledge which he has acquired in other situations, is nevertheless an *original creation* insofar as it stems from this encounter.

It is thus very difficult to say whether the child's cognitive abilities are individual characteristics, they rather appear as being the fruit of a *social co-construction* whose result does not depend entirely on the subject or on the adult.

Socio-cognitive Conflict and Intersubjectivity: Some Perspectives

The itinerary leading from the study of the role of social interaction between children in cognitive development to the study of adult-child interaction in a test situation has been briefly presented. The logical abilities which the child produces appear as being the result of an activity which is indissociably social and cognitive and in which the subject tries to interpret the situation by attempting to understand how the experimenter defines it and what he expects from him/her.

This perspective prompts questions on the results obtained in research on the role of social interaction between children in cognitive development (see Light & Perret-Clermont, 1989). As some studies in this field suggest, it could be thought that an interaction session between children is an opportunity for them not only to oppose and coordinate the logical instruments which they dispose of, but also to confront their definition of the task and the situation and to construct a common definition.

Giving a central role to the intersubjectivity process (between children, or between adult and child) in the development of new logical abilities, these studies arrive, by different means, at conclusions which are similar to those of North American studies inspired by Vygotsky (see for example Rogoff, 1990; Wertsch, 1984). Considering the higher mental functions as individual interiorizations of symbolic instruments constructed socially, historically, and culturally, research in this field is firstly centered on adult-child interaction in a learning situation, in order to study the processes through which two actors with a different level of expertise construct an intersubjectivity (Ellis & Rogoff, 1982; Rogoff, 1990; Valsiner, 1984; Wertsch, Minick, & Arns, 1984). The latest work (Rogoff, 1990) has gradually become oriented towards the study of interactions between children, putting the accent on cases where the children have different levels of expertise. This research has shown that interactions between children, by reason of the symmetrical characteristics of their relationship, give rise to greater cooperation in the progressive construction of a common definition of the situation and of the task (Forman, 1987; Forman & Kraker, 1985; Rogoff, 1990).

The confrontation of these two research currents leads us to ask how the notion of *socio-cognitive conflict* ties up with that of *intersubjectivity*. For it is observed, on the one hand, that a socio-cognitive conflict is only beneficial if each child takes his/her classmate's point of view into account, and, on the other, that intersubjectivity is not a constant state, but a series of states which are continually challenged by interruptions which provoke the interactants into re-creating a new state of intersubjectivity and which, far from necessarily breaking the dialogue, on the contrary, stimulate it.

For a socio-cognitive conflict to be beneficial, it is therefore necessary, on the one hand, to create social conditions between the children which would incite them to understand each other's point of view and to construct an intersubjectivity. However on the other hand, to make the acquisition of new abilities possible, phases of socio-cognitive conflict should interrupt this intersubjectivity. The socio-cognitive conflict and the negotiation of intersubjectivity appear to be two complementary processes which make possible the display of new abilities.

Sociogenesis and Cognitive Development: The Problems of Macro- and Micro-history and of the Unit of Analysis

Through the studies of processes such as socio-cognitive conflict and intersubjectivity, we attempted in this chapter to draw attention to two different problems:

1. A problem referring to *time*, considered first as the macro-historic duration, which encompasses the individual's history and the social and cultural history of the group he belongs to, and secondly, as the micro-historical duration, which encompasses the very moment of a given situation in which a child is involved in a cognitive activity.

The studies presented in this chapter showed that children's cognitive activity depends on social and cognitive competence they have already developed, as well as on competence which they construct (or reconstruct) during the interaction itself: in other words, new cognitive abilities, which cannot be considered as merely already made abilities, are created in the here and now.

2. A problem concerning the unit of analysis taken into consideration in the observation of children's cognitive activity. At first sight, terms such as "socio-genesis" or "cognitive development" could therefore be interpreted as the development of the child's *internal* competence (possibly influenced by some social factors). Nevertheless, the studies reported showed that the problem is more complex since the social context is far more than a set of external factors which influence development: it plays an integral part in cognitive activity. This means therefore that, in order to understand and interpret children's cognitive activity, it is not sufficient to observe the child as an isolated unit of analysis; on the contrary it is necessary to consider the *interaction* between the individual

child and the social actors he interacts with. We called this interaction "inter-subjective space."

Thus, the link between social and cognitive processes should not be considered as an internal link between different kinds of competence, but as the result of immediate interactions between the individual and his social environment, as well as of the macro-history of these interactions.

References

Bearison, D.J., S. Magzamen & E.K. Filardo (1986), Socio-cognitive growth in young children. *Merill-Palmer Quarterly,* 32, 51-72.

Bell, N. (1986), *Analysis of post-experimental interviews with kindergarten children concerning the Piagetian test of the conservation of the liquids.* University of Neuchâtel (Switzerland), Séminaire de Psychologie.

Blaye, A. (1988), Mécanismes générateurs de progrès lors de la résolution à deux d'un produit de deux ensembles par des enfants de 5-6 ans. In A.N. Perret-Clermont & M. Nicolet (eds.), *Interagir et connaître,* Cousset, Switzerland: Delval, pp.41-54.

Bovet, M., S. Parrat-Dayan, & D. Deshusses-Addor (1981), Peut-on parler de précocité et de régression dans la conservation? I. Précocité. *Archives de Psychologie,* 49, 191, 289-303.

Carraher, T.N. (1989), Negotiating the results of mathematical computations. *International Journal of Educational Research,* 13, 6, 637-646.

De Paolis, P. & V. Girotto (1987), Social marking of cognitive operations. The effect of different social rules. *European Journal of Psychology of Education,* II, 3, 219-231.

Doise, W. & G. Mugny (1984), *The social development of intellect.* Oxford: Pergamon Press.

Doise, W., S. Dionnet & G. Mugny (1975), Conflit socio-cognitif, marquage social et développement cognitif. *Cahiers de Psychologie,* 21, 231-245.

Doise, W., G. Mugny, & A.N. Perret-Clermont, A.N. (1975), Social interaction and the development of cognitive operations. *European Journal of Social Psychology,* 5, 367-383.

Donaldson, M. (1978), *Children's mind,* Glasgow: Fontana.

Elbers, E. (1986), Interaction and instruction in the conservation experiment. *European Journal of the Psychology of Education,* I, 1, 77-89.

Ellis, S. & B. Rogoff (1982), The strategies and efficacy of child versus teachers. *Child Development,* 53, 730-735.

Emler, N. & G. Valiant (1982), Social interaction and cognitive conflict in the development of spatial coordination. *British Journal of Psychology,* 73, 295-303.

Forman, E.A. (1987), Learning through peer interaction: a Vygotskian perspective. *The Genetic Epistemologist,* 15, 6-15.

Forman, E.A. & M.J. Kraker (1985), The social origin of logic: the contributions of Piaget and Vygotsky. In M.W. Berkowitz (ed.), *Peer conflict and psychological growth. New directions of child development, Vol. 29.* San Francisco: Jossey Bass.

Gilly, M. & J.P. Roux (1984), Efficacité comparée du travail individuel et du travail en interaction socio-cognitive dans l'appropriation et la mise en oeuvre d'une procédure de résolution chez des enfants de 11-12 ans. *Cahiers de Psychologie Cognitive,* 4, 171-188.

Grossen, M. (1988), *L'intersubjectivité en situation de test.* Cousset, Switzerland: Delval.

Grossen, M. & N. Bell (1988), Définition de la situation de test et élaboration d'une notion logique. In A.N. Perret-Clermont & M. Nicolet (eds.), *Interagir et connaître.* Cousset, Switzerland: Delval.

Hundeide, K. (1988), Metacontracts for situational definitions and for presentation of cognitive skills. *The Quarterly Newsletter of the Laboratory of Comparative Human Cognition,* 10, 3, 85-91.

Light, P. (1986), Context, conservation and conversation. In M. Richards & P. Light (eds.), *Children of social worlds: Development in social context.* Cambridge, MA: Cambridge University Press, pp. 170-195.

Light, P., T. Foot, C. Colbourn & I. McClelland (1987), Collaborative interactions at the microcomputer keyboard. *Educational Psychology,* 7, 13-21.

Light, P. & A.N. Perret-Clermont (1989), Social context effects in learning and testing. In A. Gellatly, D. Rogers & J.A. Sloboda (eds.), *Cognition and Social Worlds.* Oxford: Oxford Science Publication, pp. 99-112.

Monteil, J.M. (1988), Comparaison sociale. Stratégies individuelles et médiations socio-cognitives. Un effet de différenciations comportementales dans le champ scolaire. *European Journal of Psychology of Education,* III, 1, 3-18.

Nicolet, M. & M. Grossen (1988), Testons-nous des compétences cognitives? Contribu tion psychosociologique à la situation de test à travers l'étude de conduites aux épreuves opératoires piagétiennes. *Revue Internationale de Psychologie Sociale,* I, 1, 72-91.

Nicolet, M. & A. Iannaccone (1988), Norme sociale d'équité et contexte relationnel dans l'étude du marquage social. In A.N. Perret-Clermont & M. Nicolet (eds.), *Interagir et connaître,* Delval, Switzerland: Cousset, pp. 139-152.

Perret-Clermont, A.N. (1980), *Social interaction and cognitive development in children.* London: Academic Press.

Perret-Clermont, A.N. & M.L. Schubauer-Leoni (1981), Conflict and cooperation as opportunities for learning. In P. Robinson (ed.), *Communication in development.* London: Academic Press, pp. 203-233.

Piaget, J. (1971), *Biology and knowledge,* Edinburgh: Edinburgh University Press.

Rogoff, B. (1990), *Apprenticeship in thinking. Cognitive development in social context.* New York: Oxford University Press.

Rommetveit, R. (1979), On common codes and dynamic residuals in human communica-tion. In R.M. Blakar & R. Rommetveit (eds.), *Studies of language, thought and verbal communication.* London: Academic Press.

Rommetveit, R. (1985), Language acquisition as increasing linguistic structuring of experience and symbolic behaviour control. In J.V. Wertsch (ed.), *Culture, communica-tion and cognition: Vygotskian perspectives,* Cambridge: Cambridge University Press.

Roux, J.P. & M. Gilly (1984), Aide apportée par le marquage social dans une procédure de résolution chez des enfants de 12-13 ans: données et réflexions sur les mécanismes. *Bulletin de Psychologie,* XXXVII, 368, 145-155.

Säljö, R. & J. Wyndhamn (1987), The formal setting as context for cognitive activities. An empirical study of arithmetic operations under conflicting premisses for communication. *European Journal of Psychology of Education,* II, 3, 247-260.

Schubauer-Leoni, M.L. (1986), *Maître-élève-savoir: analyse psychosociale du jeu et des enjeux de la relation didactique.* Doctoral dissertation. University of Geneva (Switzerland).

Schubauer-Leoni, M.L., N. Bell, M. Grossen, & A.N. Perret-Clermont (1989), Problems of assessment of learning: the social construction of questions and answers in the scholastic context. *International Journal of Educational Research,* special issue on "Social factors in learning and instruction," 13, 6, 671-684.

Taal, M. & L. Oppenheimer (1989), Socio-cognitive conflict and peer interaction: development of compensation. *European Journal of Social Psychology,* 19, 77-83.

Valsiner, J. (1984), Construction of the zone of proximal development in adult-child joint action. In B. Rogoff & J.V. Wertsch (eds.), *Children's learning in the zone of proximal development,* San Fransisco: Jossey Bass, pp. 65-76.

Wertsch, J.V., N. Minick & F.J. Arns (1984), The creation of context in joint problem solving. In B. Rogoff & J. Lave (eds.), *Everyday cognition: its development in social context,* Cambridge, MA: Harvard University Press.

Wertsch, J.V. (1984), The zone of proximal development: some conceptual issues. In B. Rogoff & J.V. Wertsch (eds.), *Children's learning in the zone of proximal development, New directions for child development 23,* San Francisco: Jossey Bass, pp. 7-18.

Vygotsky, L.S. (1962), *Thought and language,* Cambridge, MA: MIT Press.

Zhou, R.M. (1988), Normes égalitaires, conduites sociales de partage et acquisition de la conservation des quantités. In A.N. Perret-Clermont & M. Nicolet, *Interagir et connaître,* Cousset, Switerland: Delval.

Notes

1. We would like to thank the Swiss National Foundation for Scientific Research for its financial support (Grant n° 1.738.083).

2. The experiment was done by Michèle Grossen (Grossen, 1988, pp. 227-364).

3. This test was chosen because it has given rise to numerous discussions in scientific literature and because the theoretical reasons which determined its construction are very explicit.

4. The test consisted of three sequences each composed of an "equalization item" of the quantities in two glasses of equal size and a "transformation item" during which the liquid contained in one of the glasses is poured into a different glass. A countersuggestion is made between the second and the third sequence. The experimenter asks the child to justify his judgments.

5. It should be noted that out of 57 RPs only 3 were unable to play their role of experimenter.

6. The experimenter asked the child: "Have we both the same thing to drink or do you have more or less to drink? What do you think?" The expression "the same thing" is used for "the same amount" but in French this wording cannot be understood by a 6- or 7-year-old child.

14. Circumcision and Psychogenesis:
Concepts of Individual, Self, and Person in the Description and Analysis of Initiation Rituals of Male Adolescents

Jan de Wolf

Introduction

The anthropologist Grace Harris has recently sought to clarify discussions involving the concepts of "person" and "self" by restricting the use of "individual" to biologistic discourses on human beings as members of the human kind, "self" to psychologistic discourses on human beings as the locus of experience, and "person" to sociologistic discourses on human beings as agent-in-society. She argues that these three modes of conceptualization are universal, but that their scope and interrelations may differ widely (1989).

For example, among the Ifaluk, described by Lutz (1988), concepts used to denote emotional states are to be interpreted in a sociologistic framework, in contrast to American middle-class notions which stress biologistic and psychologistic aspects. Harris herself noted a striking difference between American middle-class people who believe that other "selves" are easily accessible and have a well-developed vocabulary to talk about the states of mind of others and the Taita of southern Kenya who ventured only cautious guesses based on the observation of behavior (1978: 51, cited in 1989). Barbara Levine, who carried out research among the Gusii of western Kenya, comments that the habitual mode of expression of the women with whom she worked was to describe actions and events rather than thoughts and feelings (1979, p. 358). I myself noticed the same reluctance to explicate or speculate about motives for behaviour among the Bukusu, who live several hundreds of miles to the north of the Gusii in Kenya. I found that this was characteristic of Bukusu in general, not just of women.

Harris (1989) believes that failure to make the distinctions which she proposes can lead to the wrong conclusions when comparing societies. On this account she criticizes a paper by Shweder and Bourne (1984) who argue that there are two types of persons: one who allows the individual to be treated as independent of the social context, as among middle-class Americans and the other who conceptualizes the individual as context-dependent to the extent that his characteristics can only be described by specifying the social contexts in which they appear. Oriya people from a town in Orissa (India) illustrate this latter type. However, according to Harris, they do not really deal with concepts of the person, but with ideas about the self as interpreted by others. Harris reads the evidence as suggesting that in societies like that of the Oriya, structural features cause the concept of self to be subordinated to and shaped by the concepts of person. For Americans the concept of person is subordinated conceptually to that of self (1989, p. 607).

For anthropologists who were trained in the tradition of British social anthropology, as was the author of this contribution, the concept of the person, as defined by Harris (1989), used to be strictly separated from her notions about individual and self. The latter aspects concerned physiology and psychology and were therefore not relevant to an anthropological discourse, which was presented as comparative sociology. In Britain recent anthropological interest in these matters can be traced to at least two sources. As part of the post-structuralist reaction people turned their attention to human consciousness and intention. Human beings were seen as constructing their own worlds rather than being the epiphenomena of the unalterable underlying structures of a universal human mind (cf. Parkin, 1971). This again raised the problem of adequate description. How can we present other people's ideas when we live in different worlds? The problem was not only seen as a philosophical, perhaps even metaphysical question, but was also debated as an issue which could be investigated empirically, for example by considering the applicability of the ideas of Mauss on the notion of the person and the self (Carrithers, 1985; Hollis & Lukes, 1982).

The ideas held by Grace Harris are highly relevant if we want to look at problems of sociogenesis in the light of anthropological theories and empirical research. In this paper I want to consider the case of male initiation rituals which take place at puberty and which involve circumcision. I chose two neighboring peoples in East Africa: the Gisu, because their circumcision rituals have been studied very carefully and have been interpreted in various ways, and the Bukusu, because I am familiar with these people. They are sufficiently similar to the Gisu to allow an assessment of the plausibility of different interpretations and the formulation of hypotheses which could also be valid for the Gisu.

After a description of these circumcision rituals I shall consider the various interpretations which can be given from the three perspectives which Harris (1989) distinguishes. If sociogenesis is taken to refer to the social origins of individual psychological processes, we must, however, also look at the way in which these perspectives may be combined. In my opinion the circumcision rituals which are presented here illustrate nicely Goffman's thesis that social life would be unthinkable without individuals committed to goal-directed behavior, which can be interpreted as intentional, but that it also requires a major (social) effort to endow people with such a character. Hence my contention that one can talk equally well of psychogenesis. In other words sociogenesis entails psychogenesis and vice versa. If this is so and both processes also assume a similar physical substratum, the human body, the question arises whether such distinctions may not be rather arbitrary, depending, as they do, on our culturally determined academic categories. As Harris (1989) herself also acknowledges, the contents of her theoretical notions as well as their interrelations vary in different cultures, and their universality may well be questioned.

Circumcision Among Bukusu and Gisu

Introduction

In this section I want to present an account of circumcision ceremonies for boys among the Gisu and Bukusu who live near Mount Elgon in East Africa. I did anthropological fieldwork among the Bantu-speaking Bukusu who live to the south of the mountain in Kenya. The Gisu who live to the west of the mountain in Uganda speak a language which is closely related to that of the Bukusu. This is most markedly the case with the Gisu who live along the international border next to the Bukusu. This similarity also seems to extend to many of their customs. At least their circumcision ritual resembles so much that of the Bukusu that in this account I group them together with the Bukusu.

The slopes of Mount Elgon are very fertile and receive adequate rainfall. Among the Bukusu the most important cash crops are coffee and maize and among the Gisu, coffee and cotton. Cattle rearing is also important among the Bukusu, where it is integrated into a system of mixed farming. In the 1960s there were about 400,000 Gisu and 350,000 Bukusu. The population density of the higher Gisu areas is amongst the highest in Africa (La Fontaine, 1959, pp. 9-14; de Wolf, 1977, pp. 1-10).

The material on the Bukusu circumcision rituals was collected by the author in the field during 1968 and 1969 while data on the Gisu can be found in La Fontaine (1957, 1959, pp. 41-46) and in Heald (1982, 1986). Sometimes other publications give different or more elaborate information on certain aspects of these rituals. When such data seem important to the argument, I shall refer to them specifically in the text.

Preparations

Nowadays circumcision ceremonies are held every second year. Among the Gisu the intervals may, in the past, have been longer. The age of the Gisu novices is about 18, but in the past novices could be as old as 35. Bukusu boys are circumcised when they are between 12 and 18 years old, but here again they may have been older in the past (Wagner, 1949, p. 339). The ceremonies are held after the main finger millet harvest in August.

For a period of 1 or 2 months novices march or dance along the roads in groups, although nowadays this period may be as short as a week, and at night they practice dancing and singing. Among the Gisu a song leader teaches and leads the novices during the preliminary dancing and singing. Bukusu novices do not sing themselves, but this is done by the boys and girls who accompany them. The novices travel around because they have to visit paternal and maternal relatives and invite them to attend the ceremonies. Among the Bukusu these relatives sometimes sprinkle flour or sugar on the novices. Among the Gisu they exhort the novices and ask them to show their determination by jumping high into the air.

The novices wear strings of beads across back and chest. They get these from their female relatives. In addition Gisu wear belts studded with cowries and headdresses made of colobus monkey skin. Gisu sometimes attach a hippopotamus tusk or (imitation) horns to their forehead. Other ornaments such as handkerchiefs are bought in the shops. Gisu wear thigh bells and Bukusu wear hand bells, which they beat against iron rings around their wrists. Nowadays Bukusu also blow whistles during the dancing.

Among the Bukusu, novices help to prepare ritual beer made of sorghum. First they help with grinding and on the third day before the circumcision they fetch water from a river to pour on a mixture of fried flour mixed with germinated eleusine. A piece of *lukhaafwa* grass is tied around the pot and when they return from the river *siyoyao* is sung. This song is also sung when the Bukusu novices return from the river smeared with mud before they are circumcised. Among the Gisu, the novices thresh the millet, which will be used for brewing the beer of circumcision. They also pour on water but apparently Gisu novices do not fetch it in the same elaborate manner as do the Bukusu. On the other hand the Gisu make a paste of the germinated eleusine which is used in brewing beer and which is smeared by the officiating elder all over the body of the novice. This smearing is repeated on the next day and on the day of the circumcision itself.

Gisu and Bukusu novices have to visit the mother's brother on the day before circumcision to receive his blessing. According to La Fontaine (1959, p. 43) the Gisu uncle blesses by spitting beer and gives a goat or a cow as a present. Heald (1982, p. 25) reports that he actually kills an animal and smears chyme from the stomach on the novices. In northern parts he gives the novice peeled sticks which he keeps in his hands during the operation. On the same day Gisu elders clean the ritual groves and rebuild the shrines in preparation for a blessing ceremony the next day. They offer fowl and beer. Grandfathers of the novices, or other elders who are ritually responsible for them, make similar sacrifices to the ancestors at home.

Among the Bukusu the maternal uncle often kills a bull and the novice is smeared with chyme from the stomach which is then placed in front of a shrine. A piece of breast meat with the testicles attached to it is hung around his neck. When he comes home a father's sister shaves him (Wagner, 1949, p. 343), a bull is killed, the stomach is put in front of a shrine, and the brother or father of the novice's father smears him with chyme and hangs a piece of stomach lining around his neck.

Among both Gisu and Bukusu there is much dancing during the night before the operation. The whole community takes part. Visitors are entertained generously. Gisu novices may not speak in a normal voice during the last few days before the operation. They must chant what they wish to say. They are not expected to answer when people speak to them and are thought not to be entirely responsible for their actions. Bukusu novices are scrutinized repeatedly to see whether they know how to stand properly as required during the operation.

The Gisu kill an animal (goat) early the next morning and its chyme is smeared on the novice. A wealthy father may kill a bull for his eldest son. A piece of breast meat with the testicles attached is hung around the neck of this novice. The novice is also shaved, generally by his father's sister. Then the novices of the village, together with young women and small boys, go to the grove where the elders bless them by spitting beer on them. Next the novices who belong to the same small exogamous lineage go together to a swamp or pool where they are smeared with mud. On the way home *siwoya* is sung. The archaic words of this song make it difficult to understand its meaning. They have to make a final high jump in the circumcision enclosure to show their readiness to face the circumcisor. In parts of central Bugisu, novices smash an egg placed on a plantain leaf, together with the twigs of certain trees and bushes when coming down after their jump.

Early on the day of the circumcision Bukusu novices go to a river accompanied by a large crowd. Here they are smeared completely with mud while children and women wait at a distance. However, one woman, typically an aunt, remains present in order to wash away the leftovers of the mud with which the novice has been smeared. They go home along a different road and sing *siyoyao*, which describes how a leopard (the circumcisor) is waiting for them and tells cowards to go to Luo country (where they do not circumcise). When entering the homestead they are greeted by a paternal aunt with soot on her face and a small piece of meat attached to her ear. She gives the novices some freshly made beer on a large cooking ladle.

The Operation

The operation should be endured without any signs of pain. Everybody may watch, apart from the mothers of the Gisu novices. She takes up a childbirth position and kneels down with her hands clasping the center post of the hut while those of her sisters who happen to be there support her. The operation is held outside the hut. I did not observe this happen among the Bukusu, nor did I hear about such a custom. Yet Wagner reports something quite similar among the Luyia tribes of Kenya to which the Bukusu belong (Wagner, 1949, p. 350). Among the Gisu a flimsy fence may mark the place of the operation. Among Gisu and Bukusu, close paternal relatives are often initiated together. They are circumcised in order of genealogical seniority. In some parts of Bugisu all the novices of the same lineage are initiated together. The Bukusu used to bury an axe on the spot where the operation took place.

The two parts of the operation: cutting of the stretched foreskin and removal of the inner skin layer, are completed in one go, with the exception of northern Bugisu, where boys may dance and jump in between these two stages. In central and southern Bugisu and among the Bukusu, boys may steady themselves by holding a stick across their shoulders. A root called *itianyi* or *idanyi* is used to give the boys courage. They grip it between their toes or have to chew it. Bukusu circumcisors used to wear a colobus monkey skin headdress. Bukusu spectators watch the operation in silence, but among the Gisu a deafening noise of shouts and exhortations is kept up.

Everywhere women start rejoicing when all the novices have been circumcised. Gisu women seize ladles with millet porridge with which they beat the roofs to express their joy. In some parts of Bugisu the most senior novice throws a cockerel, which he has held during the operation, onto the roof of a hut. Bukusu boys may be supported after the operation by a young female relative for a while before they sit down. In the past a girlfriend could have claimed the novice in this way as her future husband (Wagner, 1949: 352). Sometimes a novice refuses to sit down until his father has promised him a cow. Women bring baskets with food, which are put in front of the novices and many well-wishers put coins into the mud on top of their heads or bank notes into their hands.

Particular care is taken to remove foreskins, blood-soiled earth, and blood-stained clothes. Among the Gisu, in some parts, they are buried that same night. Elsewhere they are kept for 3 days at the hut of seclusion and then disposed off. Among the Bukusu a grandmother wraps them in banana fiber and after 3 days throws them somewhere into the bush.

The Seclusion

Among the Gisu, novices stay in a newly built hut during their convalescence. Novices may not use their hands for eating until the circumcisor comes back to wash the boys ritually. Normally this happens in the evening but in the past it could take 2 or 3 days before he returned. He spits beer on the novices and tells them to wash their hands in it. He gives them pieces of the most important kinds of foodstuffs. They also have to hold his knife while he tells them that they are now grown-up men. He hands them a hoe and other symbols of male labor and gives them moral instruction. If the novice is married his wife is also washed and taught the duties of a wife. If he is not married his sister acts as a stand-in. If the novice is already father of a child additional purification rites have to be performed.

Among the Bukusu the novices enter the seclusion hut backwards in the same order in which they were circumcised. Any hut will do. The first boy has to remove the soot and the piece of meat from the father's sister. After a couple of hours the circumcisor returns and gives the boys small bits of food. Now they may eat again. The circumcisor drinks the beer which the novices helped to prepare. After 3 days the novices are shaved and caustic ash used to be put on the wound (Wagner, 1949, p. 357). When the novices are sufficiently recovered to wear clothes again the circumcisor comes to bless them. The novice kneels down covered with a blanket and the circumcisor touches him with his knife while he gives moral instruction. He spurts some beer on him by way of blessing. Now the boy receives new clothes. Only his father and mother attend this ritual, but later on that day there is a beer party for neighbors and relatives.

Grown-up women have to be avoided during the period of seclusion. Bukusu novices must also avoid cows. Gisu and Bukusu novices walk around with sticks with which they may hit girls on their legs. They only stop when they are offered eggs or some money. Gisu women do not cook for the novices, but leave this to young boys or sisters. Wagner (1949, p. 364) implies that, in the past, Bukusu novices were taken care of by female nurses. Gisu novices may steal food from gardens and fields. Bukusu boys were allowed to steal chickens and were engaged in military training (Wagner, 1949, p. 361). Nowadays the favorite pastimes of the Bukusu novices are fishing and playing the flute. Until they are recovered completely they smear themselves with white clay and wear a piece of white cotton cloth around their middle, which is fastened around their neck. In the past they wore a short leather apron (Wagner, 1949, p. 359).

Coming Out Ceremonies

Among the Gisu a beer drink for the lineage members and age-mates of the father of the novice marks his readmittance to society. He is presented with a spear and a new skin garment on this occasion. In some parts of central Bugisu a final dance is held several months later. The whole village or even a larger group takes part. The novices wear garlands of silk vine made by their mothers or sisters.

Among the Bukusu the final ceremonies are celebrated in December, but nowadays many novices omit them. They put the litter of banana leaves on which they slept on fire and run with torches, which they have lit in this fire to a banana grove without looking back. Here they make a bonfire and spend the night. In the past they were allowed to cut down as many bunches as they pleased (Wagner, 1949, p. 364). The next day the novices wash themselves in a river, put on new clothes and parade up and down the yard of the homestead with a spear. Their fathers bless them with beer and the boys receive new names. Finally they eat a meal of boiled bananas with which they may play around, trying to hit each other with balls of food.

Symbolic Meanings

Many symbols and sequences which occur in circumcision rituals are also typical of other life crisis rituals. As noted, among the Gisu the mother of the novice takes up the posture of a woman in labor "inside the hut outside which her son is being circumcised and hence 'reborn'" (La Fontaine, 1972, p. 177). After childbirth Bukusu and Gisu women are secluded for some days. Bukusu women may not touch food with their hands, and they sleep on a mattress of banana leaves and may only use the side door. At the end of the period they are shaved, take a bath, and have their hands washed ceremonially by an unmarried brother-in-law (Wagner, 1949, pp. 303-308). Gisu women are also shaved after the seclusion. Gisu girls must eat with sticks during their first menstruation (La Fontaine, 1959, pp. 39, 41). During funeral rites Bukusu widows and sisters of a deceased man may cut down a banana grove and widows are also smeared with white clay (Wagner, 1949, pp. 453, 484; 1939, p. 93). Among the Bukusu, a bride is smeared with soot and her ears are decorated with pieces of meat, like the paternal aunt who meets the novices before the operation (Wagner, 1949, p. 421).

Wagner has pointed out that the novices can be compared with women after childbirth and widows. But they are also thought to be like newborn children and recently deceased persons (1939, pp. 92-95). This interpretation is strengthened by the fact that among the Bukusu, the seclusion hut is called *li-kombe*, and the place where the dead are supposed to be is called *e-ma-kombe*, which also means "at the seclusion huts." On the other hand among the Gisu, onlookers shout after the operation: "He [the circumcisor] has spoiled you." The verb used here is also used when talking about the consummation of marriage, where it means "deflower" (La Fontaine, 1972, p. 180). Thus the novices are also like brides.

It is undoubtedly true that many symbols and activities characteristic of circumcision rituals acquire part of their meaning from the fact that they also occur in other life crisis rituals. There are also other ritual acts and objects which add meaning to the circumcision ceremonies without being restricted to life crisis rituals. Shaving, washing, anointing, and putting on new clothes are very usual to mark new stages in rituals. To mark ritual status the silk vine creeper is often used. Blessing by spitting various liquids or by applying chyme from sacrificed animals is also common.

Interpretations of Circumcision Rituals

Biologistic Interpretations

Anthropologists who focus on individuals as members of aggregates of human organisms direct their attention to society seen as a collectivity. The features of this collectivity are seen as resulting from the interaction of human beings as a certain kind of psychobiological entity, viz. natural atomistic units. Culture is seen as a resource available to the human units to change the patterns of interaction and to bind the units together into larger and larger collectivities (Harris, 1989). An anthropologist who has attempted to approach male circumcision rituals in this way is John Whiting. He combines an interest in behaviouristic learning theory with a Freudian perspective which stresses the importance of early experience for the development of personality (Whiting & Whiting, 1978, p. 41-4).

Whiting and Whiting (1978) started by supposing that societies in which mother and infant sleep together separated from other family members and in which sexual relations should not be resumed by the mother until at least a year after the child was born, encourage the establishment of a strong, exclusive tie of affection and dependency between mother and child. These factors increased the intensity of later Oedipal conflicts. Initiation at puberty was needed in such cases to suppress a potential Oedipal rebellion and to establish a firm masculine identity. Later Whiting and Whiting came to stress more strongly the establishment of a strong male identity, rather than the threat of Oedipal rebellion.

In the most complex causal model Whiting and Whiting (1978) begin with a presumed protein deficiency in tropical environments. Extended nursing is therefore necessary and to ensure this a second pregnancy of a mother should be avoided. Hence the prohibition on sexual intercourse. Husbands are then motivated to take other wives and patrilocal residence develops to facilitate the control of the polygynous co-wives. In patrilocal societies, particularly those with patrilineal descent, a strong masculine identity and a loyalty to the patrilineal kin group are necessary. Genital mutilation serves to break the strong bond with the mother fostered by exclusive mother-child sleeping arrangements to strengthen male kin ties and build up local male loyalties (cf. Paige & Paige, 1981, pp. 9-11; La Fontaine, 1985, pp. 105-106).

These hypotheses were tested cross-culturally, using samples based on the HRAF data. This is not the place to discuss this research strategy but it may be of interest to see whether Gisu and Bukusu societies conform in some measure to the interpretation by Whiting and Whiting. Both societies are characterized by polygyny, patrilocal residence, and patrilineal descent. Among the Gisu, patrilineal descent is also used as a principle for the organization of solidary groups with a common territory. Among the Bukusu the corporate entity of clans and lineages is less pronounced. However, there are no reports of post-partum taboos. Among the Bukusu it is even thought a bad thing if parents have not resumed sexual relations before the child can smile. Breastfeeding among the Bukusu may last several years but is terminated when women become pregnant again (Wagner, 1949, pp. 322-323).

From the native point of view there is no emphasis on increasing male solidarity through circumcision in order to counteract matrifocal tendencies. What is stressed at the conscious level is that circumcision is absolutely necessary for boys in order to be able to function as grown-ups. All male individuals have to be marked in this way, at least when they belong to the tribes in question. Of course, they know that other peoples do not circumcise, but for themselves there is no escaping from such an operation. Sex and age are not sufficient criteria. For men these biological indicators have to be marked by bodily signs in order to become operative in social life. On the ideological level it is justified as a custom inherited from the ancestors which is obligatory for all their descendants without exception. Men who shrink from this obligation will be circumcised forcibly. Without such a mark a man is not a "normal" individual.

It is tempting to apply a nature-culture dichotomy to rituals marking physical and social maturation. In fact, La Fontaine uses this very categorization in her interpretation. According to her, the Gisu recognize in women a creative power that is *sui generis* natural. The sign of this power is a flow of blood from the genitals occurring at menstruation, defloration, and childbirth. The rituals concerned with these events control and harness the reproductive powers of women for the benefit of men, whose powers by contrast are social, not part of the natural order. She argues that Gisu male circumcision rituals can be seen as a symbolic creation in men of the inherent physical power of women. Gisu explicitly compare the pain of childbirth with that of circumcision. This supports the view that in women it is natural uncontrolled bleeding that denotes their (reproductive) power; in men it is social, controlled bleeding that both symbolizes and creates superior social power (La Fontaine, 1972, pp. 179-180).

The difficulty with this type of interpretation is that the difference between nature and culture itself is a product of a specific Western discourse. They are not categories which the Gisu themselves apply consciously. There is no evidence that circumcision is thought to be in any way less natural than childbirth. Perhaps the underlying argument in La Fontaine's (1972) explanation is that Gisu men need circumcision in order to become superior to women in the same way as Lévi-Strauss claims that human societies need incest prohibitions in order to create the social cohesion necessary for survival. On the one hand the custom is obligatory and universal, therefore natural; on the other hand it is not necessary in the way that sexual intercourse is necessary for procreation, and therefore it has to be enforced and surrounded by sanctions. In this way it belongs to culture. The main difference is, of course, that incest prohibitions are truly universal, whereas circumcision is not.

Another aspect which is stressed is the courage with which the boy is expected to face the knife of circumcision. Heald (1986, pp. 78-81) links this to the idea of "battle-proofing," which consists of enacting situations of danger, so allowing the person to become accustomed to and inured against fear. This is especially clear in the preparatory rituals of the Gisu.

> Firstly, the emphasis is put on the boy being "strong" enough....This "strength" implies both physical strength and what we would call strength of purpose. It is evidenced in the vigour with which the boy dances and in the jumps which effectively rehearse the final jump he will make to face the circumcisors. Secondly, the boy is subjected to repeated exhortations by elders and bystanders. They tell him of the ordeal he faces, and how he must stand it....[He] is continually asked if he is sure he can go through with it and urged to withdraw if he has any doubt....On the ritual level, his determination is tested by a series of smearing rites which are explicitly interpreted as mortifications—as unpleasant and abhorrent.... (Heald, 1986, pp.78-79)

In the past warfare was very common in this part of East Africa. Courage in fighting would certainly add to better chances of survival, all things being equal. Interestingly enough the Bukusu myth of origin makes courageous behavior even a precondition for the admittance of the first Bukusu to be circumcised by neighbors who already had this custom. Yet, this stress on personal courage can also be socially destructive, if people take their rights into their own hands when asserting themselves in conflicts within the community in which they live. At least among the Gisu this seems to be a problem of the first order (Heald, 1986, pp. 72-73).

Sociologistic Interpretations

With this type of interpretation we focus on *persons* as agents-in-society. This brings properties of the social order and its cultural forms to the center of attention for these are seen as constitutive of human agency as a public fact (Harris, 1989). With regard to the Gisu, Jean La Fontaine has worked this out:

> The young man is initiated and becomes an independent member of society and a member of his lineage on equal terms with his father....[H]e is entitled to the appurte-nances of adulthood: land to cultivate and the cattle to pat bride-wealth for his wife. His father must supply these from the portion earmarked as his future inheritance. After initiation a son has a recognized right to the property which represents his economic freedom....The ceremony is the Open Sesame to independence. (1967, p.253)

Gisu fathers often resent giving political and economic independence to their sons and their reluctance to part with their property may even lead to parricide (La Fontaine, 1967, p. 256). In this connection Heald (1982, pp. 15-16) draws attention to Victor Turner's conclusion that circumcision gains its emotive force as a culturally focal symbol because "it represents an irresoluble conflict between disparate *world views*. On the one hand, the universalistic and egalitarian ethos of an age-set system; and, on the other, the localized particularism and gerontocratic authoritarianism of a narrowly patrilineal system" (Turner, 1969, p. 243). Although she thinks that the terms of this contrast seem odd, since age-set systems have a tendency towards gerontocracy, she agrees that there is an opposition between the ideals of essential equality of adult men and the system of authority that is implied in patrilineal transmission and hierarchic ranking in terms of age and genealogical seniority. "Such conflict undoubtedly enters into the situation of circumcision and accounts for some of the specific characteristics of the ritual, both formal and informal" (Heald, 1982, p. 16).

Another question which is raised by La Fontaine concerns the efficacy of the ritual. Here again she looks for an answer in sociologistic terms. She sees the ordeal of circumcision as a test of the efficacy of the preceding ritual. The events are ordered in such a way that the crucial action is a consequence of the applied knowledge of tradition. Gisu attribute power to effect subsequent events to the thing, event, or action which is identified as the antecedent. Selection of significant antecedent events in turn rests on accepted beliefs or axioms. They include ideas about what is "natural" human behavior as well as about the behavior of the observed universe. To accept them is to belong to a particular cultural community and also to accept the authority of those whose deeper knowledge guarantees that the axioms are true (1977, pp. 431-433).

The authority of the Gisu elder rests on knowledge which he has both by virtue of his closeness to the ancestors and by accumulated experience during a life in which he has qualified to *be* an ancestor by begetting sons. It is the authority of experience which justifies the subordination of women in this society, in spite of their inherent powers. Experience cannot be communicated, it can only be undergone. Initiation constitutes an intense experience which communicates the truth that traditional knowledge can exercise control over material forces, including the bodies of young men. For the experience is so construed as to prove that traditional knowledge is the cause of the successful outcome. (La Fontaine, 1977: 433)

La Fontaine concludes: "Initiation rituals create occasions in which traditional wisdom is communicated, tested and vindicated as the source of the power of rights" (1977, p. 434).

Among the Bukusu, novices are, on the whole, several years younger than among the Gisu. Therefore the rituals do not confer immediate adult status on the initiate, although they are a necessary condition on the way to achieving this status. However, Bukusu fathers have the same obligations towards their grown-up sons as Gisu fathers. They have to provide bridewealth and land for the establishment of new households. But traditionally the independence of a new household would have been delayed until at least one child had been born. Only then would the wife start cooking her own meals and no longer assist her mother-in-law in her kitchen. The father of the wife had to kill an animal to celebrate the event (Wagner, 1949: 43). Nowadays this ritual takes place when the first son has been circumcised or the first daughter has been married.

Rather than emphasizing a change in jural status, Bukusu initiation marks the sexual maturity of the novices. Initiates now have to build their own separate bachelor huts, where they can receive their girlfriends. This theme of sexual maturity is also stressed at the final coming-out ceremony, where initiates are warned against adulterous behavior. They should not enter the huts of women married to other men.

Psychologistic Interpretations

With this type of interpretation we focus on *selves* and formulate questions and direct observation with reference to posited intrapsychic structures and processes. Social structure is, as it were, taken "inside" the experiencing selves. Cultural formulations are treated as a source of goals, ideals, problems, ideas, concepts, and beliefs incorporated by selves, and as defining the contexts for the self's growth, development expression and reading by others (Harris, 1989, p. 608).

Heald (1982, 1986) has done much to make us better understand the Gisu circumcision rituals as pragmatically aiming at inducing a certain individual attitude or mental and emotional capacity. The native key concept here is *lirima*. The ritual is seen to create in the boy the capacity to experience lirima and it is this capacity which divides men from boys. There is no equivalent in English. In a way it can be typified as violent emotion, which affects the individual very strongly, dictating attitudes and actions. Lirima is especially linked to negative emotions, especially to anger, but also to jealousy, hatred, resentment, and shame, which are also seen as capable of inspiring such violent affect. But whereas in western thought such situations are interpreted as the overriding of reason by passion, Gisu do not think of reason and emotion as different forces struggling within the individual soul. Thus lirima cannot only be volitional but also an aspect of the control a man should assert over himself and the world. It is a quality or capacity to be mustered by the individual to achieve and serve his purposes. Lirima is the force which makes men courageous and determined. Thus lirima is an ambivalent capacity. It is necessary for grown-up men and therefore boys have to be circumcised, but it also makes men dangerous and is associated with violence, aggression and the disorders which disrupt the communal peace (Heald, 1986, pp. 71-74).

Lirima is also used to describe the fermentation process during the final three days of beer brewing. When the brew bubbles up, this is said to show that both the ancestors and lirima are in the beer. The boy and the beer are imbued with ancestral power and lirima and are brought into further direct association through the smearing rites (Heald, 1982, p. 28). On the one hand lirima is connected with emotions, on the other it is also a type of "'power" or aspect of creative energy. This is also apparent when the word lirima is used to describe and explain aspects of human pregnancy. It is believed that in procreation the semen of a man mixes with the placental blood of the women to form the child. As in the brewing of beer the liquids ferment and are said to bubble up inside the woman. This volatility of gestation is considered liable to spill over and affect the woman emotionally. Moreover, in gestation there is also a spiritual component, which makes the similarity with fermentation even clearer. At birth the child inherits the life force of someone in his kindred who has recently died, thus testifying to the power of the ancestors (1982, p. 30).

In circumcision lirima is positive because it gives the novice the drive to face the ordeal and helps him to overcome his anxiety and fear.

> At the beginning many boys evidence doubt and apprehension as to their ability to stand the ordeal. One way of looking at the ritual sequence and how it works to effect a change of attitudes would be to say that in the course of the rituals the boy is made to identify with the attitudes and emotions of adult men—he must present himself as a fully responsible agent freely choosing the ordeal and sticking to this resolution. From this point of view one could argue that volition and lirima are key themes in the ritual because they constitute what it is to be a man. Through identification with these, and

the constant testing for such qualities, the boy learns in the course of the ritual to experience himself and his potentialities differently, as a man rather than as a boy. Enduring the operation is thus the final proof that such a transformational process is complete (Heald, 1982, pp. 23-24).

Among the Bukusu, the concept of lirima seems to occupy a much less prominent place in the discourse about circumcision and is used less generally to explain certain aspects of (male) behavior. Personally I was struck by the emphasis which is put on the fixity of purpose which should be shown by the novices and which is apparent in the way they look. They gaze ahead and do not cast glances sideways, often appearing not even to notice bystanders. Among the Bukusu, fathers also show reluctance when boys say that they want to be circumcised as among the Gisu, but in my opinion this is not because they fear them as future competitors, but because fathers want to test their strength of resolution.

Anyone who watches the Bukusu circumcision rituals and especially the preparatory phases will be struck by the way in which people seem to empathize with the novices. In a number of situations such involvement is institutionalized. Relatives have to play definite roles in the rituals. The success of the initiation also depends on their efforts. The outcome matters to them. From a psychologistic point of view the notion of vicarious experience which this implies may well be a necessary complement to our understanding of the efficacy of ritual. How could one otherwise explain the impact of life-crisis rituals on the audience and the internalization of values which they embody for the immediate subjects of these rituals?

Discussion and Conclusion

It does seem possible to apply the threefold distinction of Harris (1989) to the description and analysis of circumcision rituals among Gisu and Bukusu. However, these rituals also seem to link her concepts in an indissoluble way. Circumcision is as necessary and natural for Bukusu and Gisu men as is breastfeeding and toilet training for people in general. Yet society demands that body and self are merged completely through self-willed genital mutilation. Nowhere is this bridging of categories clearer than in the double meaning of lirima. On the one hand it is volitional force, allowing people to constitute themselves as proper examples of the human species, on the other hand it is natural power through which people can be driven to extremes of anti-social behavior and yet it is a necessary concomitant of dynamic processes which set free creative energy.

Again during circumcision, self and society meet through the concept of character as described by Goffman (1972). In his essay, "Where the Action Is," he identifies a certain kind of activities as fateful, that is the outcome is problematic (boys may run away at the last moment) and consequential (it really matters to the individual and others connected with him). Moreover the term *action* is reserved for those activities that are apart from being consequential and problematic, undertaken for what is felt to be their own sake. Action seems most pronounced when it occurs over a period of time brief enough to be contained within a continuous stretch of attention and experience. "It is here that the individual releases himself to the passing moment, wagering his future estate on what transpires precariously in the seconds to come. At such moments a special affective state is likely to be aroused emerging transformed into excitement" (Goffman, 1972, p. 185).

If an individual is to face action successfully he has to show *character*. Some major forms that bear on the management of fateful events are various forms of courage, and gameness, that is the capacity to stick to a line of activity and continue to pour all effort into it regardless of set-backs, pain, or fatigue, and this not because of some brute insensitivity but because of inner will and determination. Constancy, in spite of everything, is what character is all about according to folk beliefs. To say that over time and across various situations the individual might not, in fact, maintain the character he currently manifests, is quite true, but beside the point. In daily life we assume that the currently expressed character is a full and lasting picture of a person and this person believes us to hold this opinion. Action has the peculiar appeal that it allows us to display or express character and at the same time to generate character. Paradoxically character is both unchanging and changeable. This is explained as follows:

> Social organization everywhere has the problem of morale and continuity. Individuals must come to all their little situations with some enthusiasm and concern for it is largely through such moments that social life occurs and if a fresh effort were not put into each of them, society would surely suffer. The possibility of effecting reputation is the spur. And yet, if society is to persist, the same pattern must be sustained from one social occasion to the next. Here is the need for rules and conventionality. Individuals must define themselves in terms of properties already accepted as theirs, and act reliably in terms of them. To satisfy the fundamental requirements of morale and continuity, we are encouraged in a fundamental illusion. It is our character. A something entirely our own that does not change, but is nonetheless precarious and mutable. Possibilities regarding character encourage us to renew our efforts at every moment of society's activity we approach, especially its social ones; and it is precisely through these renewals that the old routines can be sustained. (Goffman, 1972, p. 238)

Not only does society, through a process of psychogenesis, create people who can be held accountable for their actions because their behavior can be imputed to character, but society also allows us to do so at minimal costs. The mechanism which comes into play here is vicarious experience. In our society this possibility is exploited commercially, but among the Bukusu and Gisu it is celebrated through ritual (Goffman, 1972, pp. 262-270). In our society mass media provide an opportunity for watching action and identifying with people confronted by fateful experiences. Among the Africans considered here the biennial tribalwide circumcision ceremonies offer a similar chance to take part vicariously in the show of character performed by the initiates.

Recent trends in the philosophy of science stress the social construction of reality. In the social sciences this idea is also applied to the very instruments with which we describe such processes. Thus cognition and knowledge seem in danger of becoming sociologized. On this view concepts of individual, self, and person are typical of social scientific discourse of the 1980s. To us they appear as universal distinctions because semantically they imply each other. Sociogenesis requires a concept of self, just as psychogenesis requires a concept of person, and both cannot be imagined without what we take to be universal characteristics of individuals of the human species. This also applies to Goffman's (1972) analysis of character. After all he assumes that people are capable of vicarious experience through empathy. Yet, necessarily, other peoples have other ideas which they think to be universally valid. This makes translation a difficult and perhaps an impossible exercise.

These problems are recognized by Harris:

> The individual as human unit is the subject of divergent doctrines cross-culturally. (...) We can expect the conceptualization of capacities for and constraints on behavior to connect these various ideas in complex ways with conceptualizing the other principal modes of conceptualizing human beings.... There can, of course, be other ways of conceiving of the self without systematized ideas parallelling the self of modern Western psychologies.... As to knowledge of other selves, cross-cultural variation is striking....It is noteworthy that in many ethnographically recorded ideas about the person, not all persons are living humans or, indeed, human at all, nor are all human beings persons....The members of some societies live in a world full of non-human entities conceptualized as persons, as authors of actions affecting human life. Such a world contrasts with that of modern science, where mechanism-cause excludes the notion of personal agents from non-social contexts and, in extreme views, from social life as well. (Harris, 1989, pp. 601-603)

Yet in spite of the fact that the three concepts "are linked to a greater or lesser extent and in differing ways while they may be split or lumped terminologically in the indigenous lexicon," we should be able to identify and distinguish them ethnographically according to Harris (1989, p. 607). Probably we have no other way of presenting the ideas of people belonging to cultures very different from our own than as transformations of our own systems of thought and in this sense Harris is bound to be right. However, we cannot know either whether the people belonging to these other cultures would recognize our interpretations as valid, because they do not have similar projects regarding our own culture (cf. Strathern, 1988).

References

Carrithers, M. et al. (eds.) (1985), *The Category of the Person*. Cambridge: Cambridge University Press.

Goffman, E. (1972), *Interaction Ritual: Essays on Face-to-Face Behaviour*. Harmondsworth: Penguin Books.

Harris, G.G. (1978), *Casting Out Anger: Religion among the Taita of Kenya*. Cambridge: Cambridge University Press.

Harris, G.G. (1989), Concepts of individual, self, and person in description and analysis. *American Anthropologist* 91: 599-612.

Heald, S. (1982), The making of men: the relevance of vernacular psychology to the interpretation of a Gisu ritual. *Africa* 52: 15-36.

Heald, S. (1986), The ritual use of violence: circumcision among the Gisu of Uganda. In D. Riches (ed.), *The Anthropology of Violence*. Oxford: Blackwell. pp. 70-85.

Hollis, M. and S. Lukes (eds.) (1982), *Rationality and Relativism*. Oxford: Blackwell.

La Fontaine, J.S. (1957), *The Social Organisation of the Gisu of Uganda with Special Reference to their Initiation Ceremonies*. Unpublished Ph.D. Thesis, Cambridge.

La Fontaine, J.S. (1959), *The Gisu of Uganda*. London: International African Institute.

La Fontaine, J.S. (1972), Ritualization of Women's Life-crises in Bugisu. In J.S. La Fontaine (ed.), *The Interpretation of Ritual: Essays in Honour of A.I. Richards*. London: Tavistock. pp. 159-186.

La Fontaine, J.S. (1985), *Initiation: Ritual Drama and Secret Knowledge across the World*. Harmondsworth: Penguin Books.

LeVine, S. (1979), *Mothers and Wives: Gusii Women of East Africa*. Chicago: The University of Chicago Press.

Lutz, C.A. (1988), *Unnatural Emotions: Everyday Sentiments on a Micronesian Atoll and Their Challenge to Western Theory*. Chicago: The University of Chicago Press.

Paige, K.E. and J.M. Paige (1981), *The Politics of Reproductive Ritual*. Berkeley: University of California Press.

Parkin, D. (ed.) (1971), *Semantic Anthropology*. ASA Monographs 22. New York: Academic Press.

Shweder, R.A. & E.J. Bourne (1984), Does the concept of person vary cross-culturally? In R.A. Shweder & R.A. LeVine (eds.), *Essays on Mind, Self, and Emotion*. Cambridge: Cambridge University Press. pp. 158-199.

Strathern, M. (1988), *The Gender of the Gift: Problems with Women and Problems with Society in Melanesia*. Berkeley: University of California Press.

Turner, V.W. (1969), Symbolization and patterning in the circumcision rites of two Bantu-speaking societies. In M. Douglas & P.M. Kaberry (eds.), *Man in Africa*. London: Tavistock Press.

Whiting, J. & B. Whiting (1978), A strategy for psychocultural research. In G. Spindler (ed.), *The Making of Psychological Anthropology*. Berkeley: University of California Press.

Wagner, G. (1939), Reifeweichen bei den Bantustämmen Kavirondos und ihre hentige Bedentung. *Archive für Anthroplogie. Nene Folge*, 25, 85-100.

Wagner, G. (1949), *The Bantu of North Kavirondo*, Volume I. London: Oxford University Press for the International African Institute.

Wolf, J.J. de (1977), *Differentiation and Integration in Western Kenya: A Study of Religious Innovation and Social Change among the Bukusu*. The Hague: Mouton.

Index